Frontiers in Natural Product Chemistry

(*Volume 5*)

Edited by

Atta-ur-Rahman, *FRS*
Kings College, University of Cambridge, Cambridge, UK

Frontiers in Natural Product Chemistry

Volume # 5

Editor: Atta-ur-Rahman, *FRS*

ISSN (Online): 2212-3997

ISSN (Print): 1574-0897

ISBN (Online): 978-9-81142-377-2

ISBN (Print): 978-9-81142-376-5

Bentham Science Publishers Pte. Ltd.
80 Robinson Road #02-00
Singapore 068898
Singapore
Email: subscriptions@benthamscience.net

BENTHAM
SCIENCE

CONTENTS

PREFACE

Frontiers in Natural Product Chemistry presents recent advances in the chemistry and biochemistry of naturally occurring compounds. It covers a range of topics including important researches on natural substances. The book is a valuable resource for pharmaceutical scientists and postgraduate students seeking updated and critically important information on bioactive natural products.

The chapters in this volume are written by eminent authorities in the field and are mainly focused on inhibition of monoamine oxidase (MAO) *via* green tea extracts, cynaropicrin as an inhibitor of Bcr-Abl fusion oncogene expression, effects of dietary polyphenols on chronic diseases, taxol production, mushroom functionalities in cancer treatment, and health related enzyme inhibiting natural products.

I hope that the readers will find these reviews valuable and thought provoking so that they may trigger further research in the quest for the new and novel therapies against various diseases. I am grateful for the timely efforts made by the editorial personnel, especially Mr. Mahmood Alam (Director Publications), and Mr. Shehzad Iqbal Naqvi (Editorial Manager Publications) at Bentham Science Publishers.

Atta-ur-Rahman, *FRS*
Kings College
University of Cambridge
Cambridge
UK

List of Contributors

Athar Ata	Department of Chemistry, Richardson College for the Environmental and Science Complex, The University of Winnipeg, 599 Portage Avenue, Winnipeg, Manitoba R3B 2G3, Canada
Astrid March	Biotechnology Division, Roxbury Community College, Boston, MA02120, USA
Bilal Ahmad Asad	State Key Laboratory for Biology of Plant Diseases and Insect Pests, Institute of Plant Protection, Chinese Academy of Agricultural Sciences, Beijing, 100081, China
Bilge Sener	Department of Pharmacognosy, Faculty of Pharmacy, Gazi University, Ankara, Turkey
Chun-Tao He	State Key Laboratory for Biocontrol, School of Life Sciences, Sun Yat-Sen University, Xingang Xi Road 135, Guangzhou, 510275, China
Danijela Stanisavljević	Institute of Molecular Genetics and Genetic Engineering, University of Belgrade, Vojvode Stepe 444a, PO Box 23, 11010, Belgrade, Serbia
Dejan Stojković	Department of Plant Physiology, Institute for Biological Research "Siniša Stanković", University of Belgrade, Bulevar Despota Stefana 142, 11000, Belgrade, Serbia
Erika Cione	Department of Pharmacy Health and Nutritional Sciences, University of Calabria, Arcavacata di Rende, Cosenza, Italy
Francesca Aiello	Department of Pharmacy Health and Nutritional Sciences, University of Calabria, Arcavacata di Rende, Cosenza, Italy
Gemma R. Topaz	Biotechnology Division, Roxbury Community College, Boston, MA02120, USA Department of Biology, Boston University, Boston, MA02215, USA
Jasmina Glamočlija	Department of Plant Physiology, Institute for Biological Research "Siniša Stanković", University of Belgrade, Bulevar Despota Stefana 142, 11000, Belgrade, Serbia
Jelena Popović	Institute of Molecular Genetics and Genetic Engineering, University of Belgrade, Vojvode Stepe 444a, PO Box 23, 11010, Belgrade, Serbia
Jelena Živković	Institute for Medicinal Plant Research "Dr. Josif Pančić", Tadeuša Košćuška 1, 11000, Belgrade, Serbia
Kazuo Yamagata	Laboratory of Molecular Health Science of Food, Department of Food Bioscience and Biotechnology, College of Bioresource Sciences, Nihon University (NUBS), Fujisawa, Japan
Kenneth Friesen	Department of Chemistry, Richardson College for the Environmental and Science Complex, The University of Winnipeg, 599 Portage Avenue, Winnipeg, Manitoba R3B 2G3, Canada
Kimberly A. Stieglitz	Biotechnology Division, Roxbury Community College, Boston, MA02120, USA
Maria Cristina Caroleo	Department of Pharmacy Health and Nutritional Sciences, University of Calabria, Arcavacata di Rende, Cosenza, Italy
Maria Luisa Di Gioia	Department of Pharmacy Health and Nutritional Sciences, University of Calabria, Arcavacata di Rende, Cosenza, Italy

Marija Smiljković	Department of Plant Physiology, Institute for Biological Research "Siniša Stanković", University of Belgrade, Bulevar Despota Stefana 142, 11000, Belgrade, Serbia
Milena Stevanović	Institute of Molecular Genetics and Genetic Engineering, University of Belgrade, Vojvode Stepe 444a, PO Box 23, 11010, Belgrade, Serbia Faculty of Biology, University of Belgrade, Studentski trg 16, PO box 43, 11000, Belgrade, Serbia Serbian Academy of Sciences and Arts, Knez Mihailova 35, 11001, Belgrade, Serbia
Samavia Mubeen	State Key Laboratory for Biocontrol, School of Life Sciences, Sun Yat-Sen University, Xingang Xi Road 135, Guangzhou, 510275, China
Samina Naz	Department of Chemistry, Richardson College for the Environmental and Science Complex, The University of Winnipeg, 599 Portage Avenue, Winnipeg, Manitoba R3B 2G3, Canada
Victor Epiter-Smith	Biotechnology Division, Roxbury Community College, Boston, MA02120, USA
Zhong-Yi Yang	State Key Laboratory for Biocontrol, School of Life Sciences, Sun Yat-Sen University, Xingang Xi Road 135, Guangzhou, 510275, China

CHAPTER 1

Inhibition of Monoamine Oxidase (MAO) *via* Green Tea Extracts: Structural Insights of Catechins as Potential Inhibitors of MAO

Gemma R. Topaz[1,2], **Astrid March**[1], **Victor Epiter-Smith**[1] and **Kimberly A. Stieglitz**[1,*]

[1] *Biotechnology Division, Roxbury Community College, Boston, MA 02120, USA*

[2] *Department of Biology, Boston University, Boston, MA 02215, USA*

Abstract: MAOs perform deamination of amines, are present at high-concentration in neuronal cells, and are found bound to the outer mitochondrial membrane. MAOA oxidizes serotonin, noradrenaline, and adrenaline; and MAOB oxidizes dopamine, β-phenylethylamine (β-PEA), and benzylamine. Abnormal MAOA activity has been implicated in depression, anxiety, and other psychological or psychiatric disorders, while heightened MAOB activity in the brain occurs in Alzheimer's disease, Huntington's disease, Parkinson's disease, and normal aging. Drugs have been developed and continue to be developed with both MAOA and MAOB as targets. However, MAO inhibitors (MAOIs) have adverse side effects and serious drug interactions with some over the counter medications. MAOA is inhibited by Clorgyline and MAOB is potently inhibited by both Deprenyl and Pargyline. In addition, polyphenol green tea catechins may also target the MAO enzymes. Using these inhibitors as controls, fluorescent activity assays were performed with commercially available catechins from green tea extracts primarily composed primarily of EGCG. MAOs were utilized as targets to investigate and confirm recent studies suggesting that green tea catechin polyphenols may be preventative for certain degenerative diseases, psychiatric disorders, and emotional disabilities. Of the tested green tea extracts (confirmed EGCG), commercial catechins exhibited half-maximal inhibitory concentration (IC_{50}) values in the low-to-mid μM range, at approximately 50-750 μM. Molecular docking of specific catechins into the MAOA and MAOB active sites resulted in binding constants in the low μM range. Docking studies as such provide structural insights into possible binding models of EGCG catechin to MAOs. Efforts to understand the effect of catechins on MAO targets are currently underway, and a survey of the literature is provided.

Keywords: Catechins, EGCG, Green tea extracts, MAOA, MAOB, NDRIs, SNRIs.

* **Corresponding author Kimberly A. Stieglitz:** Biotechnology Division, Roxbury Community College, Boston, MA 02120, USA; E-mail: kastieglitz@rcc.mass.edu

Atta-ur-Rahman (Ed.)

1. INTRODUCTION

1.1. The Potential of Green Tea for Health and Disease Prevention

Investigation of Traditional Chinese Medicine is fairly recent within the scope of interest to comparative studies in Western Medicine. Chinese botanical medicine in the form of green tea continues to be a highly desired good for consumption. Green tea as an herbal medicine supports long-standing theories regarding the potential benefits of green teas for improved physical health. Tea is generally consumed not only for its taste but also for its reliable alleviative properties. Catechins, bioactive compounds known to possess medicinal benefits [1], are found in high quantities in green tea, more so than any other consumable. Previous research pertaining to green tea catechins and their potential medicinal properties has spanned many areas of study including cancer, obesity, atherosclerosis, diabetes, and gum disease, with a special emphasis on certain disorders affecting the central nervous system, notably, neurodegenerative diseases [2 - 4].

The primary motivation for this study stems from an increased interest in exploring the possible benefits of green tea to better understand its potential impact on health and disease prevention. This chapter not only seeks to gain structural insights of catechins, but also to survey literature focusing on the various mechanisms of MAO activity and inhibitor actions for the purpose of providing functional knowledge of how catechins may act as potent inhibitors of MAO.

2. CHARACTERIZATION OF CATECHINS

2.1. Characteristics and Types

On a molecular level, catechin compounds are comprised of four groups of polyphenols (flavonoid compounds) and are commonly found in plants. The primary catechin flavonoids focused herein are epicatechin (EC), epigallocatechin (EGC), epicatechin gallate (ECG), and epigallocatechin gallate (EGCG) [5]. Polyphenols as such are further characterized as flavan-3-ols, or flavanols. Catechins are secondary metabolites (not essential for survival) with a 15-carbon skeleton containing two phenyl rings and a heterocyclic ring (Fig. **1**). In green tea, plant polyphenols (of catechins) are of special significance due to their antioxidant properties [6].

Polyphenolic plant compounds display scavenger-like behavior. This scavenging activity is important for the removal of potentially toxic chemical products or reactants, thereby enabling the elimination of molecular impurities. Nakagawa and Yokozawa [7] found that flavan-3-ols-which serve as antioxidants and aid in the process of reduction-enhance the scavenging activity of polyphenolic plant compounds (gallic acids) compared to the scavenging activity of gallic acids independently. A study by Hirun and Roach [8] found that the structure of EGCG is consistent with the type of molecule that performs scavenging activity. EGCG was also evaluated for its ability to act as a neuroprotecting agent and was found to have the highest protection values against the process of DNA excision, compared to other catechin compounds [5]. In contrast, however, ECG was evaluated for having the highest potential for its scavenging abilities [9].

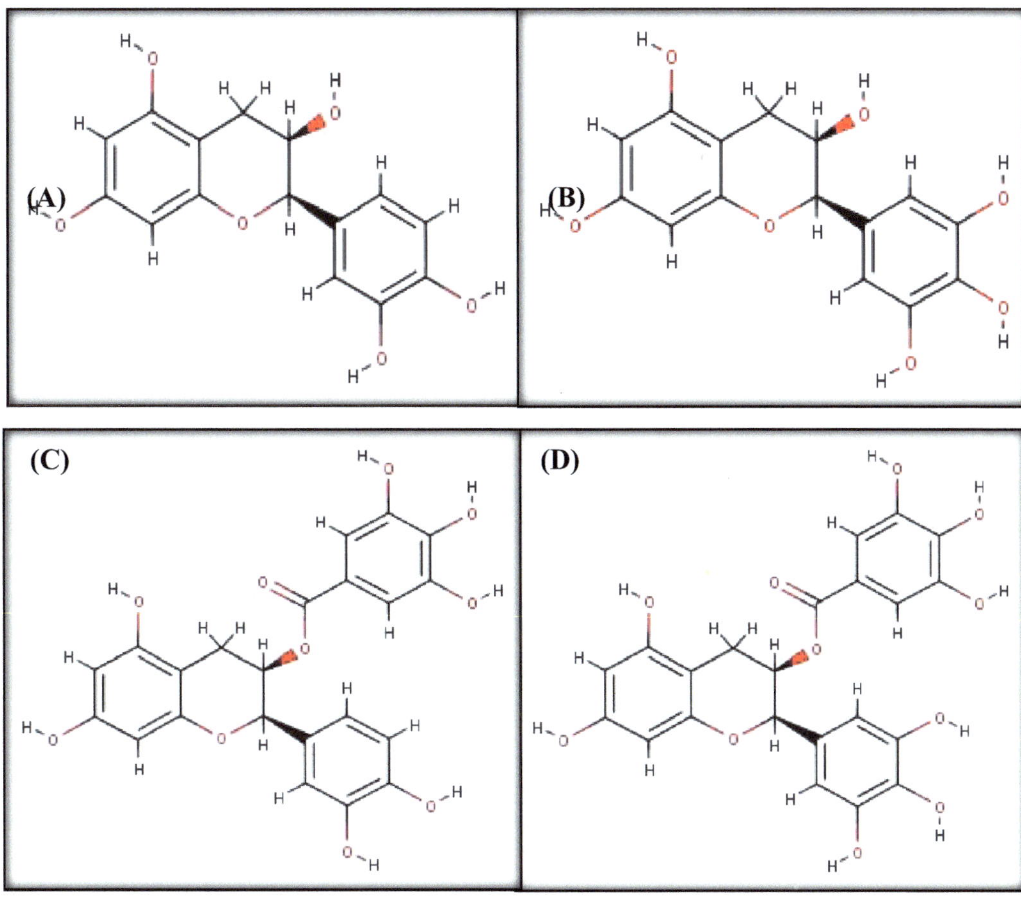

Fig. (1). Structure of Catechins. The four major types of catechins and their structures, from top-left to top-right and bottom-left to bottom-right. (**A**) Structure of Epicatechin (EC). **(B)** Structure of Epigallocatechin (EGC). **(C)** Structure of Epicatechin Gallate (ECG). **(D)** Structure of Epigallocatechin Gallate (EGCG).

2.2. Catechins as Inhibitors

Green tea catechins (especially (-) Epigallocatechin-3-gallate (EGCG)), exert multiple effects on signaling pathways and cellular proteins [1]. A study by Dulloo *et al.* [10] found that green tea catechins can inhibit Catechol-O-methyltransferase (COMT), an enzyme responsible for the degradation of neurotransmitters including norepinephrine. Similarly, EGCG has demonstrated high inhibition levels of pure catalase inhibition and increased suppression of viable cell types such as cancer cells, with IC_{50} levels of 54.5 μM [4]. This study proposes a great potential for patenting the use of gallated catechins such as EGCG, in anticancer drug treatment against the spread of cancerous cells. Moreover, studies conducted *in vitro* found that EGCG exhibits an inhibitory effect on certain signal transduction pathways such as Notch, Wnt, JAK/STAT, MAPK and P13K/Akt, where the disruption of these pathways may prevent carcinogenesis (the initiation of cancer formation) from occurring [11]. Additionally, Singh and his colleagues [11] also found that the prevention of sequential damage which occurs in response to oxidation could serve as a promising first defense mechanism against carcinogens, thereby combatting cancer progression. Some general mechanisms proposed for the biological activities of EGCG include cell cycle arrest, apoptosis, modulation of cell signaling, inhibition of DNA methylation, altered miRNA expression, protease activity, and telomerase activity [11]. Furthermore, the study in focus [11] also examines the effect of EGCG on several signal transduction pathways including the inhibition of protein kinase.

As previously mentioned, EGCG inhibits mitogen-activated protein kinase (MAPK) pathways, though it has also been shown to have an inhibitory effect on other molecular mechanisms including cyclin-dependent kinases (CDKs) which contribute to the cell cycle, DNA methyltransferase (with epigenetic applications), proteosomes (significant to proteases and the ubiquitin pathway), and the pathway for receptor tyrosine kinase (RTK) [12]. Moreover, EGCG prevents the spread of several malignant conditions (*e.g.,* cancer) as it targets mechanisms such as those aforementioned, and specifically RTK pathways [12].

2.3. Effects of Catechins on Depression

Depression can be debilitating in many ways, however, when present in combination with other underlying and thus, overlapping psychiatric and/or emotional or affective disorders, can greatly impact one's quality of life. In this circumstance, depression can be extremely dangerous and may drastically increase patient vulnerability to the risk of suicide. Furthermore, neuronal tissue is particularly prone to oxidative damage compared to other tissues in the body.

Catechins serve as natural antioxidants which aid in the prevention of neuronal damage and therefore, protect neurons during increased oxidative stress-which, notably, is higher during depressive states [13]. Interestingly, oxidative stress has previously been ascribed a contributor not only to cardiovascular disease, but is also implicated in the development of certain psychiatric disorders [13].

A recent study examining post-stroke depression identified the antioxidant activity of polyphenol catechins as the active ingredient of green tea that helps aid in the regulation of depressive symptoms, thereby reducing oxidative stress, restoring proper functioning, and partially repairing antioxidant endogenous defense mechanisms [13]. Similarly, another study found that green tea reduces symptoms of depression in non-human animal subjects by inhibiting monoamine oxidase (MAO) [14]. Likewise, a study conducted by Mähler *et al.* [15] found that neurotransmitter activity in rats decreases with age. Additionally, researchers found that upon the administration of EGCG, rats showed an increase in neurotransmitter activity, specifically of acetylcholine (ACh), dopamine, and serotonin, thereby exhibiting fewer depressive symptoms [15]. Furthermore, a meta-analysis involving 11 cohorts demonstrated that in 13 cases covering upwards of 22 thousand participants, a negative correlation existed between tea consumption and the risk of depression, resulting in a 37% reduction in symptoms among participants who drank 3 or more cups of green tea per day [16]. These findings further elucidate the potential medicinal benefits of green tea catechins and present a promising approach to the therapeutic treatment of depression and associated psychiatric disorders by means of natural products.

3. CHARACTERIZATION OF MONOAMINE OXIDASES

3.1. Functional Characteristics

Monoamine oxidase (MAO) performs deamination of amines by catalyzing the oxidation/inactivation of primary monoamines (Fig. **2**). MAOs are bound to the outer mitochondrial membrane with higher activity localized in neuronal cells, and are active in the CNS, PNS, and peripheral organs. MAO oxidizes freely accessible monoamine neurotransmitters that have not already been taken up and stored in vesicles in a presynaptic cell. In the brain, MAO primarily targets serotonin, dopamine, and norepinephrine for functional removal. Consequently, several psychological, psychiatric, and/or mental health disorders may develop as a result of the function of MAOs in brain activity.

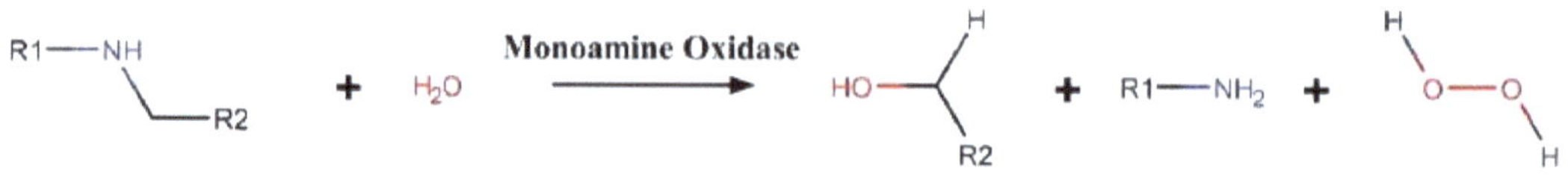

Fig. (2). The Monoamine Oxidase Mechanism. Monoamine oxidases are a group of enzymes that catalyze the oxidative deamination of monoamines. The above mechanism illustrates the oxidation of a secondary amine (into an imine) followed by hydration, resulting in the generation of an aldehyde and a primary amine.

3.2. Mechanistic Comparison of Monoamine Oxidases

MAOs are a type of amine-oxidizing flavoenzyme that serve as catalysts in the enzyme-catalyzed reaction of flavin-dependent amine oxidation. There are two forms of the MAO enzyme, collectively known as isozymes. These include type A which is further characterized as MAOA, and type B, characterized as MAOB [17]. Both monoamine oxidase isoenzymes contain highly conserved active sites and demonstrate 70% homogeneity. Substrates for MAOA predominantly include epinephrine, norepinephrine, and serotonin, whereas substrates for MAOB include phenylethylamine, phenylethanolamine, tyramine, and benzylamine [18]. However, there are substances that are metabolized by both enzymes, such as dopamine and tryptamine. Although each MAO isozyme is abundantly expressed in the brain, MAOA is also present in the liver, heart, and pancreas, while MAOB is found in the liver, posterior pituitary, renal tubules, and endocrine pancreas [17]. MAOA is a gene found in catecholaminergic neurons, in this case norepinephrine and dopamine [19]. MAOA metabolizes several different monoamine neurotransmitters and is selectively inhibited by Clorgyline, an MAO inhibitor (MAOI) that is structurally similar to the antidepressant Pargyline (Table **1**) [19]. Li and his colleagues [19] reveal that MAOB is found mostly in astrocytes as well as in some serotonergic neurons that specifically act on dopamine and β-phenylethylamine (β-PEA) monoamines, and is selectively, and irreversibly, inhibited by Selegiline (Deprenyl) (Table **1**) [19 - 21]. Both MAOA and MAOB enzymes maintain homoeostasis in the brain, with functional roles in the regulation of neurotransmitters to ensure proper neurological and psychological functioning [19]. Li and colleagues [19] also found that the excessive activation of MAOA and/or MAOB produces neurotoxic byproducts which, in turn, can trigger the development of psychiatric disorders, and may ultimately result in irreversible neurodegeneration.

3.3. Diseases of the Nervous System: Fluctuations in MAO Activity

Altered MAO activity was found to be an occurrence of some central and peripheral nervous system diseases. For instance, elevated levels of MAOA leading to heightened MAOA activity has found to be associated with episodes of major depressive disorder [22]. Interestingly, these occurrences have shown to persist even after treatment with a Selective Serotonin Reuptake Inhibitor (SSRI), a substance which functions to inhibit the reuptake of the neurotransmitter serotonin [22].

In contrast, heightened MAOB activity in the brain has been shown to occur in Alzheimer's disease, Huntington's disease, Parkinson's disease, and is a result of normal aging. Medical intervention, treatment, and therapy for these disorders is widely available, although a common form of intervention includes routine dosing of pharmaceutical agents using MAOA, MAOB, or both isozymes as targets. Alternatively, some studies have demonstrated that catechins may serve as potent inhibitors of MAO [18]. This is of special importance in that catechins, and particularly green tea catechins-using MAOs as targets-may present a new therapeutic approach to treating MAO-associated disorders using natural products as a substitute for synthetic pharmaceutical medications. These findings further suggest that, with the use of MAOs as targets, catechins may also be preventative for certain disease progression with respect to degenerative diseases and emotional disorders [19].

3.4. Monoamine Oxidase Inhibitors: A Pharmaceutical Approach

Monoamine oxidase inhibitors (MAOIs) are a class of drugs generally used as antidepressants and are effective in treating depression, although they are also used to treat Bipolar disorder as well as various Panic disorders. MAOIs functionally inhibit the actions of the MAO enzymes. As the MAO isoenzymes catalyze the breakdown of monoamine neurotransmitters through the process of oxidative deamination, methods of inhibition as such enable a steady increase in the level of monoamine neurotransmitter accumulation at the synapse, thereby enhancing the docking potential of monoamines onto postsynaptic cells. This activity ultimately results in the steady firing of action potentials which, in turn, maintains neuronal amine homeostasis.

3.5. Current Pharmacological Agents as MAOIs

As presented in Table **1** below, the most common MAO inhibitors (from DrugBank.com) are shown. There are many types of pharmacological agents currently on the market as MAOIs. Despite molecular variations, these drugs share similar function in that they mimic monoamine neurotransmitters such as dopamine, serotonin, epinephrine (adrenaline), norepinephrine (noradrenaline), and β-phenylethylamine (β-PEA), for inhibition and inactivation of the target MAO enzymes. However, the effects of these drugs are not solely confined to the central nervous system. In fact, pharmaceutical agents in the form of MAOIs are often administered in the treatment of neurodegenerative diseases for the purpose of targeting the peripheral nervous system. As previously mentioned, the overall objective of MAOIs is to regulate the accumulation of neurochemicals (specifically, monoamine neurotransmitters) between presynaptic and postsynaptic cells. As certain neurochemicals, neurotransmitters, and neuromodulators, such as those aforementioned, are primarily responsible for many aspects pertaining to emotion (including the perception of mood and feelings) and are crucial for proper cognitive functioning, an imbalance of any such chemical can play a critical role in the pathogenesis of many psychological and/or neurological conditions. MAOIs therefore serve as a means to offset the impact of chemical imbalances on mood and behavior, while also temporarily restoring impaired cognitive functioning in response to neurodegeneration as a result of such imbalances.

3.6. Pharmacotherapy of Monoamine Oxidase-Associated Disorders

Table **1** presents a display for elements of (or pertaining to) current, developmental, experimental, and investigational pharmacological treatments for MAOA- and MAOB-related disorders by means of monoamine oxidase inhibitors. The table details various properties of MAOIs in terms of chemical classification, pharmacological classification, their known side effects, and current status, in accordance with the Food and Drug Association (FDA). Depending on whether the drug is an inhibitor of MAOA or MAOB can determine the way in which the inhibitor treats the condition for the patient.

Table 1. Pharmacotherapy of Monoamine oxidase-related disorders *via* MAOIs [20, 21].

Inhibitors of MAOA					
Medication	**Chemical Classification**	**Pharmacological Classification**	**Comments**	**Side Effects**	**Status**
BEFLOXATONE	*Unclassified* **Super Class**: N/A **Class**: N/A **Sub Class**: N/A	Neuropsychiatric agent and Antidepressant-used to mitigate panic disorders.	Selective. Prescription information currently unavailable.	Increased sleep latency (REM sleep), decreased sleep duration (SEM sleep).	Experimental
BROFAMINE	*Benzenofurans* **Super Class:** Organoheterocyclic compounds **Class:** Benzenofurans **Sub Class**: N/A	No further information is available at this time.	Used to make Abediterol, Acarbose, and Accebutolol.	N/A	Experimental

(Table 1) cont.....

Medication	Chemical Classification	Pharmacological Classification	Comments	Side Effects	Status
CLORGILINE (CLORGYLINE)	*Dichlorobenzenes* **Super Class**: Benzenoids **Class**: Benzene & Substitute Derivatives (SDs) **Sub Class**: Halobenzenes	Antidepressant.	Related to Pargyline. Used to make Clorgiline Hydrochloride and Moclobemide.	Anxiety, dizziness, headache, nausea, vomiting, dry mouth, sleep disturbances, constipation, liver damage, sexual dysfunction.	Experimental
MINAPRINE	*Phenylpyridazines* **Super Class:** Organoheterocyclic compounds **Class:** Diazines **Sub Class:** Pyridazines and derivatives	Psychoactive drug. Also used as an antidepressant to treat depression.	Used to make Cantor and Minaprine Dihydro-chloride.	N/A	Approved
MOCLOBEMIDE	*4-halobenzoic acids & Derivatives* **Super Class:** Benzenoids **Class:** Benzene & SDs **Sub Class:** Benzoic acids & derivatives	Antidepressant-used to treat depression (Major Depressive Disorder) and is more effective in the acute form.	Selective and reversible. Used to make Manerix; also used to make Moclobemide 100 and PMS Moclobemide.	Agitation, dizziness, drowsiness, muscle rigidity, headache, confusion, seizures, and hypertension.	Approved, Under Investigation
PHENELZINE	*Benzene* **Super Class:** Benzenoids **Class:** Benzene & SDs **Sub Class:** N/A	Antidepressant and anxiolytic agent used to treat depression and social anxiety disorder. Also used as a panic disorder treatment option.	Nonselective and irreversible. Used to make Nardil and Phenelzine Sulfate.	Elevation in aminotransferase levels; injury to liver.	Approved
PIRLINDOLE	*Carbazoles* **Super Class:** Organoheterocyclic compounds **Class:** Indoles & Derivatives **Sub Class:** Carbazoles	Antidepressant. Also used to treat fibromyalgia.	Reversible. Elevates mood by regulating levels of available catecholamines and norepinephrine.	Seizures, agitation, and hyperthermia. Tremors and death when coupled with SSRIs, TCAs, tyramine-rich foods, and sympathomimetic drugs.	Approved
PYRAZOLINE DERIVATIVES	*Alkaloids / Pyrazoles* **Super Class:** Organoheterocyclic compounds **Class:** Azoles **Sub Class:** Pyrazoles	Anticancer, antipyretic, antiviral, anticonvulsant, anti-inflammatory, and analgesic agent.	Reversible.	N/A	Experimental

(Table 1) cont.....

Medication	**Chemical Classification**	**Pharmacological Classification**	**Comments**	**Side Effects**	**Status**
TOLOXATONE	*Toluenes* **Super Class:** Benzenoids **Class:** Benzene & SDs **Sub Class:** Toluenes	Antidepressant.	Selective and reversible.	Constipation, dysuria, nausea, insomnia, vertigo and fulminant hepatitis.	Approved
TRANYL-CYPROMINE (PARNATE)	*Aralkylamines* **Super Class:** Organic Nitrogen Compounds **Class:** Organo-nitrogen compounds **Sub Class:** Amines	Psychoactive drug used as an antidepressant or anxiolytic agent to treat major and atypical depression, panic and phobia-based disorders, and dysthymic disorder.	Nonselective and irreversible. Used to make Tranyl-cypromine Sulfate and Parnate.	Anxiety, mental incoherence, insomnia, feeling of drowsiness or dizziness, and hypotension.	Approved, Under Investigation
TYRIMA	*Unclassified* **Super Class**: N/A **Class**: N/A **Sub Class**: N/A	Used to treat anxiety and depression.	Catalyzes biogenic and xenobiotic amines.	N/A	Under Investigation
3,5-DIARYL PYRAZONE	*Alkaloids / Pyrazoles* **Super Class:** Organoheterocyclic Compounds **Class:** Azoles **Sub Class:** Pyrazoles	Potential anticancer and anti-inflammatory agent. Potential tyrosinase inhibitor.	Selective and reversible.	N/A	Experimental
		Inhibitors of MAOB			
Medication	**Chemical Classification**	**Pharmacological Classification**	**Comments**	**Side Effects**	**Status**
3,5-DIARYL PYRAZONE	*Alkaloids / Pyrazoles* **Super Class:** Organoheterocyclic Compounds **Class:** Azoles **Sub Class:** Pyrazoles	Potential anticancer and anti-inflammatory agent. Potential tyrosinase inhibitor.	Selective and reversible.	N/A	Experimental
CATECHIN / EPICATECHINS	*Catechins* **Super Class**: Phenylproponoids & Polyketides **Class**: Flavonoids **Sub Class**: Flavans	Unclassified.	Used in studies for pre-diabetes treatment.	N/A	Under Investigation
CHALCONE DERIVATIVES *Derivatives:* Hesperidin	*Chalcanoids* **Super Class**: Polyphenols **Class**: Chalcanoids **Sub Class**: N/A	Potential anticancer agent.	Potential MAOB inhibitor.	Hepa, Nephra, neuro and ototoxicity.	Under Investigation

(Table 1) cont.....

Medication	Chemical Classification	Pharmacological Classification	Comments	Side Effects	Status
COURAMINE *Derivatives:* Photovoltaic sensitizers, Warfarin, laser dye gain medium, edema modifier.	*Phenylpropanoids (see Geiparvarin)* **Super Class**: Benzopyrones **Class**: Lactones **Sub Class**: Coumarin	Antidepressant.	Potential anti-inflammatory, antibacterial, anticoagulant, antifungal and antitumor properties.	Anxiety, nausea, vomiting, dry mouth, dizziness, headache, sleep disturbances, constipation, sexual dysfunction, and liver damage.	Under Investigation
DESMETHOXY-YANGONIN	*Kavalactones* **Super Class**: N/A **Class**: N/A **Sub Class**: N/A	Potential MAOB inhibitor.	Used to make Kava.	Liver damage, apoptosis.	Experimental
GEIPARVARIN *Derivatives:* Couramin-derived treatments.	*Phenylpropanoids* **Super Class**: Benzopyrones **Class**: Lactones **Sub Class**: Coumarin	Used to treat lymphedema and is under study for its antitumor properties.	Sometimes used to make organic blue-green laser dyes.	Moderate toxicity in humans, mainly liver and kidneys.	Under Investigation
ISATIN	*Indolines* **Super Class**: Organoheterocyclic compounds **Class**: Indoles & Derivatives **Sub Class**: Indolines	Potential MAOB inhibitor. Biosynthesizes pigments, hormones, and neurotransmitters.	Found in Schiff bases and certain plants. Used to make Isatin-based derivatives.	N/A	Experimental
PARGYLINE	*Phenylmethylamines* **Super Class**: Benzenoids **Class**: Benzene & Substitute Derivatives **Sub Class**: Phenylmethylamine	Antidepressant. Also used to reduce hypertension and hypertensive properties.	Used to make Abediterol, Acarbose, and Acebutolol.	Increased hypertension, increased blood pressure, increased heart rate, and increased levels of glucose in the bloodstream.	Approved, Under Investigation
PHTHALIMIDES/ THALIDOMIDE	*Phthalimides* **Super Class**: Organoheterocyclic compounds **Class**: Isoindoles & Derivatives **Sub Class:** Isoindolines	Non-barbiturate hypnotic-used for treatment of immunological and inflammatory disorders. Potential tumor suppressive properties.	Used to make Thalomid and Thalidomide Celgene.	Teratogenic side effects.	Approved, Under Investigation, Withdrawn
PYRAZOLINE DERIVATIVES	*Alkaloids / Pyrazoles* **Super Class:** Organoheterocyclic compounds **Class:** Azoles **Sub Class:** Pyrazoles	Anticancer, antipyretic, antiviral, anticonvulsant, anti-inflammatory, and analgesic agent.	Reversible.	N/A	Experimental

(Table 1) cont.....

Medication	Chemical Classification	Pharmacological Classification	Comments	Side Effects	Status
RASAGILINE	*Propargylamine* **Super Class:** Benzenoids **Class:** Indanes **Sub Class:** Unavailable	MAOB Inhibitor used to treat Parkinson's disease. Treatments also available for Alzheimer's disease, ALS and MSA.	Irreversible. Used to make aporasagiline, Rasagiline Mesylate, and Azilect.	Irregular pulse, agitation, feeling of drowsiness or dizziness, coma, hyperactivity, convulsions, migraines, irritability.	Approved
SAFINAMIDE	*Alpha amino acid amines* **Super Class:** Organic Acids & Derivatives **Class:** Carboxylic Acid & Derivatives **Sub Class:** Analogues, Amino acids & Peptides	Amino acid amide used to treat Parkinson's disease.	Used to make Xadago.	Insomnia, involuntary movement, high blood pressure, hallucinations, nausea, vomiting.	Approved, Under Investigation
SELEGILINE (DEPRENYL)	*Amphetamines & Derivatives* **Super Class:** Benzenoids **Class:** Benzene & Substitute Derivatives **Sub Class:** Phenylethylamines	MAOB inhibitor used towards making treatments for Parkinson's Disease.	Selective and irreversible. Prolongs dopamine. Used to make Atapryl, Carbex, and Eldepryl.	Heartburn, nausea, dry-mouth, insomnia, dizziness. Confusion, nightmares, hallucinations, headaches.	Approved, Under Investigation, Vet-Approved

3.7. Monoamine Reuptake Inhibitors: Mechanisms of Inhibitor Action

Although synthetic drugs employ a variety of different mechanistic approaches for the ways in which they exert their effects, the pharmacological agents discussed herein primarily alter-*e.g.,* enhance (by means of activation), disrupt (through methods of interference), or inhibit (*via* inactivation)-synaptic transmission (*i.e.,* neurotransmission) by targeting either neurotransmitter-receptor interactions or neurotransmitter-transporter interactions on pre- and postsynaptic cells. Monoamine reuptake inhibitors (MARIs), in particular, constitute a category of inhibitory agents which act on monoamine transporters directly, and functionally prevent the reuptake of monoamine neurotransmitters by blocking access of transporters to their respective neurotransmitters [23]. In other words, MARIs block the transporters for monoamine neurotransmitters. This action further prevents the transport of neurotransmitters from pre- to postsynaptic cells. Examples of monoamine transporters include serotonin transporters (SERT), noradrenaline/norepinephrine transporters (NET), and the selective dopamine transporter (DAT). Upon the inhibition of such transporters, an increase in the amount of neurotransmitter able to accumulate in the synapse is observed [24]. As more neurotransmitters accumulate, they are redistributed further along the synapse before being metabolized [24]. Moreover, upon the binding of neurotransmitters to transporters such as SERT or DAT, an event known as colocalization typically occurs, generally with PICK1 (Protein Interacting with C Kinase-1; a protein encoded by the PICK1 gene in humans) *via* a PDZ domain [24]. The PDZ domain serves as an anchoring protein bound to the membrane which colocalizes the SERT or DAT neurotransmitter-transporter complex to the metabotropic glutamate receptor (mGluR7a), which then mediates endocytosis on the postsynaptic cell [25, 26]. However, the binding of an inhibitor to the transporters SERT or DAT functionally prevents this mechanistic sequence of events.

There are selective and nonselective MARIs, where the former selectively binds a single, specific type of transporter, and the latter binds two or more different kinds of monoamine transporters. Examples of pharmaceutical MARIs include Tricyclic Antidepressants (TCAs), Tetracyclic Antidepressants, Selective Serotonin Reuptake Inhibitors (SSRIs), Noradrenaline Reuptake Inhibitors (NARIs), Serotonin-Noradrenaline Reuptake Inhibitors (SNRIs), Noradrenaline-Dopamine Reuptake Inhibitors (NDRIs), and Nonselective MARIs [27, 28].

3.8. MAOIs: Mechanisms of Inhibitor Action-Nonselective and Selective Inhibition

MAOIs act on both mitochondrial-bound MAO isozymes adjacently located to receptor sites for neurotransmitters in postsynaptic cells. While MAOs function in the catabolism of ingested monoamines, they are also responsible for the inactivation of monoamine neurotransmitters through a process of deamination in which the amine group of an incoming monoamine neurotransmitter is oxidized by an MAO enzyme.

MAOIs, however, serve to inhibit the actions of MAOs which, in turn, prevent the process of deamination. As a result, receptors become saturated with neurotransmitters. These actions enable neurotransmitters to remain in the synapse for longer durations, thereby maintaining psychological homeostasis. The development and use of MAOIs marks an important feat in pharmacology as the first pharmacological treatment to combat symptoms of depression. MAOIs provide a means to correct an imbalance of neurotransmitters (due to insufficiency, deficiency, or excessive levels) in response to MAO activity, and synthetic MAOIs have been manufactured as antidepressants for decades. As with MARIs, MAO enzyme inhibitors can also be selective or nonselective. Nonselective MAOIs are irreversible, while selective MAOIs can be either reversible or irreversible. Examples of nonselective MAOIs include Phenelzine, and Tranylcypromine (Table **1**), although these are traditionally used as MAOA inhibitors rather than MAOB inhibitors. These nonselective MAOIs interact with the flavin N5 atom in the active site of each MAO enzyme.

Previous structural studies of inhibitor-MAOB complexes provide electron density maps which show that various clinically used inhibitors of MAOB may also interact with the flavin N5 atom of the FAD cofactor [27]. The active site of MAOB consists of a hydrophobic substrate cavity interconnected to an entrance cavity in the active site by Ile199 which acts like a 'hinge' connecting these two sites. The recognition site for the substrate amino group(s) is an aromatic cage partly formed by Tyr398 and Tyr435 [27].

Moreover, of the selective inhibitors, there are also two types of MAOIs: reversible and irreversible. Selective, reversible MAOIs for the MAOA isozyme include MoclobemideBlue; and examples of irreversible MAOIs for the MAOB isoenzyme are Rasagiline and Selegiline (Deprenyl) (Table **1**) [20, 21, 27]. Selective, irreversible drugs which act on MAOB are typically used for the treatment of neurological disorders (*e.g.,* Parkinson's disease) as they target cells in the PNS, thereby prolonging the presence of dopamine in the synapse [28]. Drugs of this type therefore serve as a reliable means to combat symptoms brought on by the progression of the disease. In contrast, drugs which inhibit MAOA are more commonly used to treat psychological disorders, such as depression and anxiety, by targeting neuronal cells in the CNS [29].

3.9. Adverse Effects of Conventional MAOIs: Clinical Considerations and Toxicity

Selective MAOIs are currently used more frequently than nonselective MAOIs as they pose less risk for the occurrence of adverse side effects. Nonselective MAOIs display a broader systemic effect, while selective MAOIs exhibit more specificity. However, MAOIs have a higher degree of toxicity compared to other forms of antidepressants, as apparent by the increased risk of adverse side effects for which these drugs impose. The more pronounced side effects of MAOIs generally include dry mouth, nausea, diarrhea, constipation, headache, drowsiness, insomnia, and dizziness (or lightheadedness) from possible postural hypotension [28].

In addition to the adverse reactions caused by the drugs themselves, MAOIs tend to be less favorable compared to other forms of antidepressants, as they are often accompanied by many hazardous food-drug and drug-drug interactions. The most common side effect of a food-drug interaction with MAOIs is the inhibition of tyramine breakdown. This results in a buildup of tyramine, increasing tyramine toxicity, and may ultimately cause increased hypertension and possible hypertensive crisis. Tyramine is derived from the amino acid tyrosine, which helps regulate blood pressure. Tyramine is often found in foods such as aged cheese, cured/smoked meats, fish, beer, red wines, certain beans, pickles, olives, some soy products, teriyaki sauce, and is sometimes found in chocolate, caffeine, yogurt, avocados, and raspberries. Because of this, the consumption of these food types with the use of MAOIs is usually prohibited. Consequently, dietary limitations as extensive and restrictive as these typically result in lower patient compliance [29].

Concerning drug-drug interactions, the action of MAOIs in conjunction with any other drug affecting the metabolism, release, synthesis, or reuptake of monoamine neurotransmitters, can cause an increase in MAOI toxicity by increasing the risk of potentially dangerous side effects. Examples of drugs that pose such risks include Dextromethorphan, SSRIs, and serotonergic agents [29]. Furthermore, because pharmacological agents are metabolized more effectively over time, an increase in metabolism (or tolerance) generally requires a subsequent-and perhaps continuous-increase in dosage to compensate for diminishing effects, thereby maintaining the overall efficacy of the drug. Although a constant increase in dosage may seem like an easy solution in a therapeutic context, indeed such increases actually pose great risk to patients in a clinical setting. For example, in addition to the many possible harmful interactions as well the various negative side effects associated with MAOIs, the need for frequent dosage increases can also introduce an array of complications and other concerning factors which contribute to the overall toxicity of the drug and ultimately affect one's overall health. These risks can include drug dependency as well as overdose, but when taken in considerable amounts over particularly extended durations, may also pose significant threat to physiological systems and individual organs such as the heart, liver, and kidneys, and may result in chronic disease-possibly accompanied by organ failure-all of which can be a contributor to premature death [29 - 34].

With respect to potentially life-threatening adverse reactions, there is also the possibility, although rather uncommon and somewhat rare, of developing various potentially fatal conditions, such as Serotonin Syndrome (SS) or Neuroleptic Malignant Syndrome (NMS), which arise in response to excessive and prolonged use of, for example, antidepressants or antipsychotics-used in the treatment of depression, manic depressive disorder, and bipolar disorder, among many other debilitating neurological disorders. Such conditions arise unexpectedly and can take the form of an unintentional drug-induced overdose, regardless of the appropriate and responsible use of the prescription medication.

3.10. The Need for Additional (natural) Inhibitors of MAO

Although MAOIs are continuously reliable for their intended purpose, particularly for atypical symptoms associated with certain disorders, the popularity and use of MAOIs has waned for decades. As previously mentioned, the most common reasons for not prescribing MAOIs include drug-drug interactions, drug-food interactions, negative adverse effects, preference for alternative treatment, and dietary restrictions [29 - 34]. Therefore, substantial research efforts have been set forth to investigate the potential medicinal benefits of natural products-a widely explored topic recently-as natural products may demonstrate comparable impact and effectiveness as MAOIs on neurotransmitters and surrounding mechanisms, but without the increased probability of harsh adverse effects. A natural inhibitor of MAO can have the same impact as a synthetic pharmaceutical agent, yet with minimal side effects and far fewer, if any, restrictions due to potentially harmful interactions. Thus, a significant amount of research has been conducted with efforts currently underway for the purpose of identifying additional natural methods to treat psychological disorders and neurodegenerative diseases.

3.11. The Proposed Benefits of Catechins as Natural Inhibitors of MAO

For the above reasons, catechins could serve as potentially powerful, minimal-to-no-risk alternatives to MAOIs. For instance, the aforementioned meta-analysis of 11 studies involving over 22 thousand participants concluded that an inverse, linear relationship exists between routine tea consumption and the risk of depression [16, 35]. However, these studies account for only a small fraction of the many available studies which demonstrate a pharmacological potential for the bioactive constituents found in various natural products. Catechins, for example, have been shown to display similar actions as a multitude of synthetic drugs used in the treatment of certain neurological disorders. Likewise, catechins have shown to exert the same inhibitory actions as MAOIs, and can be a safer alternative to the medications which hinder the lives of many individuals Each year, studies continue to confirm the effectiveness of green tea catechins as natural, yet potent substitutes for certain pharmaceutical drugs that are frequently accompanied by hazardous drug-drug and drug-food interactions, in addition to unwanted side effects [36]. These findings are in further support of the notion that green tea may serve as a safer alternative to MAOIs.

4. HIGH THROUGHPUT SCREENING STRATEGIES

4.1. Non-Fluorescence-based Assays

There are many different types of assays that use various techniques to monitor and measure the progress of the MAOA and MAOB reactions. As shown in Fig. (**2**), an imine is generated from the oxidative deamination of monoamines, and the following hydration produces an aldehyde and hydrogen peroxide. This provides several efficient approaches to monitor MAO activity using various detection methods: either by tracking the absence of substrate or by probing the presence of specific products in the reaction. One of the original approaches to high throughput assays utilized radiolabeling (^{14}C labeling) of selective substrates Serotonin (for MAOA) and Benzylamine (for MAOB) [37]. Another approach (developed by Promega) called the MAO-GLO™ Assay makes use of a bioluminescent-coupled assay. This is particularly advantageous in that it is not susceptible to interference, as fluorescent assays may be due to endogenous fluorescent molecules in cell lysate and tissue homogenates. Promega developed an assay that couples the activity of MAO to the production of light by luciferase. Briefly, the non-selective substrate aminopropyl ether (analog of luciferin methyl ester) is cleaved to generate light.

This occurs in a two-step process. Once the MAO enzyme oxidizes the amine of the substrate to an imine—which is quickly hydrolyzed to an aldehyde—the specific aldehyde product in the MAO-GLO™ assay undergoes a spontaneous β-elimination reaction to form luciferin methyl ester. In the second step of the assay, the luciferin detection reagent inactivates the MAO enzyme, and the esterase and luciferase enzymes in the reagent hydrolyze the methyl ester, thus oxidizing the luciferin to produce light. The reactions are rapid and the amount of light produced in the second step is proportional to the activity of MAO in the first part of the reaction [38].

4.2. Fluorescence-based Assays: The Role of the Fluorescent Probe

A fluorescent probe is introduced to the reaction where it reacts with either a reactant, product, or byproduct of the initial reaction and fluoresces. These probes are generally designed to exhibit a high-degree of specificity for a target molecule (the stimulus). Upon interaction with the target, fluorescence emission (the signal) is generated and released by a fluorophore, thereby becoming measurable. Because of this, fluorescent assays serve as a useful method to detect and quantify the presence of specific components within a reaction. Redox-sensitive probes are one of several examples in which a probe can be sensitized to different stimuli, but react and respond via the same process of fluorescence. These assays thus serve as effective methods to not only measure the presence of a known reactant or product within a reaction, but also to study certain aspects of a reaction itself, with the ability to monitor specific enzymatic activity of a given reaction.

Fluorescent probes have therefore played a crucial role in the study of biological reactions and have greatly expanded the ways in which reactions can be quantitatively assessed-through the use of kinetic studies. Furthermore, the convenience of using fluorescence as a means to study kinetics has largely enabled the ease of drug design in addition to the study of natural products, but has also proven quite useful in studying the particular pharmacokinetics of proposed medications within the scope of pharmacology. This is largely due to the ability to not only measure enzymatic activity, but to also examine specific enzymatic activity in response to pharmacological agents which modulate this activity, such as an inhibitor.

As indicated by Youdim and a multitude of fellow colleagues who have since referenced him [39 - 43], the use of fluorescence-based methods to probe for the detection of MAO activity is most beneficial. Fluorescent assays now include (but are by no means limited to) bioimaging with either near-infrared or two-photon techniques [19], as well a plethora of assays performed in combination with ELISA methods, fluorescent probe kits (example: Amplex Red kit), and a multitude of synthetic MAOA and MAOB substrates that cleave to fluorescent molecules such as kynuramine assays which utilize kynuramine to form 4-hydroxyquinoline (a fluorescent product) [41].

4.3. Fluorescence-based Assays: Inhibition Assays

Fluorescent assays provide a reliable means to assess certain components of a reaction, such as the effectiveness of an inhibitor and its effect on enzymatic activity. The ability of reaction-sensitive probes to sense changes in enzymatic activity (assessed *via* concentration levels) as a result of pharmacological manipulation has proven most valuable when investigating the pharmacokinetics of potential drug inhibitors.

Fluorescent assays for MAO generally make use of a non-fluorescent probe exhibiting high-affinity for hydrogen peroxide, a byproduct of the MAO oxidation reaction, and are typically coupled with a peroxidase. Following oxidation, the non-fluorescent probe is converted to a fluorophore, enabling fluorescence emission to be quantitatively measured. The specific enzymatic activity of MAO can be assessed as a measure of the resulting fluorescence. However, in the presence of a MAO inhibitor, fluorescence emission is greatly reduced. Since the purpose of an MAOI is to functionally block the actions of the MAO enzyme(s), the use of a fluorescent probe which exhibits preferential selectivity for a product of the MAO reaction further enables a precise confirmation for the particular efficacy of the inhibitor being assessed. The presence of a potent MAO inhibitor would result in an absence of the hydrogen peroxide byproduct, which, in turn, would be reflected by a substantial reduction in fluorescent activity. In contrast, the presence of the hydrogen peroxide byproduct as reflected *via* enhanced fluorescence activity, would suggest that either a MAO inhibitor was absent in the reaction (a positive control), or, if present, that the inhibitor used was unable to effectively target either one (or both) of the MAO enzymes-*i.e.,* is selective and therefore only compatible with MAOA or MAOB.

4.4. High Throughput Screening with Enzyme-Linked Fluorescent Assays

High throughput screening for the inhibition of MAOs by smallest molecules makes use of fluorescent assays and can assess both kinetic and endpoint measurements of MAO activity. The source of MAO can be either purified enzyme or an extract from specific tissue homogenate, however, the total protein content should be known so that the assay parameters can be optimized. Additionally, p-tyramine substrate is generally used in these assays since it can be used for both of the MAO isozymes. Recall that in general, MAO reacts with specific monoamines and generates a hydrogen peroxide byproduct. In the presence of horse radish peroxidase (HRP), a weakly fluorescent-otherwise referred to as non-fluorescent-fluorometric probe, called resazurin, reacts with H_2O_2 (the hydrogen peroxide byproduct) to produce highly fluorescent Resorufin. The Resorufin product can be easily read by a fluorescence microplate reader, with excitation ranging from 530-560 nm, and an emission of 580-590 nm [42, 43]. Fluorescence values are proportional to the amine oxidase levels within the samples, and unknown samples can be determined and identified by comparison with a hydrogen peroxide standard curve. The absence of the hydrogen peroxide product (in the presence of a potent MAO inhibitor), yields results which reflect a substantial reduction in fluorescent activity compared to that observed in the presence of hydrogen peroxide (no inhibitor). Thus, the interaction of MAO with an effective inhibitor, such as Clorgyline or Deprenyl (as depicted in Fig. **3**), would result in a reduction in enzyme activity as determined by fluorescent assay as the concentration of the inhibitor increases. The convention is to assess the activity at 50% that of the positive control. This value is known as the IC_{50} value which reflects the inhibitor concentration at 50% activity of the control sample.

More specifically, Clorgyline (a specific inhibitor of MAOA) and Pargyline (a specific inhibitor of MAOB) are convenient controls to use in fluorescent assay kits, since the samples that contain these inhibitors will have minimal hydrogen peroxide and will thus yield a low fluorescent signal compared to a positive control in the absence of an inhibitor. Furthermore, fluorescent activity units can be calculated by comparing the test compounds with other known inhibitors, which can then be quantified by the slope of the hydrogen peroxide standard curve [42]. In contrast, an alternative method to assess inhibition normalizes the activity of the contents of each well in the presence of the inhibitor by subtracting the fluorescent intensity from the control with no inhibitor, divided by the control with no inhibitor [43].

These assays are simple yet highly sensitive, and are easily adaptable to a high throughput testing model. Thus, fluorescent assays as such can be ideal for screening experiments as they allow for the specific, selective, and reliable detection of the activity certain substances and compounds within a reaction, and in this case, hydrogen peroxide.

5. EGCG AS AN INHIBITOR OF MAOA AND MAOB

5.1. EGCG Content in Green Tea and Recommended Dosage

Catechins are bioactive compounds which serve as plant secondary metabolites, flavonoids, and natural antioxidants. For many years, catechins and specifically green tea catechins (primarily composed of EGCG) have been speculated to exhibit various medicinal properties. For example, catechins have been shown to act as neuroprotecting agents which aid in the prevention of neuronal damage, particularly during states of oxidative stress [13]. This is especially true during increased states of depression. Moreover, catechins are comprised of polyphenols which have been identified as the active ingredient in green tea and for which its antioxidant activity is attributed to. These polyphenolic catechin compounds which are abundantly found in green tea have been further implicated in the regulation of depressive symptoms and in the reduction of oxidative stress [13]. Additionally, catechins have also been shown to temporarily aid in the repair of antioxidant endogenous defense mechanisms [13]. These findings, among many others, greatly support the notion that green tea catechins are natural products which may aid in an array of medical conditions due to their potential medicinal benefits. According to a 2007 USDA report [44], a cup of green tea has variable amount of EGCG ranging from 5 to 450 mg. Dosage of green tea has been determined to be safe below 800 mg/day as a nutritional supplement. Above this concentration, however, there is general concern of adverse effects in the medical community that toxicity to hepatocytes may occur (as serum transaminases increase). The European Food and Safety Authority (EFSA) reports that there is negligible evidence of side effect with green tea infusions when catechins absorbed in natural state; but food supplements (green tea catechin tablets) are a concern for adverse side effects [45]. Many popular health websites recommend ~ 300 mg/day of dietary supplements of EGCG for putative "fat burning properties" for maximum effectiveness.

Therefore, in order to assess whether green tea catechin polyphenols, specifically EGCG-the most abundant of the four catechin forms (Fig. **1**) found in green tea-can also act as an inhibitor of MAO within physiological range (low micromolar high nanomolar range), fluorescent kinetic assays were performed for MAOA and MAOB in the presence of control inhibitors and catechin EGCG. Preliminary studies were performed in which catechins were isolated from commercially available green tea extracts, and were tested for monoamine oxidase inhibition of MAOA and MAOB. The assay utilized is described in detail above in section 4.4 of this chapter.

5.2. Preliminary Studies

Consistent with previous studies testing catechin inhibition of MAOB and MAOA [11, 15, 46], our analysis showed direct inhibition of MAOs by purified catechins. In preliminary studies reported here, catechins were purified from commercially available green tea products *via* extraction in water at 80°C for 1 hour, and the crude product was checked with Thin Layer Chromatography (TLC). The following procedure outlines the process more specifically:

- Commercially available green teas were prepared (using water as a solvent) by initial incubation of tea extract (or leaves) in water for 60 minutes at 80°C.
- Extract was concentrated by either rotary evaporation or simple evaporation (steeping tea at 80°C), before being cooled on ice and incubated at 4°C for 24-48 hours, to precipitate catechins.
- Catechin precipitant was then isolated by centrifugation at 3500 rpm for 15-30 minutes, and liquid was decanted and incubated at 4°C for 24-48 hours to precipitate additional catechins (repeated 2x).
- Pellets were analyzed by Thin Layer Chromatography in dichloromethane / methanol at a 10:1.5 volume ratio, and catechins were visualized under U/V short wavelength light. R_f values were calculated and compared among the different commercially available green teas.
- For commercially available green tea extracts (capsules), preparative TLC was performed. Catechin bands were first visualized under U/V light before being scraped off the plate and incubated in acetone to extract the purified catechin for further kinetic study.

- The composition of recrystallized catechin was identified and confirmed as EGCG through powder X-Ray analysis (studies currently underway).

Preliminary kinetic data is represented (Fig. **3**) by a high throughput fluorescent assay for MAOA and MAOB with control inhibitors, reflecting a reduction in enzyme activity, confirming the inhibition of the MAO enzymes. Fig. (**3A**) depicts the inhibition of MAOA by known inhibitor Clorgyline; Fig. (**3B**) illustrates the inhibition of MAOB by known inhibitor Deprenyl.

5.3. Inhibition of MAO *via* Green Tea Extracts

Moreover, the inhibition of MAOA and MAOB by catechins-isolated and recrystallized from commercially available green tea products-is presented in Fig. (**4**). Furthermore, results from curve-fitting analyses performed *via* Origin software [47] showed catechin EGCG to inhibit MAOB with an IC_{50} value in the low-micromolar (μM) range (Fig. **4B**) between 50 and 750 μM. Likewise, MAOA was found to be inhibited by catechin EGCG (Fig. **4A**), but in the high-micromolar/low-millimolar (μM/mM) range, with IC_{50} values between 0.95 and 1.5 mM. The results of these assays are therefore in agreement with literature values [48 - 52].

5.4. Molecular Docking Studies

To better understand the effects of catechin EGCG on MAO, molecular docking studies were performed in order to establish a precise prediction for the particular binding models of EGCG in the active sites of the MAO enzymes. The use of molecular docking as a molecular modeling technique has proven particularly valuable in the scope of drug design. Such methods allow for the construction and visual representation of molecule-molecule interactions, and typically micromolecule-macromolecule complexes. Notably, docking frequently enables predictions for the distinct molecular conformations and orientations at which optimal binding occurs-such that the micromolecule-macromolecule complex (or in this study, the enzyme-inhibitor complex) is stable and in ideal conditions (*i.e.,* the preferred conformation and orientation of the various binding models of the complex). In addition, the ability to establish optimal binding conditions further enables predictions for the specific association strength and relative stability of such interactions, as well as corresponding binding affinities-all of which are reasons for why molecular docking has, understandably, become a very useful tool in structural and molecular biology, and has aided in the fields of drug design and drug discovery.

(A)

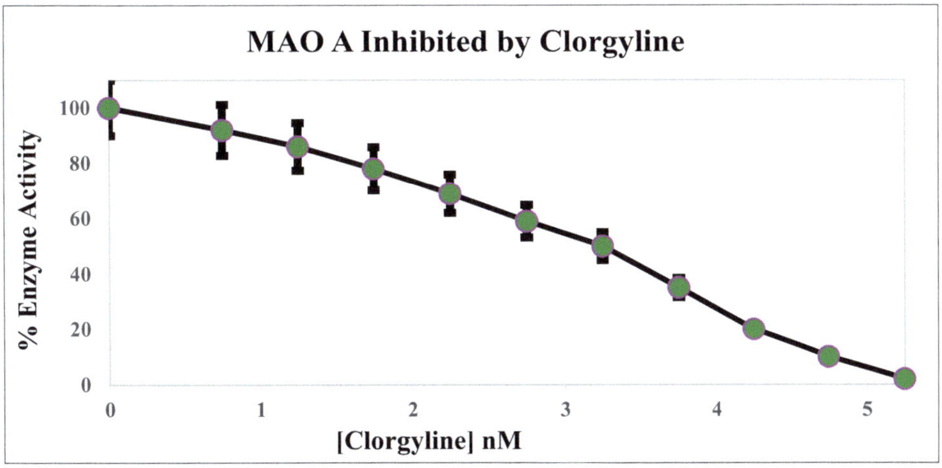

(B)

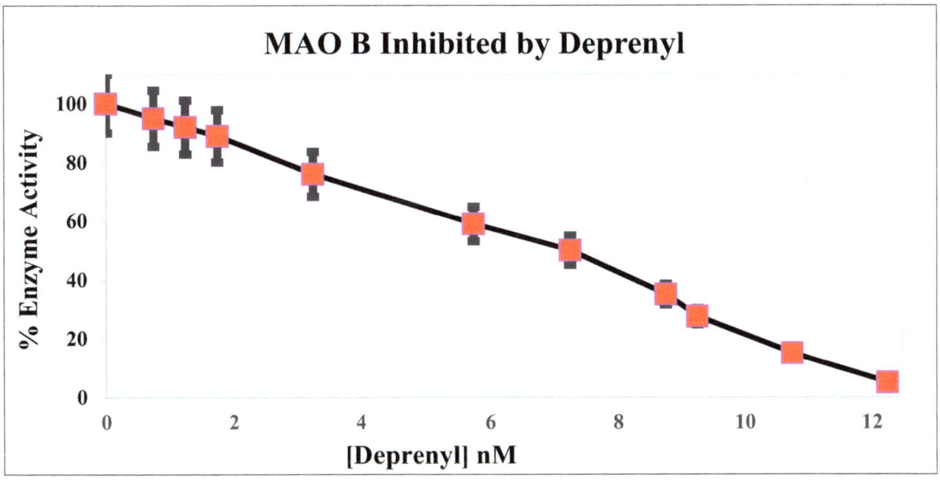

Fig. (3). Fluorescent Kinetic Assays of MAO Inhibition. (**A**) Inhibition of MAOA by control inhibitor Clorgyline. (**B**) Inhibition of MAOB by control inhibitor Deprenyl.

In the present study, molecular structures for the MAO enzymes (proteins) were retrieved from the Protein Data Bank (PDB) archives [53] using PDB code 2BXR [54] for MAOA, and PDB code 2BYB [54] for MAOB. Coordinates were visualized using UCSF Chimera crystallographic software [55]. Docking actions for the corresponding enzyme-catechin complexes-referred to herein as receptor-ligand complexes-of MAO with catechin EGCG inhibitor (prepared with PRODRG software [56]) (Fig. **6**) were predicted and simulated using AutoDockVina [57, 58].

(A)

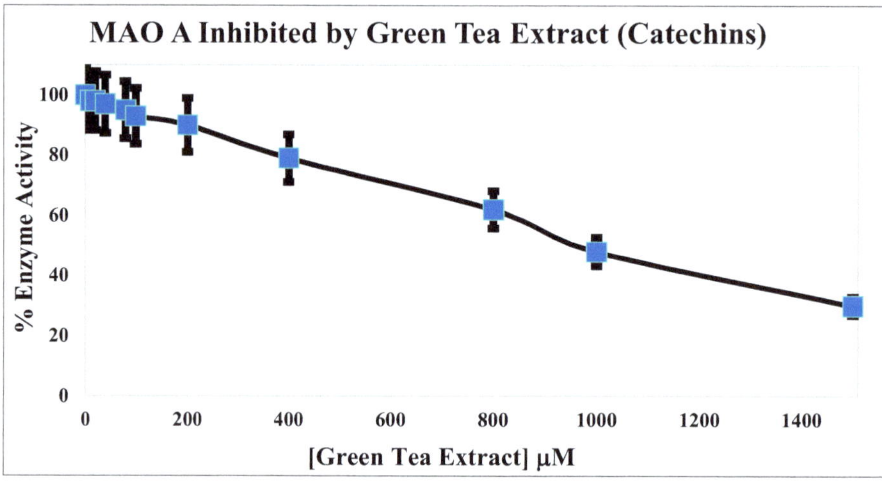

(B)

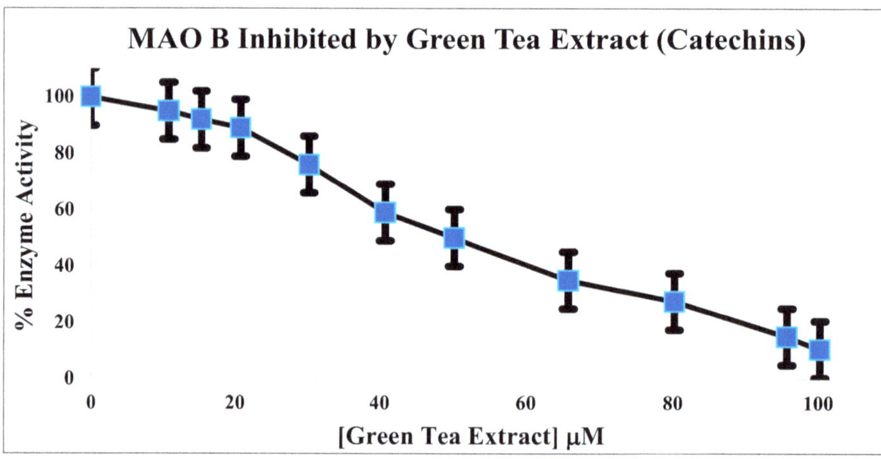

Fig. (4). Fluorescent Kinetic Assays of MAO Inhibition. (**A**) Inhibition of MAOA by catechin green tea extract. (**B**) Inhibition of MAOB by catechin green tea extract.

5.5. Molecular Docking of Control Inhibitors

The preferred active site binding mode of MAOA (PDB code 2BXR) with the crystallographic ligand inhibitor, Clorgyline, is shown (Fig. **5A**) in close proximity to the site where reduction occurs upon reaction with substrate-at one of two reactive nitrogen atoms within the heterocyclic ring of the FAD cofactor (an important coenzyme for the MAO mechanism). TYR60 and TYR435 residues are predicted to interact with Clorgyline *via* hydrogen bonding with a Clorgyline nitrogen atom. Additionally, LEU337 and TYR69 residues appear to stabilize the Clorgyline inhibitor by means of hydrophobic interactions.

Moreover, the preferred active site binding mode of MAOB (PDB code 2BYB) with the crystallographic ligand inhibitor, Deprenyl, is shown (Fig. **5B**) as a crystallographic protein-inhibitor complex. Deprenyl shares similar interactions with MAOB as Clorgyline with MAOA in that hydrophobic interactions are predicted for the flavin ring in close proximity to the nitrogen on the ring where the reduction occurs. Additionally, hydrogen bonding is predicted for Deprenyl with TYR60 and TYR435, as also predicted for Clorgyline. Furthermore, PHE343 and LEU171 may promote the stabilization of the phenyl ring of Deprenyl.

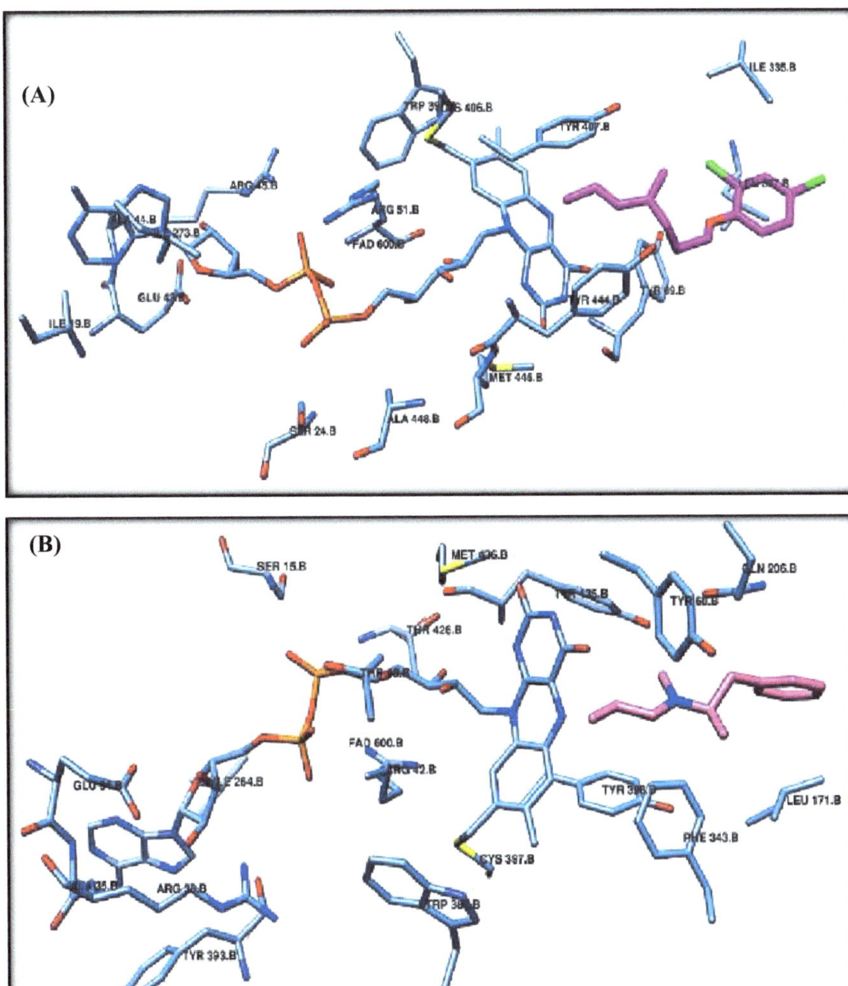

Fig. (5). Molecular Docking of Control Inhibitors into MAOA and MAOB Active Sites. (A) PDB code 2BXR MAOA (Blue) with crystallographic ligand inhibitor Clorgyline (magenta). **(B)** PDB code 2BYB MAOB (blue) with crystallographic ligand inhibitor Deprenyl (pink).

(A)

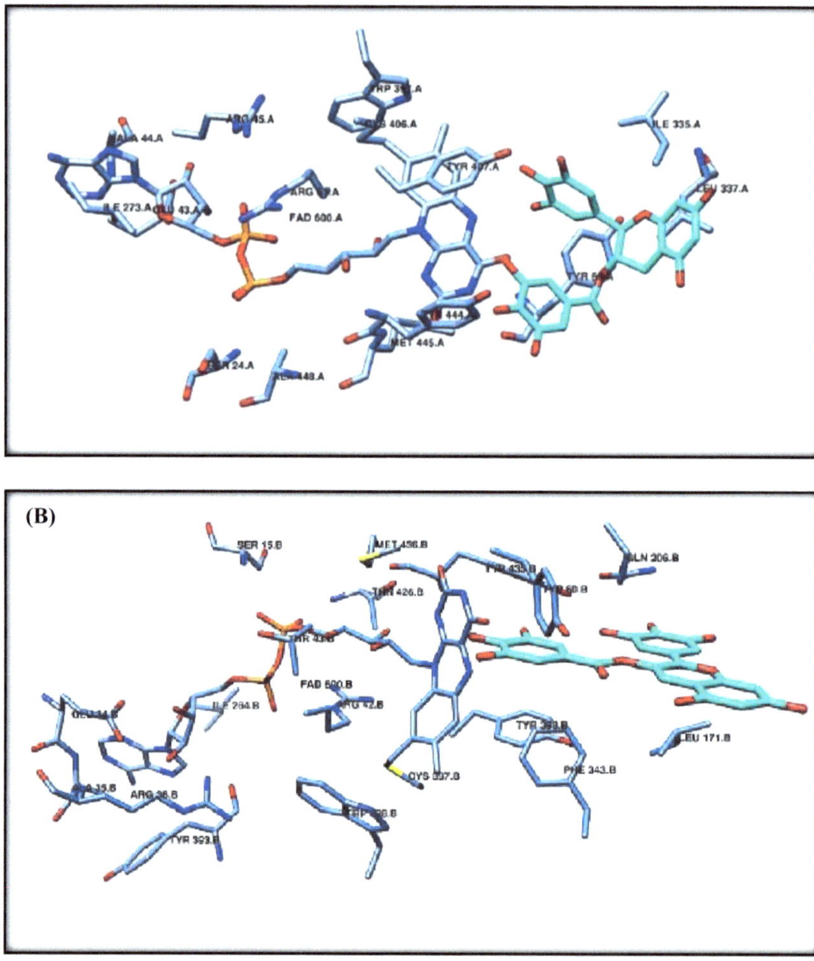

Fig. (6). Molecular Docking of Catechin EGCG into MAOA and MAOB Active Sites. (A) PDB code 2BXR MAOA (blue) with docked EGCG (cyan). **(B)** PDB code 2BYB MAOB (blue) with docked EGCG (cyan).

5.6. Molecular Docking of Catechin EGCG

The docking of catechin EGCG in the MAOA active site (Fig. **6A**) is predicted to hydrogen bond with TYR407 and TYR444, as well as with the backbone of LEU337, the OH moiety of TYR69 and-as seen with control inhibitors Clorgyline and Deprenyl-with nitrogen atoms on the flavin ring of the FAD cofactor. These predictions provide further convincing evidence for the occurrence of hydrophobic interactions between TYR69, LEU337, and ILE335. Similarly, TYR398, PHE343 and LEU171 also seem to stabilize the phenol rings on EGCG.

Finally, the predicted binding of EGCG in the MAOB active site (Fig. **6B**) (PDB code 2BYB) reflects extensive hydrogen bonding with the flavin ring of FAD, TYR60, GLN206, and TYR435, as well as hydrophobic interactions with LEU171, TYR60, TYR398, and PHE343. The predictions obtained from these docking experiments therefore yielded promising results for the interactions of ligand EGCG with target receptor proteins MAOA and MAOB. Similarities in the interactions between MAO with control inhibitors, and MAO with catechin EGCG suggests that the latter may suffice as a potential potent inhibitor of the MAO enzymes.

Computer molecular docking methods for small molecules docked into proteins (Figs. **5** - **6**) was performed in AutoDockVina using a previously described protocol [45]. The catechin EGCG was drawn in PRODRG [56] then run through MGLTools-a more recent version of AutoDockTools or ADT for file formatting [57]. The Protein Data Bank (PDB) codes for 3D coordinates of the MAO proteins 2BXR (MAOA) and 2BYB (MAOB) were downloaded from the RCSB database [53] and prepared for docking in MGLTools.

6. PHARMACOKINETICS AND ADVERSE EFFECTS OF GREEN TEA CATECHINS

6.1. Absorption, Distribution, Metabolism, and Excretion of Green Tea Catechins

Catechins are water soluble in low doses and because they are phenolic in nature, they are weakly acidic. Under physiological conditions, catechins may exist in equilibrium with unionized forms at neutral pH. As with many compounds, solubility of protonated functional groups is greatly reduced in the aqueous environment, and therefore prevents absorption by the GI tract. Moreover, the galloyl groups of EGCG and ECG may bind to cell membranes via proteins that have open, random and coil-type conformations. These types of proteins are abundant in saliva and mucous, and the formation of these catechin-protein complexes may hinder their absorption by lowering catechin aqueous solubility. In addition, the variable chemical structures of catechins cause heterogeneity of absorption [59]. Certain proteins such as milk and whey proteins are ideal carriers for delivering catechins. Other proteins confirmed to improve the stability, bio-accessibility, and permeability of catechins are corn zein, soy, and rice bran protein isolate [60]. Moreover, the bioavailability of catechin compounds EGC and EGCG was reported to be significantly enhanced when presented as a mixture of green tea extract (GTE), sucrose, and ascorbic acid, or GTE and stachyose, compared to green tea alone [61, 62]. Additionally, several studies have concluded that an accumulation of EGCG, EGC, and ECG were significantly increased by Caco-2 cells when formulations contained ascorbic acid and sucros3 [60]. Furthermore, intestinal uptake of total catechins increased up to ~ten times when administering green tea with xylitol and citric acid or with xylitol and ascorbic acid, when compared to the green tea control [61]. Despite effects of drug and food interaction discussed in the next section, catechin absorption can, ultimately, be significantly enhanced when presented in combination with other substances.

After the oral administration of green tea, EGCG present in the gastric juice of the stomach is neutralized by bicarbonate ions. EGCG is slightly acidic and more stable in the stomach while unstable at a higher pH as in the intestines, and therefore, degraded rapidly. Within the small intestine, catechins are conjugated by o-methylation and glucuronic acid. Catechins are absorbed by the small intestine with excess catechins continuing on to the colon. The catabolized phenolic acids are reabsorbed into circulation and excreted into the urine. In the colon, they are degraded into different flavonoid rings by endogenous microorganisms. Absorbed catechins have been reported in high concentrations in various ocular tissues, as well as in the prostate and liver. It's currently accepted that, after passage through the liver, the metabolized catechins would be available to other organs and tissues [61].

Since catechins undergo extensive metabolism, a wide variety of catechin breakdown products have been found in the plasma and urine following the consumption of green tea. The majority of the metabolism of catechins does not happen in the intestine, but after methylation, glucuronidation, and sulfation in the liver [61].

Catechins are rapidly degraded and metabolized due to the hydroxyl groups on their phenol rings. After degradation, catechins are further metabolized and shortened to C6-C1 phenolic and aromatic acid and reabsorbed to enter circulation or excreted through the urine. Although up to 37% of catechins metabolized may be excreted through the urine, there is evidence that more hydrophobic gallated catechins bind stronger to serum proteins and exist in unconjugated free form, and thus not excreted via the renal system. This would imply that a significant amount of catechins may be available to various organs and tissues depending on dosage [61].

There is a disparity between superior catechin *in vitro* biological activity and low activity in *in vivo* studies. This may be attributed to the low stability of the absorbed catechins, leading to the degradation of products and oxidized molecules. Therefore, it remains uncertain if the intact catechin compound is the bioactive species causing the effects seen in *in vivo* studies. However, in *in vitro* studies, cell cultures may have a specific expression profile such that researchers can postulate how the catechin may be metabolized, if not eliciting an effect as an intact molecule. Be that as it may, within the complexity of the *in vivo* system, catechin processes are unfortunately more difficult to track [60].

6.2. Adverse Effects of Green Tea Consumption: Toxicity and Drug Interactions

It is believed that an overconsumption of highly concentrated green tea extracts could have adverse effects, potential toxic capabilities, and drug interactions. Toxic effects could be due to possible trace amounts of pesticides, such as organochlorines, organophosphates, and pyrethrins found in GTE. The proportions of these pesticides and the four main catechin components found in green tea is dependent on cultivation, clonal variation, and the age of leaves. For instance, older leaves have a higher number of total catechins components when compared to younger leaves.

Original studies of pharmacokinetic green tea constituents in humans done by Yang and colleagues involved healthy volunteers given various doses of GTE from 282 to 846 mg, equivalent to 3-9 cups of green tea. Plasma levels of catechins peaked between 1.5-2.5 hours in all subjects, and declined after 24 hours with no apparent adverse effects. The half- life of EGCG was 5 hours and EGC, 2.7 hours. In terms of toxicity, the major dose limiting ingredients in GTE has been suggested to be caffeine, which can range from 10-50 mg per cup of green tea and up to 10% of GTE [63, 64]. However, several studies also suggest, caffeine may contribute to the beneficial effects of green tea as an anticancer agent, as studied *in vivo*. The effective, biologically active concentrations of catechins in many *in vitro* studies is five to 50 times more effective than the plasma concentration in *in vivo* studies. In terms of administration, several studies have reported that EGCG showed elevated plasma levels several fold higher when given after an overnight fast as compared to the same dose given with food. This high plasma content could lead to adverse effects, such as hepatotoxicity. Although GTE and green tea infusions have been reported as beneficial for various cancers, several ongoing clinical trials have shown adverse side effects patients with chronic lymphocytic leukemia ingesting 200-400 mg of GTE. Side effects included dysphagia and intestinal problems, respectively. What is unknown is if this dosage is beyond the threshold of human consumption and potential toxicity. The multiplicity of ingredients in GTE and green tea makes it difficult to establish a definitely causal relationship between green tea extracts, caffeine, and toxicity, such as hepatotoxicity. Some studies argue green tea has hepatoprotective effects in lesser concentrations [63, 65 - 67].

Potential drug interactions of GTE have also been reported. It is known, however, that components of green tea, other than catechins, react with various drugs. For instance, the tannins in GTE cause decreased absorption of iron supplements, warfarin, codeine, atropine, ephedrine, pseudoephedrine, theophylline, and aminophylline. GTE may interfere with MDR1 transmembrane proteins which has been known to pump various drugs out of cells. This could be beneficial for cancer treatment because since GTE inhibits the MDR1 pump, the cancer drug is prevented from exiting that cell. Although there is a desired effect of increasing chemosensitivity to multidrug resistant cancer cells, there are adverse effects. A transmembrane glycoprotein pump that is inhibited by catechins may also result in interference with drug excretion (into the biliary tract) and, thus result in an increased amount of drug compound bioavailability and increased risk for systemic toxicity. This occurred in the administration of EGCG and the cancer drug Irinotecan (Cpt-11) and its active metabolite (SN-38). There have been conflicting reports in the literature whether isolated catechins or GTE is more beneficial for anticancer effects and potential drug interactions. The situation has been complicated by the fact that catechins have been shown to block the therapeutic efficacy of certain protease inhibitors used for multiple myeloma, stromal tumors, and advanced renal cell carcinoma. For instance, catechins have been reported to completely block the efficacy of Bortezomib, a protease inhibitor, and Sunitinib, a multikinase inhibitor.

There is a natural tendency for healthy individuals to retain their healthy state by ingesting nutritional dietary supplements, such as GTE and other herbal products. It has recently emerged in the literature that EGCG is impacted by other herbal supplements and can also exacerbate adverse effects in combination with other herbal supplements. For instance, the combination of EGCG and the flavonoid Genistein, present in soy, *in vitro* and *in vivo* produced anti-tumorigenesis-like effects. Genistein seemed to maintain concentrations of EGCG in the tumor cell's cytosol, ultimately causing greater inhibition of tumor cell growth, a result due to this combination of herbal drugs more than EGCG alone. Simultaneously, however, this combination also proved to display cancer promoting effects in tumor-prone adenomatous polyposis coli, specifically.

The adverse effects of GTE are just starting to emerge, and are complex and somewhat contradictory at this time. One unifying theme is the idea of dosage control. In regards to *in vitro* studies with both purified MAO recombinant enzyme assays and cell culture studies, it is difficult to assess the potential physiological relevance to results obtained when dosages of EGCG are higher than 10 micromolar. *In vivo,* this elevated level of EGCG could easily lead to toxic effects, such as hepatotoxicity [63]. According to pharmacokinetic studies of EGCG *in vivo*, 8 μM is the peak plasma catechin concentration limit in humans. Future research should be done with different combinations with ECGC or components of GTE to understand what threshold can be sustained with minimal to no toxicity.

CONCLUDING REMARKS

Monoamine oxidase (MAO) enzymes are a class of amine oxidizing flavoenzymes which catalyze the reaction of flavin-dependent amine oxidation. More specifically, MAOs catalyze the oxidation and deamination of monoamine neurotransmitters. MAOs are found in two isoforms: MAOA and MAOB. Both MAO isoenzymes function in brain homeostasis and play a major role in the regulation of neurotransmitters, thereby maintaining proper psychological and neurological functioning [17]. MAOA acts on serotonin-a natural substrate of MAOA-in addition to epinephrine (adrenaline) and norepinephrine (noradrenaline). Abnormal MAOA activity is implicated in various psychological and/or psychiatric disorders including depression and anxiety. In contrast, MAOB acts on dopamine and benzylamine-a natural substrate of MAOB. Abnormal MAOB activity is implicated in numerous neurodegenerative diseases, such as Parkinson's disease and Alzheimer's disease. This is partially due to the presence of neurotoxic byproducts produced in response to the excessive activation of MAOA and/or MAOB [17].

Monoamine oxidase inhibitors (MAOIs) are a class of pharmaceutical drugs which target the MAO isozymes for regulation. MAOIs functionally regulate the activity of MAO, thereby preventing the oxidation and deamination of the monoamine neurotransmitters that are essential to maintaining neurological stability. MAOIs therefore serve a very critical function and have played an important role in the manner in which psychiatric disorders have been treated for decades. However, despite being quite the milestone, the use of MAOIs has decreased dramatically, especially in younger generations. The once uniform use of MAOIs has been replaced by a multitude of pharmacotherapies involving various alternative drug methods. The development of these new alternative methods marked a turning point in the way in which psychiatric disorders are treated, just as MAOIs did. This is because MAOIs have an extremely high-degree of toxicity compared to other forms of antidepressants, and this makes them much less tolerable and certainly less favorable than safer alternatives.

Although newer forms of antidepressants pose less risk to patients, are more agreeable in terms of adverse effects, and carry far fewer limitations and restrictions, the emergence of natural product chemistry marks another new turning point in the pharmacotherapy of certain emotional illnesses and psychiatric disorders. While we have many natural products to thank for the origin of countless medications, the mass production and manufacturing of synthetic pharmaceutical agents has trumped the use of natural products for decades. As a result, efforts have been set forth to confirm the medicinal potential of several natural products as safer alternatives to synthetic agents.

Among the many natural products currently in focus are green tea catechins, which exhibit antioxidant properties due to their polyphenolic composition [6], but also have been shown to exert similar effects as MAOIs by targeting the MAO enzymes [18]. Catechins appear to improve cognitive functioning as well as mental and emotional stability, and may serve as potential potent inhibitors of monoamine oxidase [2, 5, 10, 11, 13 - 17, 21, 22, 29, 32, 50, 51]. This is of particular significance in that catechins, and specifically green tea catechin EGCG, may provide a new therapeutic method to treating MAO-associated disorders using natural products as a substitute for synthetic pharmaceutical medications. This, in turn, would eliminate potential hazards of drug-drug and drug-food interactions accompanying the use of MAOIs (in addition to various other forms of antidepressants), but would also substantially reduce the risk of pharmaceutical dependence, and would have a colossal impact on the number of drug-induced overdoses affiliated with the regular use of antidepressants. Although additional research is required to fully understand possible catechin-drug interactions and associated side effects when ingested as food supplements, the use of natural products would mark another great milestone in the treatment of psychiatric and neurological disorders. Ongoing research pertaining to green tea catechins could elucidate other possible solutions that are natural, healthy, and effective alternatives to the use of risky pharmaceuticals. Natural products as such are especially relevant as the demand for cures abiding by these descriptors is high in demand.

ABBREVIATIONS

βPEA β-phenylethylamine

CDK cyclin–dependent kinase

CNS central nervous system

DAT selective dopamine transporters

EFSA European Food and Safety Authority

EGCG epigallocatechin gallate

EC epigallocatechin

ECG epicatechin gallate

EGC	epigallocatechin
GTE	green tea extract
HRP	horse radish peroxidase
MRI	monoamine reuptake inhibitors
MAOI	monoamine oxidase inhibitor
MDR1	multiple drug resistant-1 gene product
MAOB	monoamine oxidase B
MAOA	monoamine oxidase A
MAPK	mitogen activating protein kinase
NET	noradrenaline/norepinephrine transporter
NDRI	noradrenaline-dopamine reuptake inhibitors
NMS	neuroleptic malignant syndrome
PICK1	protein interacting with C kinase-1
PNS	peripheral nervous system
RTK	receptor tyrosine kinase
SSRI	selective serotonin reuptake inhibitor
SERT	serotonin transporter
SNRI	serotonin-noradrenaline reuptake inhibitors
SS	serotonin syndrome
TCA	tricyclic antidepressant
USDA	Unites States Department of Agriculture

CONSENT FOR PUBLICATION

Not applicable.

CONFLICT OF INTEREST

The authors declare no conflict of interest, financial or otherwise.

ACKNOWLEDGEMENT

The authors wish to thank Jimmy Tran for isolating the Green tea catechin and providing it for the preliminary kinetic studies.

REFERENCES

[1] Ye, F.; Yang, C.; Kim, J.; MacNevin, C.J.; Hahn, K.M.; Park, D.; Ginsberg, M.H.; Kim, C. Epigallocatechin gallate has pleiotropic effects on transmembrane signaling by altering the embedding of transmembrane domains. *J. Biol. Chem.*, **2017**, *292*(24), 9858-9864. [http://dx.doi.org/10.1074/jbc.C117.787309] [PMID: 28487468]

[2] Suzuki, T.; Pervin, M.; Goto, S.; Isemura, M.; Nakamura, Y. Beneficial effects of tea and the green tea catechin Epigallocatechin-3-gallate on obesity. *Molecules,* **2016**, *21*(10), 1305. [http://dx.doi.org/10.3390/molecules21101305] [PMID: 27689985]

[3] Miao, M.; Jiang, H.; Jiang, B.; Li, Y.G.; Cui, S.W.; Zhang, T. Structure elucidation of catechins for modulation of starch digestion. *Lebensm. Wiss. Technol.,* **2014**, *57*(1), 188-193. [http://dx.doi.org/10.1016/j.lwt.2014.01.005]

[4] Pal, S.; Dey, S.K.; Saha, C. Inhibition of catalase by tea catechins in free and cellular state: a biophysical approach. *PLoS One,* **2014**, *9*(7)e102460 [http://dx.doi.org/10.1371/journal.pone.0102460] [PMID: 25025898]

[5] Gupta, J.; Siddique, Y.H.; Beg, T.; Ara, G.; Afza, M. A review on the beneficial effects of tea polyphenols on human health. *Int. J. Pharmacol.,* **2008**, *4*(5), 314-338. [http://dx.doi.org/10.3923/ijp.2008.314.338]

[6] Park, Y.H.; Han, D.W.; Suh, H.; Ryu, G.H.; Hyon, S.H.; Cho, B.K.; Park, J.C. Protective effects of green tea polyphenol against reactive oxygen species-induced oxidative stress in cultured rat calvarial osteoblast. *Cell Biol. Toxicol.,* **2003**, *19*(5), 325-337. [http://dx.doi.org/10.1023/B:CBTO.0000004986.51081.c5] [PMID: 14703119]

[7] Nakagawa, T.; Yokozawa, T. Direct scavenging of nitric oxide and superoxide by green tea. *Food Chem. Toxicol.,* **2002**, *40*(12), 1745-1750. [http://dx.doi.org/10.1016/S0278-6915(02)00169-2] [PMID: 12419687]

[8] Hirun, S.; Roach, P.D. A study of stability of (-)-Epigallocatechin gallate (EGCG) from green tea in a frozen product. *Int. Food Res. J.,* **2011**, *18*(4), 1261-1264.

[9] Pillai, S.P.; Mitscher, L.A.; Menon, S.R.; Pillai, C.A.; Shankel, D.M. Antimutagenic/antioxidant activity of green tea components and related compounds. *J. Environ. Pathol. Toxicol. Oncol.,* **1999**, *18*(3), 147-158. [PMID: 15281227]

[10] Dulloo, A.G.; Duret, C.; Rohrer, D.; Girardier, L.; Mensi, N.; Fathi, M.; Chantre, P.; Vandermander, J. Efficacy of a green tea extract rich in catechin polyphenols and caffeine in increasing 24-h energy expenditure and fat oxidation in humans. *Am. J. Clin. Nutr.,* **1999**, *70*(6), 1040-1045. [http://dx.doi.org/10.1093/ajcn/70.6.1040] [PMID: 10584049]

[11] Singh, B.N.; Shankar, S.; Srivastava, R.K. Green tea catechin, epigallocatechin-3-gallate (EGCG): mechanisms, perspectives and clinical applications. *Biochem. Pharmacol.,* **2011**, *82*(12), 1807-1821. [http://dx.doi.org/10.1016/j.bcp.2011.07.093] [PMID: 21827739]

[12] Lemmon, M.A.; Schlessinger, J. Cell signaling by receptor tyrosine kinases. *Cell,* **2010**, *141*(7), 1117-1134. [http://dx.doi.org/10.1016/j.cell.2010.06.011] [PMID: 20602996]

[13] Di Lorenzo, A.; Nabavi, S.F.; Sureda, A.; Moghaddam, A.H.; Khanjani, S.; Arcidiaco, P.; Nabavi, S.M.; Daglia, M. Antidepressive-like effects and antioxidant activity of green tea and GABA green tea in a mouse model of post-stroke depression. *Mol. Nutr. Food Res.,* **2016**, *60*(3), 566-579. [http://dx.doi.org/10.1002/mnfr.201500567] [PMID: 26626862]

[14] Nabavi, S.M.; Daglia, M.; Braidy, N.; Nabavi, S.F. Natural products, micronutrients, and nutraceuticals for the treatment of depression: A short review. *Nutr. Neurosci.,* **2017**, *20*(3), 180-194. [http://dx.doi.org/10.1080/1028415X.2015.1103461] [PMID: 26613119]

[15] Mähler, A.; Mandel, S.; Lorenz, M.; Ruegg, U.; Wanker, E.E.; Boschmann, M.; Paul, F. Epigallocatechin-3-gallate: a useful, effective and safe clinical approach for targeted prevention and individualised treatment of neurological diseases? *EPMA J.,* **2013**, *4*(1), 5. [http://dx.doi.org/10.1186/1878-5085-4-5] [PMID: 23418936]

[16] Dong, X.; Yang, C.; Cao, S.; Gan, Y.; Sun, H.; Gong, Y.; Yang, H.; Yin, X.; Lu, Z. Tea consumption and the risk of depression: a meta-analysis of observational studies. *Aust. N. Z. J. Psychiatry,* **2015**,

49(4), 334-345.
[http://dx.doi.org/10.1177/0004867414567759] [PMID: 25657295]

[17] Saura, J.; Kettler, R.; Da Prada, M.; Richards, J.G. Quantitative enzyme radioautography with 3H-Ro 41-1049 and 3H-Ro 19-6327 *in vitro*: localization and abundance of MAO-A and MAO-B in rat CNS, peripheral organs, and human brain. *J. Neurosci.*, **1992**, *12*(5), 1977-1999. [http://dx.doi.org/10.1523/JNEUROSCI.12-05-01977.1992] [PMID: 1578281]

[18] Finberg, J.P.M.; Rabey, J.M. Inhibitors of MAOA and MAOB in psychiatry and neurology. *Front. Pharmacol.*, **2016**, *7*, 340. [http://dx.doi.org/10.3389/fphar.2016.00340] [PMID: 27803666]

[19] Li, L.; Zhang, C.W.; Chen, G.Y.; Zhu, B.; Chai, C.; Xu, Q.H.; Tan, E.K.; Zhu, Q.; Lim, K.L.; Yao, S.Q. A sensitive two-photon probe to selectively detect monoamine oxidase B activity in Parkinson's disease models. *Nat. Commun.*, **2014**, *5*(3276), 3276. [http://dx.doi.org/10.1038/ncomms4276] [PMID: 24522637]

[20] https://www.drugbank.ca/documentation/search / Last accessed 1/15/19.

[21] Youdim, M.B.H. Monoamine oxidase inhibitors, and iron chelators in depressive illness and neurodegenerative diseases. *J. Neural Transm.*, **2018**, *125*(11), 1719-1733. [http://dx.doi.org/10.1007/s00702-018-1942-9] [PMID: 30341696]

[22] Meyer, J.H.; Wilson, A.A.; Sagrati, S.; Miler, L.; Rusjan, P.; Bloomfield, P.M.; Clark, M.; Sacher, J.; Voineskos, A.N.; Houle, S. Brain monoamine oxidase A binding in major depressive disorder: relationship to selective serotonin reuptake inhibitor treatment, recovery, and recurrence. *Arch. Gen. Psychiatry*, **2009**, *66*(12), 1304-1312. [http://dx.doi.org/10.1001/archgenpsychiatry.2009.156] [PMID: 19996035]

[23] Huot, P.; Fox, S.H.; Brotchie, J.M. Monoamine reuptake inhibitors in Parkinson's disease. *Parkinsons Dis.*, **2015**, *2015*609428 [http://dx.doi.org/10.1155/2015/609428] [PMID: 25810948]

[24] Hinz, M.; Stein, A.; Uncini, T. Monoamine depletion by reuptake inhibitors. *Drug Healthc. Patient Saf.*, **2011**, *3*, 69-77. [http://dx.doi.org/10.2147/DHPS.S24798] [PMID: 22171164]

[25] Marcora, E.; Carlisle, H.J.; Kennedy, M.B. The Role of the Postsynaptic Density and the Spine Cytoskeleton in Synaptic Plasticity.*Learning & Memory: A Comprehensive Reference*; Academic Press: Oxford, **2008**, Vol. 4, pp. 649-673. [http://dx.doi.org/10.1016/B978-012370509-9.00036-X]

[26] Boudin, H.; Craig, A.M. Molecular determinants for PICK1 synaptic aggregation and mGluR7a receptor coclustering: role of the PDZ, coiled-coil, and acidic domains. *J. Biol. Chem.*, **2001**, *276*(32), 30270-30276. [http://dx.doi.org/10.1074/jbc.M102991200] [PMID: 11375398]

[27] Binda, C.; Hubálek, F.; Li, M.; Herzig, Y.; Sterling, J.; Edmondson, D.E.; Mattevi, A. Binding of rasagiline-related inhibitors to human monoamine oxidases: a kinetic and crystallographic analysis. *J. Med. Chem.*, **2005**, *48*(26), 8148-8154. [http://dx.doi.org/10.1021/jm0506266] [PMID: 16366596]

[28] Non-Selective and Selective Monoamine Reuptake Inhibitors. Drug Bank Home Page. https://www.drugbank.ca/categories [Accessed on: January 4, 2019]

[29] Agius, M.; Bonnici, H. Antidepressants in use in clinical practice. *Psychiatr. Danub.*, **2017**, *29* Suppl. 3, 667-671. [PMID: 28953850]

[30] Fookes, C. BPharm. Monoamine oxidase inhibitors. Drugs.com Home Page. https://www.drugs.com/drug-class/monoamine-oxidaseinhibitors.html?condition [Accessed on: January 4, 2019].

[31] Garcia, E.; Santos, C. Toxicity, monoamine oxidase inhibitor. In: *StatPearls [Internet]*; Eds.; StatPearls Publishing; Treasure Island (FL), **2017**; pp. 1-17.

[32] Fiedorowicz, J.G.; Swartz, K.L. The role of monoamine oxidase inhibitors in current psychiatric practice. *J. Psychiatr. Pract.,* **2004**, *10*(4), 239-248. [http://dx.doi.org/10.1097/00131746-200407000-00005] [PMID: 15552546]

[33] Boyer, E.W.; Shannon, M. The serotonin syndrome. *N. Engl. J. Med.,* **2005**, *352*(11), 1112-1120. [http://dx.doi.org/10.1056/NEJMra041867] [PMID: 15784664]

[34] Attaway, A.; Sroujieh, L.; Mersfelder, T.L.; Butler, C.; Ouellette, D. "Ping-pong gaze" secondary to monoamine oxidase inhibitor overdose. *J. Pharmacol. Pharmacother.,* **2016**, *7*(1), 34-37. [http://dx.doi.org/10.4103/0976-500X.179360] [PMID: 27127395]

[35] Dong, X.; Yang, C.; Cao, S.; Gan, Y.; Sun, H.; Gong, Y.; Yang, H.; Yin, X.; Lu, Z. Tea consumption and the risk of depression: a meta-analysis of observational studies. *Aust. N. Z. J. Psychiatry,* **2015**, *49*(4), 334-345. [http://dx.doi.org/10.1177/0004867414567759] [PMID: 25657295]

[36] Chow, H.H.; Cai, Y.; Hakim, I.A.; Crowell, J.A.; Shahi, F.; Brooks, C.A.; Dorr, R.T.; Hara, Y.; Alberts, D.S. Pharmacokinetics and safety of green tea polyphenols after multiple-dose administration of epigallocatechin gallate and polyphenon E in healthy individuals. *Clin. Cancer Res.,* **2003**, *9*(9), 3312-3319. [PMID: 12960117]

[37] Yu, P.H. Studies on the pargyline-binding site of different types of monoamine oxidase. *Can. J. Biochem.,* **1981**, *59*(1), 30-37. [http://dx.doi.org/10.1139/o81-005] [PMID: 6784898]

[38] https://www.promega.com/resources/pubhub/cellnotes/the-mao-glo-assay-a-bioluminescent-c-upled-assay-for-monoamine-oxidase-activity/ Last accessed 1/14/19.

[39] Matsukawa, M.; Hirai, T.; Karita, S.; Akizawa, T.; Pan-Hou, H.; Yoshioka, M.; Goto, G.; Parvez, H.; Youdim, M.B. A screening system of prodrugs selective for MAO-A or MAO-B. *Neurotoxicology,* **2004**, *25*(1-2), 293-302. [http://dx.doi.org/10.1016/S0161-813X(03)00108-6] [PMID: 14697904]

[40] Youdim, M.B.; Finberg, J.P. New directions in monoamine oxidase A and B selective inhibitors and substrates. *Biochem. Pharmacol.,* **1991**, *41*(2), 155-162. [http://dx.doi.org/10.1016/0006-2952(91)90471-G] [PMID: 1989626]

[41] Santillo, M.F.; Liu, Y.; Ferguson, M.; Vohra, S.N.; Wiesenfeld, P.L. Inhibition of monoamine oxidase (MAO) by β-carbolines and their interactions in live neuronal (PC12) and liver (HuH-7 and MH1C1) cells. *Toxicol. In Vitro,* **2014**, *28*(3), 403-410. [http://dx.doi.org/10.1016/j.tiv.2013.12.006] [PMID: 24373881]

[42] Guang, H.M.; Du, G.H. High-throughput screening for monoamine oxidase-A and monoamine oxidase-B inhibitors using one-step fluorescence assay. *Acta Pharmacol. Sin.,* **2006**, *27*(6), 760-766. [http://dx.doi.org/10.1111/j.1745-7254.2006.00336.x] [PMID: 16723097]

[43] Mazzio, E.; Deiab, S.; Park, K.; Soliman, K.F. High throughput screening to identify natural human monoamine oxidase B inhibitors. *Phytother. Res.,* **2013**, *27*(6), 818-828. [http://dx.doi.org/10.1002/ptr.4795] [PMID: 22887993]

[44] https://www.ars.usda.gov/ARSUserFiles/80400525/Data/Flav/Flav02-1.pdf Last accessed 1/15/19

[45] https://www.efsa.europa.eu/en/press/news/180418 Last accessed 1/15/19 Last accessed 1/15/19

[46] Bandaruk, Y.; Mukai, R.; Kawamura, T.; Nemoto, H.; Terao, J. Evaluation of the inhibitory effects of quercetin-related flavonoids and tea catechins on the monoamine oxidase-A reaction in mouse brain mitochondria. *J. Agric. Food Chem.,* **2012**, *60*(41), 10270-10277. [http://dx.doi.org/10.1021/jf303055b] [PMID: 23009399]

[47] Origin Lab Home Page. https://www.originlab.com/ [Accessed on: June 2018].

[48] Herraiz, T.; Flores, A.; Fernández, L. Analysis of monoamine oxidase (MAO) enzymatic activity by high-performance liquid chromatography-diode array detection combined with an assay of oxidation with a peroxidase and its application to MAO inhibitors from foods and plants. *J. Chromatogr. B Analyt. Technol. Biomed. Life Sci.*, **2018**, *1073*, 136-144. [http://dx.doi.org/10.1016/j.jchromb.2017.12.004] [PMID: 29268246]

[49] Ademosun, A.O.; Oboh, G. Comparison of the inhibition of monoamine oxidase and butyrylcholinesterase activities by infusions from green tea and some citrus peels. *Int. J. Alzheimers Dis.*, **2014**, *2014*(586407)586407 [http://dx.doi.org/10.1155/2014/586407] [PMID: 25243093]

[50] Oboh, G.; Ogunruku, O.O.; Oyeleye, S.I.; Olasehinde, T.A.; Ademosun, A.O.; Boligon, A.A. Phenolic extracts from *Clerodendrum volubile* leaves inhibit cholinergic and monoaminergic enzymes relevant to the management of some neurodegenerative diseases. *J. Diet. Suppl.*, **2017**, *14*(3), 358-371. [http://dx.doi.org/10.1080/19390211.2016.1237401] [PMID: 27753518]

[51] Zheng, H.; Gal, S.; Weiner, L.M.; Bar-Am, O.; Warshawsky, A.; Fridkin, M.; Youdim, M.B.H. Novel multifunctional neuroprotective iron chelator-monoamine oxidase inhibitor drugs for neurodegenerative diseases: *in vitro* studies on antioxidant activity, prevention of lipid peroxide formation and monoamine oxidase inhibition. *J. Neurochem.*, **2005**, *95*(1), 68-78. [http://dx.doi.org/10.1111/j.1471-4159.2005.03340.x] [PMID: 16181413]

[52] Pan, T.; Fei, J.; Zhou, X.; Jankovic, J.; Le, W. Effects of green tea polyphenols on dopamine uptake and on MPP^+ -induced dopamine neuron injury. *Life Sci.*, **2003**, *72*(9), 1073-1083. [http://dx.doi.org/10.1016/S0024-3205(02)02347-0] [PMID: 12495785]

[53] Berman, H.M.; Westbrook, J.; Feng, Z.; Gilliland, G.; Bhat, T.N.; Weissig, H.; Shindyalov, I.N.; Bourne, P.E. The Protein Data Bank. *Nucleic Acids Res.*, **2000**, *28*(1), 235-242. [http://dx.doi.org/10.1093/nar/28.1.235] [PMID: 10592235]

[54] De Colibus, L.; Li, M.; Binda, C.; Lustig, A.; Edmondson, D.E.; Mattevi, A. Three-dimensional structure of human monoamine oxidase A (MAO A): relation to the structures of rat MAO A and human MAO B. *Proc. Natl. Acad. Sci. USA,* **2005**, *102*(36), 12684-12689. [http://dx.doi.org/10.1073/pnas.0505975102] [PMID: 16129825]

[55] Pettersen, E.F.; Goddard, T.D.; Huang, C.C.; Couch, G.S.; Greenblatt, D.M.; Meng, E.C.; Ferrin, T.E. UCSF Chimera--a visualization system for exploratory research and analysis. *J. Comput. Chem.*, **2004**, *25*(13), 1605-1612. [http://dx.doi.org/10.1002/jcc.20084] [PMID: 15264254]

[56] Schüttelkopf, A.W.; van Aalten, D.M.F. PRODRG: a tool for high-throughput crystallography of protein-ligand complexes. *Acta Crystallogr. D Biol. Crystallogr.*, **2004**, *60*(Pt 8), 1355-1363. [http://dx.doi.org/10.1107/S0907444904011679] [PMID: 15272157]

[57] Trott, O.; Olson, A.J. AutoDock Vina: improving the speed and accuracy of docking with a new scoring function, efficient optimization, and multithreading. *J. Comput. Chem.*, **2010**, *31*(2), 455-461. [PMID: 19499576]

[58] Morris, G.M.; Huey, R.; Lindstrom, W.; Sanner, M.F.; Belew, R.K.; Goodsell, D.S.; Olson, A.J. AutoDock4 and AutoDockTools4: Automated docking with selective receptor flexibility. *J. Comput. Chem.*, **2009**, *30*(16), 2785-2791. [http://dx.doi.org/10.1002/jcc.21256] [PMID: 19399780]

[59] Zhu, M.; Chen, Y.; Li, R.C. Oral absorption and bioavailability of tea catechins. *Planta Med.*, **2000**, *66*(5), 444-447. [http://dx.doi.org/10.1055/s-2000-8599] [PMID: 10909265]

[60] Cai, Z-Y.; Li, X.M.; Liang, J.P.; Xiang, L.P.; Wang, K.R.; Shi, Y.L.; Yang, R.; Shi, M.; Ye, J.H.; Lu, J.L.; Zheng, X.Q.; Liang, Y.R. Bioavailability of tea catechins and its improvement. *Molecules,* **2018**,

23(9), 2346.
[http://dx.doi.org/10.3390/molecules23092346] [PMID: 30217074]

[61] Chu, K.O.; Pang, C.P. *Pharmacokinetics and disposition of green tea catechins.*, https://cdn.intechopen.com/pdfs/60659.pdf Last accessed 1/16/19.
[http://dx.doi.org/10.5772/intechopen.74190]

[62] Wenfeng, L.; Yalong, L.; Huang, D.; Han, X.; Yang, X. Effects of stachyose on absorption and transportation of tea catechins in mice: Possible role of phase II metabolic enzymes and efflux transporters inhibition by stachyose. *Food & Nutrtion Research,* **2016**, *60*, 32783.
[http://dx.doi.org/10.3402/fnr.v60.32783]

[63] Schönthal, A.H. Adverse effects of concentrated green tea extracts. *Mol. Nutr. Food Res.,* **2011**, *55*(6), 874-885.
[http://dx.doi.org/10.1002/mnfr.201000644] [PMID: 21538851]

[64] Yang, C.S.; Chen, L.; Lee, M.J.; Balentine, D.; Kuo, M.C.; Schantz, S.P. Blood and urine levels of tea catechins after ingestion of different amounts of green tea by human volunteers. *Cancer Epidemiol. Biomarkers Prev.,* **1998**, *7*(4), 351-354.
[PMID: 9568793]

[65] Mahmoud, M.F.; Fahmy, A.; Auf, M.A. Evaluation of the hepatoprotective effect of green tea extract ad selenium on CCL4-induced fibrosis. *ESPEN J.,* **2012**, *7*, E23-E29.
[http://dx.doi.org/10.1016/j.eclnm.2011.12.004]

[66] El-Beshbishy, H.A. Hepatoprotective effect of green tea (Camellia sinensis) extract against tamoxifen-induced liver injury in rats. *J. Biochem. Mol. Biol.,* **2005**, *38*(5), 563-570.
[PMID: 16202236]

[67] Anudeep Reddy, M.; Kala Kumar, B. Boobalan, G., Kasi Reddy, M., Satish Kumar, C.S.V., Gopala Reddy, A., Lakshman, M. Hepatoprotective potential of green tea extract against experimental hepatotoxicity in rats. *Indian J. Pharm. Sci.,* **2017**, *79*(1), 58-64.

CHAPTER 2

Sesquiterpene Lactone Cynaropicrin as Novel Inhibitor of Bcr-Abl Fusion Oncogene Expression

Maria Cristina Caroleo[*], **Francesca Aiello, Erika Cione** and **Maria Luisa Di Gioia**

Department of Pharmacy Health and Nutritional Sciences, University of Calabria, Arcavacata di Rende, Cosenza, Italy

Abstract: Chronic Myeloid Leukemia (CML) is a progressive myeloproliferative disorder accounting for about 20% of all leukemia cases in adults. The hallmark of the disease is a genetic translocation at the level of the long arms of chromosomes 9 and 22 resulting into the formation of BCR/ABL fusion oncogene, that in turn translates into the Bcr-Abl p210 oncoprotein. The expression and the aberrant function of Bcr-Abl p210 trigger both hematopoietic cell transformation and disease maintenance as established by experimental and clinical studies. The Bcr-Abl p210 chimeric protein is targeted by the kinase inhibitor (TKI) imatinib and its use has substantially improved the prognosis in CML patients however, the development of mutations in the ABL kinase domain often result in drug resistance. In most of the patients showing mutation the shift to second-generation of TKIs such as dasatinib and nilotinib can overcome imatinib resistance unless the occurrence of the gatekeeper T315I mutation in ABL domain, thus strategies in association with TKI, are currently being studied. In the past few years, natural products gained attention because of its potential effects to prevent cancer or to diminish the risk of tumor development and in this concern, the antioxidant and the anti-proliferative properties of bioactive components of Cynara cardunculus extracts are well known. This chapter is a focus on the medicinal chemistry and pharmacology of the sesquiterpene lactone cynaropicrin and its deacyl derivate that allows these compounds to negatively regulate bcr BCR/ABL fusion oncogene expression, thus paving the way for a novel therapeutic strategy aimed to both potentiate the effectiveness of imatinib or of its analogues and to delay or overcome the occurrence of resistance CML chemotherapy.

Keywords: Cynara Carduncuius, Chronic Myeloid Leukemia, Bcr-Abl p210 oncoprotein, K562 cell line, CML drug-resistance.

[*] **Corresponding author Maria Cristina Caroleo:** Department of Pharmacy Health and Nutritional Sciences, University of Calabria, Arcavacata di Rende, Cosenza, Italy; Tel: +390984 493455; E-mail: mariacristinacaroleo@virgilio.it

Atta-ur-Rahman (Ed.)

INTRODUCTION

Chronic myeloid leukemia (CML) is a progressive and often deadly myeloproliferative disease accounting for about 20% of all leukemia cases in adult age. [1]. The disorder typically progresses into three phases namely chronic (CP), accelerated (AP) and blast crisis (BC) [2]. Subjects in the chronic phase are relatively asymptomatic or show mild symptoms and the diagnosis often occurs during blood tests or a medical routine. Most patients develop AP prior to BC, a condition identical to acute myelogenous leukemia or acute lymphoblastic leukemia, but 20% evolve into BC without AP clinical signals. Of note, the blast phase is unresponsive to therapy with a median survival rate of 3-5 months. The disease stems from the aberrant transformation of the pluripotent hematopoietic stem cells and is characterized by a stable cytogenetic defect, the so-called Philadelphia (Ph) chromosome, and the presence of Bcr-Abl fusion gene which in turn encodes the Bcr-Abl chimeric protein [3]. Of note, three translocation breakpoints were mapped at the level of the Bcr gene [4] accounting for the expression of proteins with apparent molecular weight of 210 kDa (so called Bcr-Abl p210), 185/190 kDa (so called Bcr-Abl p185), and 230 kDa (so called Bcr-Abl p230) [5]. These chimeric products are expressed in several hematologic malignancies, however among these Bcr-Abl p210 represents the molecular signature of CML. The expression of the Bcr-Abl p210 fusion protein has related implications: i) the Abl kinase domain becomes catalytically active and phosphorylates different substrate proteins; ii) the Bcr-moiety of the fusion protein provides key domains and sequence motifs that drive activation of downstream signaling pathways; iii) Bcr-Abl p210 has a constitutively augmented tyrosine kinase activity because the lack of auto-inhibitory *N*-terminal myristoylation at the level of Abl protein. Therefore, Bcr-Abl p210 works as a docking scaffold for PTB (phosphotyrosine- binding) domain-containing proteins and SH2 (Src Homology 2) that assemble a multiprotein complex and induces the phosphorylation of various downstream signaling molecules such as PI3K, MAPK, NF-kB, RAS and STAT-5 thus promoting proliferative and anti-apoptotic activities. Until 2000 therapeutic arsenal for CML comprised non-specific drugs such as busulfan, hydroxyurea, and interferon-alfa (IFN-α) [6]. This immunobiological agent led to disease regression and improved survival, however its use was hampered by low efficacy and substantial side-effects. Allogenic stem cell transplantation is the only option still considered curative, but it entails risks of morbidity and mortality. In addition, this procedure is influenced by patient's general status and by transplantation procedures. The occurrence of tyrosine kinase inhibitors changed dramatically the CML therapeutic approach. These small molecules strongly affected the interaction between the Bcr-Abl p210 oncoprotein and adenosine triphosphate (ATP) ultimately leading to the block of cellular proliferation in the aberrant clone. This "tailored" approach has profoundly changed the outcome of CML, improving the 10-year survival rate from approximately 20% to up 80% [1, 7, 8].

Tyrosine Kinase Inhibitors (TKIs)

Imatinib mesylate (IM) was the first TKIs approved by FDA for the treatment of patients with CML-CP. It binds to inactive configuration domain of Bcr-Abl p210 kinase and competitively inhibits the adenosine triphosphate-binding site of the Bcr-Abl p210 oncoprotein, thereby avoiding tyrosine autophosphorylation and, in turn, phosphorylation of its substrates. This event results in switching-off the phosphorylation of downstream proteins involved in cell signal transduction cascade with a direct effect on the molecular mechanisms underlying the proliferative and anti-apoptotic activities. Of note, IM also blocks the C-KIT tyrosine kinase and the platelet-derived growth factor receptor [9]. By directly targeting the Bcr-Abl p210 kinase, IM yields to long lasting cytogenetic response and to a dramatic survival improvement especially in CP CML patients. Indeed, treatment with IM alone in early phase of CML has been shown to improve the overall survival (OS) rate of 88% after 5 years, compared to the OS rate of 57% observed with previous nonspecific treatment such as hydroxyurea and interferon [10, 11]. In addition to IM, other TKIs have been developed and are commercially available for CML treatment such as dasatinib, nilotinib, bosutinib and ponatinib. Unlike IM and nilotinib, dasatinib binds the kinase domain of Bcr-Abl p210 in the open conformation while bosutinib is a dual SRC/ABL kinase inhibitor. All of these compounds are endorsed by current guidelines as choices for initial treatment of CML in CP patients although dasatinib and nilotinib were originally devoted to CML patients showing resistance to IM as well as bosutinib, which was the drug first approved for patients with CML resistant and/or intolerant to prior therapy. Most TKIs are well-tolerated even if adequate monitoring and supportive care are recommended. The toxicological profile for each compound should be also taken into account. Indeed, for patients with cardiac and lung diseases or uncontrolled hypertension TKIs other than dasatinib should be selected since this compound has been shown to induce pulmonary arterial hypertension [12]. Dasatinib also inhibits platelets function [13] and patients underwent to therapy with anticoagulants may be prone to hemorrhagic complications [14]. Nilotinib has been linked with hyperglycemia and vasospastic or vaso-occlusive events [15, 16]. Therefore, the drug should be avoided or prescribed with caution in diabetic patients or with clinical history of vascular diseases or pancreatitis. Conversely IM produces far fewer side effects, hence it still remains the frontline choice of drug for the disease treatment [17, 18]. Although the precision therapy with IM shows high efficacy in the majority of CML patients, a substantial proportion of these subjects may not achieve the desired response or may eventually lose an adequate response to IM. Treatment failure is often related to the development of resistance owing to Bcr-Abl-p2-0-dependent mechanism, emergence of additional chromosome abnormalities or BCR/ABL independent mechanisms. The most commonly identified Bcr-Ab--p210-dependent mechanisms associated with relapse involves point mutations in the kinase domain of oncoprotein which impair the activity of the available TKIs. In this frame BCR/ABL mutation screening is a relevant tool for optimization of therapeutic response or selection of subsequent therapy because certain specific Bcr-Abl-p210 mutations have been related with poor prognosis. It is worth mentioning that mutations in discrete regions of Bcr-Abl-p210 tyrosine kinase domain yields to different modality of resistance. Accordingly, the type of harboring mutation can address both the alternative use of TKI belonging to the second or third generation in such IM resistant patients and the timely identification of those who need IM dosing escalation [19]. The use of dasatinib or nilotinib overcomes most of the mutations conferring resistance to IM, even though novel mutations making the leukemia resistant to these second generation TKIs have emerged. Among these the so-called the "gatekeeper" mutation T315I, displays resistance to all currently available TKIs except ponatinib [20]. A novel treatment option in CML patients harboring the T3151 mutation is the tyrosine kinase inhibitor TKI asciminib. This molecule is an effective and selective BCR-ABL1 inhibitor that binds to the myristoyl pocket of ABL1 and switches kinase configuration in the inactive state, furthermore the different binding site enables ascyminib to preserve its activity against BCR-ABL1 mutants conferring resistance to canonical TKIs [21]. The peculiar pharmacodynamic profile of ascyminib also provides the opportunity of a combination therapy with second generation ATP-binding site TKIs, thus avoiding the occurrence of resistance in the first line setting [21]. Moreover, advanced clinical trials comparing the efficacy of ascyminib *vs* bosutinib are ongoing. Beside Bcr-Abl-p210-dependent mechanism of resistance, pharmacokinetic variability as a result of genetic polymorphisms in genes related to the binding, metabolism and transport of IM may also influence the intracellular delivery, bioavailability and effectiveness of IM and hence affect clinical response to IM. The impact of candidate SNPs in genes such as ABCB1, ABCG2, ABCC1, ABCC2, SLC22A1, CYP3A4, CYP3A5, CYP2C8, GSTM1, GSTT1, GSTP, ORM1, and BIM have been widely studied, but the results obtained have been conflicting. Few potential genotypes and haplotypes of the above genes underlying inter-individual pharmacokinetic variability and clinical response to IM in CML patients have been identified but the data are not yet conclusive enough to be translated into tailored IM dosing in CML patients [22]. Noteworthy, the lack of adherence to TKI therapy paves also the way to the occurrence of IM resistance. Generally, non-adherence or non-compliance are due to drug reactions, dose changes or in some cases to unavailability of the medication. All these factors can have an impact to IM treatment and can result in an increase in the mortality rate related with CML progression [23, 24].

Sesquiterpene Lactone Cynaropicrin Extraction

Traditionally natural products from medicinal plants have found many applications in the fields of medicine, pharmacy and biology and in recent years they gained attention because of their putative effects to prevent cancer or to reduce the risk of carcinogenesis. *Cynara cardunculus* L. (Asteraceae), commonly named "cardoon" is a Mediterranean species typical of arid and semi-arid region throughout the world [25] encompassing three varieties, namely var. sylvestris (L.) Fiori (wild cardoon), var. scolymus (L.) Fiori (globe artichoke), and var. altilis (DC) (cultivated cardoon) [26]. Several bioactive compounds such as saponins, flavones, sterols, coumarins and lignans in *C. cardunculus* leaves and seeds were previously identified [27]. Apart from their nutritive value, cynara cardunculus species are recognized for the bitterness of leaves due to the presence of guaianolide-type sesquiterpenes lactones [28]. In 1960 for the first time Šorm and co-workers isolated from *Cynara scolymus L* Cynaropicrin. This molecule is the most representative sesquiterpenes lactone, accounting for about 80% of the plant typical bitter taste and showing a variety of biological properties [29]. These comprise antispasmodic, anti-inflammatory and proapoptotic activities [30 - 32]. Considering the pharmacological and chemical biology potential of the sesquiterpene lactone natural products it is of particular interest the development of more efficient strategies concerning the extraction and recovery of cynaropicrin from cardoon. The improvement of methodology is also important with a view to its use in nutraceutical formulations [33]. Classified as a guaianolide sesquiterpene lactone, cynaropicrin has a 5-7-5 fused tricyclic skeleton with six carbon stereocenters, four exo-olefins, and two hydroxyl groups (Fig. **1**). The highest concentration of cynaropicrin is found in plant leaves (especially in trichomes), while low levels of the molecule are detected in roots, stems and in completely developed inflorescences [34].

Presently, cynaropicrin is extracted from different types of biomass through volatile and often toxic organic solvents, such as dichloromethane and chloroform [35, 36] yielding to human health risks and environmental damage. Additional procedures for the extraction of cynaropicrin are performed using water at elevated temperatures, methanol or supercritical CO_2, or rely on the use of co-solvents to improve the extraction yields [37, 38]. Cynaropicrin can be isolated in gram-scale using counter current chromatography [39]. Most of the conventional methods are time or energy consuming and in some cases they require the use of sophisticated equipment resulting in low cynaropicrin yields [40]. Recently, several efforts have been devoted to the development of eco-friendlier processes for the extraction of value-added compounds from biomass. These approaches encompass mainly the use of green solvents such as deep eutectic solvents (DES) and ionic liquids (ILs) [41]. DES are constituted of at least a hydrogen bond donor (HBD) and a hydrogen bond acceptor (HBA) species, which upon mixing create strong hydrogen bond interactions yielding to the formation of eutectic mixtures, that became liquid at room temperature. In a recent study the use of organic acids and quaternary ammonium salts-based DES, as substitute solvents for the extraction of cynaropicrin from *Cynara cardunculus L.* leaves was highlighted, revealing the usefulness of DES aqueous solutions for both the extraction of value-added compounds from biomass and the recovery of the desired compounds and solvents [42]. Among alternate solvents, ILs are the most studied for the extraction of bioactive compounds from biomass and in recent study de Faria and co-workers [43] clearly demonstrated the remarkable ability of aqueous solutions of surface-active ILs in extracting cynaropicrin from the leaves of *C. cardunculus L.*

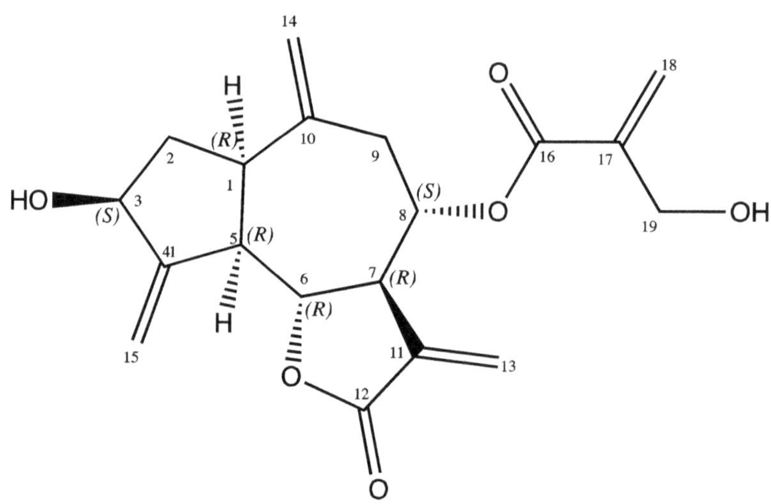

Fig. (1). Chemical structure of cynaropicrin.

Sesquiterpene Lactone Cynaropicrin Derivatives and Structure–Activity Relationship (SAR) Studies

The α-methylene-γ- and δ -lactones and lactams motif is recurrent in numerous biologically attracting natural compounds used in traditional medicine, due to their anti-inflammatory activity, robust inhibitory effects [44] on the expression of tumor necrosis factor (TNF)-α and cyclooxygenase anti-bacterial and cytotoxic and/or anticancer properties, this latter nowadays extensively studied [45]. It is well known that, compounds containing an exo-methylene moiety conjugated with α-carbonyl group work as Michael-type acceptors reacting with mercapto groups in cysteine residues of enzymes, free intracellular glutathione and functional proteins, by the formation of covalent adducts. Such alkylation reaction, results in the interruption of principal living process of the cells. This kind of action is mainly present in potent anticancer agents [46]. For these reasons, various synthetic analogues have been synthesized and assayed for their cytotoxicity and structure activity relationship (SAR) studies were performed [47]. Moreover, all the Michael-type acceptors are defined "multi-targeted" and as consequence, their therapeutic value is less compared to compounds with a single target only, and some of them are toxic toward normal cells. One more, the chemical environment of the target plays a central role in the selectivity of their biological activity. The sesquiterpenelactones (SLs), are one of the largest categories of secondary metabolites major retrieved in *Asteraceae* family. SLs are 15-carbon terpenoids, containing three isoprene (5C) units, a lactone ring that is either cis- or trans-fused to the carbocyclic skeleton. At this SLs group belong eremophilanolides, eudesmanolides, germacranolides, guaianolides, pseudo-guaianolides, xanthanolides and carabranolides [48]. Among these, cynaropicrin and deacyl-cynaropicrin, are classified as guaianolide sesquiterpene lactones. Both molecules, show many biological actions, such as inhibition of NF-kB, anti-inflammatory and immunomodulatory properties [49], anti-hyperilipidemic [50] other than bitterness mediated action due to the activation of bitter sensory receptors. Structurally, cynaropicrin could be viewed as a potential drug candidate since it shows no violation of Lipinski rules, so it is water soluble. The preparation of cynaropicrin derivatives by chemical modification of its skeleton has enabled to conduct studies on the SAR. Cravotto *et al.* produced different cynaropicrin derivatives by esterification reactions, redox reactions on the oxygenated functions, chemo-selective reduction of the exomethylene double bonds and ring opening of the lactone. A sensorial study of these compounds showed the influence of the chemical modification on the taste of this sesquiterpene lactone [51]. The acylation of both hydroxyls and the deacylation of cynaropicrin, abate the bitterness; the opening of the lactone ring has the same result; finally, the exomethylene groups play a critical role in defining bitterness. This effect decreases in parallel with the number of exomethylenes converted to methyl groups by reduction and it seemed to be especially pronounced with the exomethylene placed on the γ -lactone ring [51]. Other synthetic cynaropicrin derivatives were recently prepared to study the antitrypanosomal structure-activity-relationship against T. brucei. The two hydroxyl groups (OH-3 and OH-19) were the main target of the modifications to obtain new derivatives with reduced hydrophilicity. To this end the introduction of a methoxymethyl (MOM) group or an acetyl group on the two OH functional groups was performed. Furthermore, the esterification of the primary alcohol using methacrylic acid afforded a different derivative. Several synthetic compounds, *in vitro* assayed for activity against T. b. rhodesiense [52, 53], and for cytotoxicity in cell lines (rat skeletal myoblasts, L6 cells) showed interesting SAR results confirming that: i) an acyl side chain at OH-8 is crucial for antitrypanosomal activity; ii) changes in the hydrophilicity of the OH-3 substituent move neither antitrypanosomal activity nor cytotoxicity; iii) by varying the hydrophilicity of OH-19 group it affects the cytotoxic activity; iv) esterification of OH-19 position reduces both the antitrypanosomal and cytotoxic activities while the introduction of Ac groups at OH-19 and OH-3 positions yields to a decrease of both actions [51]. The synthesis of a cynaropicrin deuterated derivative, cynaropicrin-d_4, bearing four deuterium atoms on the side-chain [54]. The synthesis of cynaropicrin-d_4 was performed through esterification of hydrolyzed cynaropicrin and deuterated side chain. In performing pharmacokinetic study on cynaropicrin this molecule could be employed as an internal standard for liquid chromatography–mass spectrometry analysis, thus advancing the knowledge of cynaropicrin-d_4 as a therapeutic tool. Research are still ongoing to better understand the selectivity of α-methylene-γ- and δ -lactones with selective activities to realize specific lead compounds.

Cynaropricrin as Co-adjuvant CML Therapy

Undoubtedly, the advent in CML management of ABL kinase inhibitor IM improved the outcome in CML patients, nevertheless some evidence shows that it cannot eradicate the disease [55]. In addition, the development of resistance in patients who remain on IM therapy is still a clinical challenge, thus several strategies in association with TKI are currently under investigation. Phytochemicals, which are non-nutritive chemicals found in plants and food, have been found to modulate key cellular signaling pathways exerting proven anticancer effects [56]. In this frame, sesquiterpene lactones are assessed as major classes of natural products with a wide range of biological activities and among them cynaropicrin, has been reported to modulate cytokine release and nitric oxide production [57, 58]. *In vitro* studies on leukocyte lineage cancer cell [58] showed how methanol extract of CCL flower and/or cynaropicrin had a notable anti-proliferative activity. Both reactive oxygen species and protein kinase (PK) Cδ are involved in mediating the pro-apoptotic activity of cynaropicrin, as suggested by pharmacological and biochemical evidence [59]. In this concern, SAR studies conducted regarding the cytotoxicity and anti-proliferative activity of cynaropicrin revealed that the exo-methylene group on the lactone seems to be crucial for cytotoxicity, in fact its saturation or addition reactions, exhibit a drastic loss of activity. On the other hands, the presence of additional alkylating groups improves cytotoxicity. The α-methylene-γ-lactone and α, β-unsaturated cyclopentenone moieties are pivotal for their *in vivo* anti-proliferative effect and their absence abolishes this property [60]. Through the conventional *in vitro* model for dissecting the molecular mechanisms in CML and for screening new pharmacological approaches, a recent report [38] highlighted how lipophilic extracts of CCL dose-dependently and time independently, inhibited cell proliferation in both K562 and K562 IM resistant (IMAR) cell lines. Molecular approach unveiled that this effect was related to a considerable decrease of Bcr-Abl-p210 oncoprotein kinase expression indicating that the antiproliferative activity of CCL lipophilic fraction is likely due to the inhibition at transcriptional level of BCR/ABL fusion gene in both cell lines. The same authors identified among the biocomponents of CCL cynaropicrin and its deacyl derivative as the molecules having the capability to down-regulate the Bcr-Abl-p210 oncoprotein. The effect of these compounds on transcriptional activity of BCR/ABL fusion gene is of relevance in view of the occurrence of resistance in patients on IM therapy. In most cases the use of second-generation TKIs such as dasatinib and nilotinib can overcome imatinib resistance, however the presence of the T315I gatekeeper mutation makes ineffective these drugs and drug resistance also occurs when they are used as second line options [20]. In this frame, the inhibition at transcriptional level of Bcr-Abl-p210 expression induced by cynaropicrin and its deacyl derivative may be a novel strategy for potentiating the capability Tk_is to induce tumor growth arrest and for avoiding or counteracting the resistance to chemotherapy in CML. However, further *in vivo* and clinical studies are required to validate this hypothesis and ascertain the efficacy and safety of cynaropicrin and its deacyl derivative. An emerging target in CML clinical setting is treatment-free remission (TFR), that is achieved when a CP patient maintains a deep molecular response after discontinuing TKis therapy and without restarting treatment [61]. Effective TFR constitutes the paradigm of "functional cure" in which the risk of disease relapse is negligible although BCR-ABL1 transcripts may be detectable. Several clinical studies aimed at evaluating the feasibility and safety of discontinuing TKI therapy have been performed and to date the bulk of evidence concerning TFR is based on patients who underwent long-term therapy with imatinib [62 - 66]. However, subsequent investigations have also established the feasibility of TFR after discontinuing dasatinib or nilotinib, used as either first-line or second line treatment, in CP CML patients showing a DMR for 12 months after two years or more of TKI therapy [67 - 70]. As data from TFR studies continue to growing up, questions remain about molecular monitoring as well as the proper selection of patients and longer-term outcome [71]. This issue is particularly relevant since about 40% of patients who achieved deep molecular responses loose TFR showing a recurrence. Typically, molecular relapses occurred within 6 months, however the immediate restoration of therapy with the same TKIs results in the achievement of undetectable disease in almost all patients [72]. Innovative treatment approaches that may enable more patients to achieve TFR are therefore needed and in this frame the capability of cynaropicrin and its deacyl derivate to down regulate the Bcr-Abl p210 oncoprotein kinase could be useful tool in improving TFR rate, as it positively correlates with lasting DMR.

CONCLUDING REMARKS

The BCR-ABL1 fusion protein is perhaps the most investigated oncogenic tyrosine kinase. Being it the hallmark in CML pathogenesis, switching off BCR-ABL1 kinase activity with TKIs results in optimal clinical responses in most of patients. Although the tailored molecular therapy has changed the outcome of CML the occurrence of drug resistance and the maintenance of lasting deep molecular response are still a clinical challenge. The presence of new mutations required further development of inhibitors and novel therapeutic approaches. In this frame, the use of cynaropicrin or its deacyl derivative in combination therapy with TKIs might be a new therapeutic strategy for both synergize with IM and or its analogues in cancer growth arrest and to retard or overcome the TKIs resistance in CML. Moreover, the inhibition of BCR-ABL1 gene expression induced by these molecules could be an added value considering that the varied levels of the Bcr-Abl oncoprotein expressed by CD34+ CML reflect the degree and extent of their response to imatinib and the fairly high levels of oncoprotein may underlie the rapid occurrence of resistance observed in advanced-phase of the disease [73]. Finally, cynaropicrin and its derivative consist of complex structures, therefore traditional systematic structure function studies could ameliorate their properties as is already shown for vinblastine and vincristine (Vinca alkaloids) often regarded as prototypical members of natural products.

CONSENT FOR PUBLICATION

Not applicable.

CONFLICT OF INTEREST

The authors confirm that this chapter contents have no conflict of interest.

ACKNOWLEDGMENT

Declared none.

REFERENCES

[1] American Cancer Society. *Cancer Facts & Figures 2017*; American Cancer Society: Atlanta, **2017**.

[2] Hehlmann, R.; Hochhaus, A.; Baccarani, M. Chronic myeloid leukaemia. *Lancet,* **2007**, *370*(9584), 342-350.
[http://dx.doi.org/10.1016/S0140-6736(07)61165-9] [PMID: 17662883]

[3] Rowley, J.D. Chromosomal translocations: revisited yet again. *Blood,* **2008**, *112*(6), 2183-2189.
[http://dx.doi.org/10.1182/blood-2008-04-097931] [PMID: 18779403]

[4] Deininger, M.W.; Goldman, J.M.; Melo, J.V. The molecular biology of chronic myeloid leukemia.

Blood, **2000**, *96*(10), 3343-3356.
[PMID: 11071626]

[5] Wong, S.; Witte, O.N. The BCR-ABL story: bench to bedside and back. *Annu. Rev. Immunol.,* **2004**, *22*, 247-306.
[http://dx.doi.org/10.1146/annurev.immunol.22.012703.104753] [PMID: 15032571]

[6] Silver, R.T.; Woolf, S.H.; Hehlmann, R.; Appelbaum, F.R.; Anderson, J.; Bennett, C.; Goldman, J.M.; Guilhot, F.; Kantarjian, H.M.; Lichtin, A.E.; Talpaz, M.; Tura, S. An evidence-based analysis of the effect of busulfan, hydroxyurea, interferon, and allogeneic bone marrow transplantation in treating the chronic phase of chronic myeloid leukemia: developed for the American Society of Hematology. *Blood,* **1999**, *94*(5), 1517-1536.
[PMID: 10477676]

[7] Huang, X.; Cortes, J.; Kantarjian, H. Estimations of the increasing prevalence and plateau prevalence of chronic myeloid leukemia in the era of tyrosine kinase inhibitor therapy. *Cancer,* **2012**, *118*(12), 3123-3127.
[http://dx.doi.org/10.1002/cncr.26679] [PMID: 22294282]

[8] Deininger, M.; O'brien, S.G.; Guilhot, F. International randomized study of interferon *vs.* STI571 (IRIS) 8-year follow up: sustained survival and low risk for progression of events in patients with newly diagnosed chronic myeloid leukemia in chronic phase (CMLCP) treated with imatinib. *Blood,* **2009**, 114.

[9] Druker, B.J.; Lydon, N.B. Lessons learned from the development of an abl tyrosine kinase inhibitor for chronic myelogenous leukemia. *J. Clin. Invest.,* **2000**, *105*(1), 3-7.
[http://dx.doi.org/10.1172/JCI9083] [PMID: 10619854]

[10] von Bubnoff, N.; Duyster, J. Chronic myelogenous leukemia: treatment and monitoring. *Dtsch. Arztebl. Int.,* **2010**, *107*(7), 114-121.
[PMID: 20221270]

[11] Allan, N.C.; Richards, S.M.; Shepherd, P.C. UK Medical Research Council randomised, multicentre trial of interferon-α n1 for chronic myeloid leukaemia: improved survival irrespective of cytogenetic response. The UK Medical Research Council's Working Parties for Therapeutic Trials in Adult Leukaemia. *Lancet,* **1995**, *345*(8962), 1392-1397.
[http://dx.doi.org/10.1016/S0140-6736(95)92596-1] [PMID: 7760609]

[12] Montani, D.; Bergot, E.; Günther, S.; Savale, L.; Bergeron, A.; Bourdin, A.; Bouvaist, H.; Canuet, M.; Pison, C.; Macro, M.; Poubeau, P.; Girerd, B.; Natali, D.; Guignabert, C.; Perros, F.; O'Callaghan, D.S.; Jaïs, X.; Tubert-Bitter, P.; Zalcman, G.; Sitbon, O.; Simonneau, G.; Humbert, M. Pulmonary arterial hypertension in patients treated by dasatinib. *Circulation,* **2012**, *125*(17), 2128-2137.
[http://dx.doi.org/10.1161/CIRCULATIONAHA.111.079921] [PMID: 22451584]

[13] Quintás-Cardama, A.; Han, X.; Kantarjian, H.; Cortes, J. Tyrosine kinase inhibitor-induced platelet dysfunction in patients with chronic myeloid leukemia. *Blood,* **2009**, *114*(2), 261-263.
[http://dx.doi.org/10.1182/blood-2008-09-180604] [PMID: 19414863]

[14] Quintás-Cardama, A.; Kantarjian, H.; Ravandi, F.; O'Brien, S.; Thomas, D.; Vidal-Senmache, G.; Wierda, W.; Kornblau, S.; Cortes, J. Bleeding diathesis in patients with chronic myelogenous leukemia receiving dasatinib therapy. *Cancer,* **2009**, *115*(11), 2482-2490.
[http://dx.doi.org/10.1002/cncr.24257] [PMID: 19280591]

[15] Quintás-Cardama, A.; Kantarjian, H.; Cortes, J. Nilotinib-associated vascular events. *Clin. Lymphoma Myeloma Leuk.,* **2012**, *12*(5), 337-340.
[http://dx.doi.org/10.1016/j.clml.2012.04.005] [PMID: 22633167]

[16] Giles, F.J.; Mauro, M.J.; Hong, F.; Ortmann, C.E.; McNeill, C.; Woodman, R.C.; Hochhaus, A.; le Coutre, P.D.; Saglio, G. Rates of peripheral arterial occlusive disease in patients with chronic myeloid leukemia in the chronic phase treated with imatinib, nilotinib, or non-tyrosine kinase therapy: a retrospective cohort analysis. *Leukemia,* **2013**, *27*(6), 1310-1315.

[http://dx.doi.org/10.1038/leu.2013.69] [PMID: 23459450]

[17] Jabbour, E.; Cortes, J.; Ravandi, F.; O'Brien, S.; Kantarjian, H. Targeted therapies in hematology and their impact on patient care: chronic and acute myeloid leukemia. *Semin. Hematol.*, **2013**, *50*(4), 271-283.
[http://dx.doi.org/10.1053/j.seminhematol.2013.09.006] [PMID: 24246694]

[18] Cortes, J.E.; Gambacorti-Passerini, C.; Deininger, M.W.; Mauro, M.J.; Chuah, C.; Kim, D.W.; Dyagil, I.; Glushko, N.; Milojkovic, D.; le Coutre, P.; Garcia-Gutierrez, V.; Reilly, L.; Jeynes-Ellis, A.; Leip, E.; Bardy-Bouxin, N.; Hochhaus, A.; Brümmendorf, T.H. Bosutinib *Versus* Imatinib for Newly Diagnosed Chronic Myeloid Leukemia: Results From the Randomized BFORE Trial. *J. Clin. Oncol.*, **2018**, *36*(3), 231-237.
[http://dx.doi.org/10.1200/JCO.2017.74.7162] [PMID: 29091516]

[19] Bixby, D.; Talpaz, M. Mechanisms of resistance to tyrosine kinase inhibitors in chronic myeloid leukemia and recent therapeutic strategies to overcome resistance. *Hematology (Am. Soc. Hematol. Educ. Program)*, **2009**, 461-476.
[http://dx.doi.org/10.1182/asheducation-2009.1.461] [PMID: 20008232]

[20] Jabbour, E.; Kantarjian, H. Chronic myeloid leukemia: 2018 update on diagnosis, therapy and monitoring. *Am. J. Hematol.*, **2018**, *93*(3), 442-459.
[http://dx.doi.org/10.1002/ajh.25011] [PMID: 29411417]

[21] Wylie, A.A.; Schoepfer, J.; Jahnke, W.; Cowan-Jacob, S.W.; Loo, A.; Furet, P.; Marzinzik, A.L.; Pelle, X.; Donovan, J.; Zhu, W.; Buonamici, S.; Hassan, A.Q.; Lombardo, F.; Iyer, V.; Palmer, M.; Berellini, G.; Dodd, S.; Thohan, S.; Bitter, H.; Branford, S.; Ross, D.M.; Hughes, T.P.; Petruzzelli, L.; Vanasse, K.G.; Warmuth, M.; Hofmann, F.; Keen, N.J.; Sellers, WR. The allosteric inhibitor ABL001 enables dual targeting of BCR-ABL1. *Nature,* **2017**, *543*(7647), 733-737.
[http://dx.doi.org/10.1038/nature21702] [PMID: 28329763]

[22] Ankathil, R.; Azlan, H.; Dzarr, A.A.; Baba, A.A. Pharmacogenetics and the treatment of chronic myeloid leukemia: how relevant clinically? An update. *Pharmacogenomics.*, **2018**, *19*(5), 393-475.
[http://dx.doi.org/10.2217/pgs-2017-0193] [PMID: 29569526]

[23] Noens, L.; van Lierde, M.A.; De Bock, R.; Verhoef, G.; Zachée, P.; Berneman, Z.; Martiat, P.; Mineur, P.; Van Eygen, K.; MacDonald, K.; De Geest, S.; Albrecht, T.; Abraham, I. Prevalence, determinants, and outcomes of nonadherence to imatinib therapy in patients with chronic myeloid leukemia: the ADAGIO study. *Blood,* **2009**, *113*(22), 5401-5411.
[http://dx.doi.org/10.1182/blood-2008-12-196543] [PMID: 19349618]

[24] Eliasson, L.; Clifford, S.; Barber, N.; Marin, D. Exploring chronic myeloid leukemia patients' reasons for not adhering to the oral anticancer drug imatinib as prescribed. *Leuk. Res.*, **2011**, *35*(5), 626-630.
[http://dx.doi.org/10.1016/j.leukres.2010.10.017] [PMID: 21095002]

[25] Kelly, M. Cynara cardunculus.*Invasive Plants of California's Wildlands*; Bossard, C.C.; Randall, J.M.; Hoshovsky, M.C., Eds.; University of California Press: Berkeley, CA, USA, **2000**, pp. 139-145.

[26] Wiklund, A. The genus Cynara L. (Asteraceae-Cardueae). *Bot. J. Linn. Soc.*, **1992**, *109*(1), 75-123.
[http://dx.doi.org/10.1111/j.1095-8339.1992.tb00260.x]

[27] Lerna, A.; Mauromicale, G. Cynara cardunculus L. genotypes as a crop for energy purposes in a Mediterranean environment. *Biomass Bioenergy,* **2010**, *34*, 754-760.
[http://dx.doi.org/10.1016/j.biombioe.2010.01.018]

[28] Pinelli, P.; Agostini, F.; Comino, C.; Lanteri, S.; Portis, E.; Romani, A. Simultaneous quantification of caffeoyl esters and flavonoids in wild and cultivated cardoon leaves. *Food Chem.*, **2007**, *105*, 1695-1701.
[http://dx.doi.org/10.1016/j.foodchem.2007.05.014]

[29] Suchý, M.; Herout, V.; Šorm, F. On terpenes. CXVI. Structure of cynaropicrin. *Collect. Czech. Chem. Commun.*, **1960**, *25*, 2777-2782.
[http://dx.doi.org/10.1135/cccc19602777]

[30] Cho, J.Y.; Baik, K.U.; Jung, J.H.; Park, M.H. *In vitro* anti-inflammatory effects of cynaropicrin, a sesquiterpene lactone, from Saussurea lappa. *Eur. J. Pharmacol.*, **2000**, *398*(3), 399-407. [http://dx.doi.org/10.1016/S0014-2999(00)00337-X] [PMID: 10862830]

[31] Cho, J.Y.; Kim, A.R.; Jung, J.H.; Chun, T.; Rhee, M.H.; Yoo, E.S. Cytotoxic and pro-apoptotic activities of cynaropicrin, a sesquiterpene lactone, on the viability of leukocyte cancer cell lines. *Eur. J. Pharmacol.*, **2004**, *492*(2-3), 85-94. [http://dx.doi.org/10.1016/j.ejphar.2004.03.027] [PMID: 15178350]

[32] Emendörfer, F.; Emendörfer, F.; Bellato, F.; Noldin, V.F.; Cechinel-Filho, V.; Yunes, R.A.; Delle Monache, F.; Cardozo, A.M. Antispasmodic activity of fractions and cynaropicrin from Cynara scolymus on guinea-pig ileum. *Biol. Pharm. Bull.*, **2005**, *28*(5), 902-904. [http://dx.doi.org/10.1248/bpb.28.902] [PMID: 15863902]

[33] Ramos, P.A.B.; Guerra, A.R.; Guerreiro, O.; Freire, C.S.R.; Silva, A.M.S.; Duarte, M.F.; Silvestre, A.J.D. Lipophilic extracts of Cynara cardunculus L. var. altilis (DC): a source of valuable bioactive terpenic compounds. *J. Agric. Food Chem.*, **2013**, *61*(35), 8420-8429. [http://dx.doi.org/10.1021/jf402253a] [PMID: 23915287]

[34] Sato, T.; Hara, S.; Sato, M.; Ogawa, K.; Adams, M.; Usuki, T. Synthesis of cynaropicrin-d(4). *Bioorg. Med. Chem. Lett.*, **2015**, *25*(23), 5504-5507. [http://dx.doi.org/10.1016/j.bmcl.2015.10.065] [PMID: 26520660]

[35] Bhattacharyya, P.R.; Barua, N.C.; Ghosh, A.C. Cynaropicrin from Tricholepis glaberrima: a potential insect feeding deterrent compound. *Ind. Crops Prod.*, **1995**, *4*(4), 291-294. [http://dx.doi.org/10.1016/0926-6690(95)00044-5]

[36] Ramos, P.A.B.; Guerra, A.R.; Guerreiro, O.; Freire, C.S.R.; Silva, A.M.S.; Duarte, M.F.; Silvestre, A.J.D. Lipophilic extracts of Cynara cardunculus L. var. altilis (DC): a source of valuable bioactive terpenic compounds. *J. Agric. Food Chem.*, **2013**, *61*(35), 8420-8429. [http://dx.doi.org/10.1021/jf402253a] [PMID: 23915287]

[37] Sovová, H.; Opletal, L.; Sajfrtová, M.; Bártlová, M. Supercritical fluid extraction of cynaropicrin and 20-hydroxyecdysone from Leuzea carthamoides DC. *J. Sep. Sci.*, **2008**, *31*(8), 1387-1392. [http://dx.doi.org/10.1002/jssc.200700496] [PMID: 18383243]

[38] Russo, A.; Perri, M.; Cione, E.; Di Gioia, M.L.; Nardi, M.; Caroleo, M. C. Biochemical and chemical characterization of Cynara cardunculus L. extract and its potential use as co-adjuvant therapy of chronic myeloid leukemia. *J. Ethnopharmacol.*, **2017**, *18*(202), 184-191. [http://dx.doi.org/10.1016/j.jep.2017.03.026]

[39] Adekenova, A.S.; Sakenova, P.Y.; Ivasenko, S.A.; Khabarov, I.A.; Adekenov, S.M.; Berthod, A. Gram-Scale Purification of Two Sesquiterpene Lactones from Chartolepsis Intermedia Boiss. *Chromatographia,* **2016**, *79*, 37-43. [http://dx.doi.org/10.1007/s10337-015-3000-1]

[40] Kaminskii, I.P.; Krasnov, E.A.; Kadyrova, T.V.; Ivasenko, S.A.; Rakhimova, B.B.; Adekenov, S.M. Quantitative HPLC determination of cynaropicrin in Centaurea scabiosa dry extract. *Pharm. Chem. J.*, **2011**, *45*(9), 560-563. [http://dx.doi.org/10.1007/s11094-011-0679-7]

[41] Paiva, A.; Craveiro, R.; Aroso, I.; Martins, M.; Reis, R.L.; Duarte, A.R.C. Natural deep eutectic solvents - solvents for the 21st century. *ACS Sustain. Chem.& Eng.*, **2014**, *2*(5), 1063-1071. [http://dx.doi.org/10.1021/sc500096j]

[42] de Faria, E.L.P.; do Carmo, R.S.; Cláudio, A.F.M.; Freire, C.S.R.; Freire, M.G.; Silvestre, A.J.D. Deep Eutectic Solvents as Efficient Media for the Extraction and Recovery of Cynaropicrin from Cynara cardunculus L. Leaves. *Int. J. Mol. Sci.*, **2017**, *18*(11), 2276. [http://dx.doi.org/10.3390/ijms18112276] [PMID: 29084184]

[43] de Faria, E.L.P.; Gomes, M.V.; Cláudio, A.F.M.; Freire, C.S.R.; Silvestre, A.J.D.; Freire, M.G.

Extraction and recovery processes for cynaropicrin from Cynara cardunculus L. using aqueous solutions of surface-active ionic liquids. *Biophys. Rev.*, **2018**, *10*(3), 915-925. [http://dx.doi.org/10.1007/s12551-017-0387-y] [PMID: 29294260]

[44] Adams, J.D.; Haworth, I.S.; Coricello, A.; Perri, F.; Nguyen, C.; Aiello, F.; Williams, T.J.; Lien, E.J. The treatment of pain with topical sesquiterpenes. *Frontiers in Natural Product Chemistry.*, **2017**, *3*, 176-195.

[45] Hwang, D.; Fischer, N.H.; Jang, B.C.; Tak, H.; Kim, J.K.; Lee, W. Inhibition of the expression of inducible cyclooxygenase and proinflammatory cytokines by sesquiterpene lactones in macrophages correlates with the inhibition of MAP kinases. *Biochem. Biophys. Res. Commun.*, **1996**, *226*(3), 810-818. [http://dx.doi.org/10.1006/bbrc.1996.1433] [PMID: 8831694]

[46] Bruno, M.; Rosselli, S.; Maggio, A.; Raccuglia, R.A.; Bastow, K.F.; Lee, K.H. Cytotoxic activity of some natural and synthetic guaianolides. *J. Nat. Prod.*, **2005**, *68*(7), 1042-1046. [http://dx.doi.org/10.1021/np0500575] [PMID: 16038545]

[47] Coricello, A.; El-Magboub, A.; Luna, M.; Ferrario, A.; Haworth, I.S.; Gomer, C.J.; Aiello, F.; Adams, J.D. Rational drug design and synthesis of new α-Santonin derivatives as potential COX-2 inhibitors. *Bioorg. Med. Chem. Lett.*, **2018**, *28*(6), 993-996. [http://dx.doi.org/10.1016/j.bmcl.2018.02.036] [PMID: 29501395]

[48] Janecka, A.; Wyrębska, A.; Gach, K.; Fichna, J.; Janecki, T. Natural and synthetic α-methylenelactones and α-methylenelactams with anticancer potential. *Drug Discov. Today,* **2012**, *17*(11-12), 561-572. [http://dx.doi.org/10.1016/j.drudis.2012.01.013] [PMID: 22309965]

[49] Cho, J.Y.; Kim, A.R.; Joo, H.G.; Kim, B.H.; Rhee, M.H.; Yoo, E.S.; Katz, D.R.M.; Chain, B.M.; Jung, J.H. Cynaropicrin, a sesquiterpene lactone, as a new strong regulator of CD29 and CD98 functions. *Biochem. Biophys. Res. Commun.*, **2004**, *313*(4), 954-961. [http://dx.doi.org/10.1016/j.bbrc.2003.12.026] [PMID: 14706635]

[50] Shimoda, H.; Ninomiya, K.; Nishida, N.; Yoshino, T.; Morikawa, T.; Matsuda, H.; Yoshikawa, M. Anti-hyperlipidemic sesquiterpenes and new sesquiterpene glycosides from the leaves of artichoke (Cynara scolymus L.): structure requirement and mode of action. *Bioorg. Med. Chem. Lett.*, **2003**, *13*(2), 223-228. [http://dx.doi.org/10.1016/S0960-894X(02)00889-2] [PMID: 12482428]

[51] Cravotto, G.; Nano, G.M.; Binello, A.; Spagliardi, P.; Seu, G. Chemical and biological modification of cynaropicrin and grosheimin: a structure–bitterness relationship study. *J. Sci. Food Agric.*, **2005**, *85*, 1757-1764. [http://dx.doi.org/10.1002/jsfa.2180]

[52] Usuki, T.; Sato, M.; Hara, S.; Yoshimoto, Y.; Kondo, R.; Zimmermann, S.; Kaiser, M.; Brun, R.; Hamburger, M.; Adams, M. Antitrypanosomal structure-activity-relationship study of synthetic cynaropicrin derivatives. *Bioorg. Med. Chem. Lett.*, **2014**, *24*(3), 794-798. [http://dx.doi.org/10.1016/j.bmcl.2013.12.099] [PMID: 24433861]

[53] Zimmermann, S.; Fouché, G.; De Mieri, M.; Yoshimoto, Y.; Usuki, T.; Nthambeleni, R.; Christopher, J. Parkinson, C.J.; van der Westhuyzen, C.; Kaiser, M.; Hamburger, M.; Adams, M. Structure-Activity Relationship Study of Sesquiterpene Lactones and Their Semi-Synthetic Amino Derivatives as Potential Antitrypanosomal Products. *Molecules,* **2014**, *19*, 3523-3538. [http://dx.doi.org/10.3390/molecules19033523] [PMID: 24662071]

[54] Sato, T.; Hara, S.; Sato, M.; Ogawa, K.; Adams, M.; Usuki, T. Synthesis of cynaropicrin-d(4). *Bioorg. Med. Chem. Lett.*, **2015**, *25*(23), 5504-5507. [http://dx.doi.org/10.1016/j.bmcl.2015.10.065] [PMID: 26520660]

[55] Holtz, M.; Forman, S. J.; Bhatia, R. Growth factor stimulation reduces residual quiescent chronic myelogenous leukemia progenitors remaining after imatinib treatment. *Cancer Res,* **2007**, *67*(3), 1113-1120.

[56] González-Vallinas, M.; González-Castejón, M.; Rodríguez-Casado, A.; Ramírez de Molina, A. Dietary phytochemicals in cancer prevention and therapy: a complementary approach with promising perspectives. *Nutr. Rev.,* **2013**, *71*(9), 585-599. [http://dx.doi.org/10.1111/nure.12051] [PMID: 24032363]

[57] Cho, J.Y.; Park, J.; Yoo, E.S.; Baik, K.U.; Jung, J.H.; Lee, J.; Park, M.H. Inhibitory effect of sesquiterpene lactones from Saussurea lappa on tumor necrosis factor-alpha production in murine macrophage-like cells. *Planta Med.,* **1998**, *64*(7), 594-597. [http://dx.doi.org/10.1055/s-2006-957528] [PMID: 9810262]

[58] Cho, J.Y.; Kim, A.R.; Yoo, E.S.; Baik, K.U.; Park, M.H. Immunomodulatory effect of arctigenin, a lignan compound, on tumour necrosis factor-alpha and nitric oxide production, and lymphocyte proliferation. *J. Pharm. Pharmacol.,* **1999**, *51*(11), 1267-1273. [http://dx.doi.org/10.1211/0022357991777001] [PMID: 10632084]

[59] Cho, J.Y.; Kim, A.R.; Jung, J.H.; Chun, T.; Rhee, M.H.; Yoo, E.S. Cytotoxic and pro-apoptotic activities of cynaropicrin, a sesquiterpene lactone, on the viability of leukocyte cancer cell lines. *Eur. J. Pharmacol.,* **2004**, *492*(2-3), 85-94. [http://dx.doi.org/10.1016/j.ejphar.2004.03.027] [PMID: 15178350]

[60] Zhang, S.; Won, Y.K.; Ong, C.N.; Shen, H.M. Anti-cancer potential of sesquiterpene lactones: bioactivity and molecular mechanisms. *Curr. Med. Chem. Anticancer Agents,* **2005**, *5*(3), 239-249. [http://dx.doi.org/10.2174/1568011053765976] [PMID: 15992352]

[61] Mahon, F.X.; Réa, D.; Guilhot, J.; Guilhot, F.; Huguet, F.; Nicolini, F.; Legros, L.; Charbonnier, A.; Guerci, A.; Varet, B.; Etienne, G.; Reiffers, J.; Rousselot, P. Intergroupe Français des Leucémies Myéloïdes Chroniques. Discontinuation of imatinib in patients with chronic myeloid leukaemia who have maintained complete molecular remission for at least 2 years: the prospective, multicenter Stop Imatinib (STIM) trial. *Lancet Oncol.,* **2010**, *11*, 1029-1035. [http://dx.doi.org/10.1016/S1470-2045(10)70233-3] [PMID: 20965785]

[62] Rousselot, P.; Huguet, F.; Rea, D.; Legros, L.; Cayuela, J.M.; Maarek, O.; Blanchet, O.; Marit, G.; Gluckman, E.; Reiffers, J.; Gardembas, M.; Mahon, F.X. Imatinib mesylate discontinuation in patients with chronic myelogenous leukemia in complete molecular remission for more than 2 years. *Blood,* **2007**, *109*(1), 58-60. [http://dx.doi.org/10.1182/blood-2006-03-011239] [PMID: 16973963]

[63] Etienne, G.; Guilhot, J.; Rea, D.; Rigal-Huguet, F.; Nicolini, F.; Charbonnier, A.; Guerci-Bresler, A.; Legros, L.; Varet, B.; Gardembas, M.; Dubruille, V.; Tulliez, M.; Noel, M.P.; Ianotto, J.C.; Villemagne, B.; Carré, M.; Guilhot, F.; Rousselot, P.; Mahon, F.X. Long-term follow-up of the French Stop Imatinib study (STIM1) in chronic myeloid leukemia patients. *J. Clin. Oncol.,* **2017**, *35*, 298-305. [http://dx.doi.org/10.1200/JCO.2016.68.2914] [PMID: 28095277]

[64] Rousselot, P.; Charbonnier, A.; Cony-Makhoul, P.; Agape, P.; Nicolini, F.E.; Varet, B.; Gardembas, M.; Etienne, G.; Réa, D.; Roy, L.; Escoffre-Barbe, M.; Guerci-Bresler, A.; Tulliez, M.; Prost, S.; Spentchian, M.; Cayuela, J.M.; Reiffers, J.; Chomel, J.C.; Turhan, A.; Guilhot, J.; Guilhot, F.; Mahon, F.X. Loss of major molecular response as a trigger for restarting tyrosine kinase inhibitor therapy in patients with chronic-phase chronic myelogenous leukemia who have stopped imatinib after durable undetectable disease. *J. Clin. Oncol.,* **2014**, *32*(5), 424-430. [http://dx.doi.org/10.1200/JCO.2012.48.5797] [PMID: 24323036]

[65] Ross, D.M.; Branford, S.; Seymour, J.F.; Schwarer, A.P.; Arthur, C.; Yeung, D.T.; Dang, P.; Goyne, J.M.; Slader, C.; Filshie, R.J.; Mills, A.K.; Melo, J.V.; White, D.L.; Grigg, A.P.; Hughes, T.P. Safety and efficacy of imatinib cessation for CML patients with stable undetectable minimal residual disease: results from the TWISTER study. *Blood,* **2013**, *122*(4), 515-522. [http://dx.doi.org/10.1182/blood-2013-02-483750] [PMID: 23704092]

[66] Lee, S.E.; Choi, S.Y.; Song, H.Y.; Kim, S.H.; Choi, M.Y.; Park, J.S.; Kim, H.J.; Kim, S.H.; Zang, D.Y.; Oh, S.; Kim, H.; Do, Y.R.; Kwak, J.Y.; Kim, J.A.; Kim, D.Y.; Mun, Y.C.; Lee, W.S.; Chang, M.H.; Park, J.; Kwon, J.H.; Kim, D.W. Imatinib withdrawal syndrome and longer duration of imatinib have a close association with a lower molecular relapse after treatment discontinuation: the KID study. *Haematologica,* **2016**, *101*(6), 717-723.
[http://dx.doi.org/10.3324/haematol.2015.139899] [PMID: 26888022]

[67] Rea, D.; Nicolini, F.E.; Tulliez, M.; Guilhot, F.; Guilhot, J.; Guerci-Bresler, A.; Gardembas, M.; Coiteux, V.; Guillerm, G.; Legros, L.; Etienne, G.; Pignon, J.M.; Villemagne, B.; Escoffre-Barbe, M.; Ianotto, J.C.; Charbonnier, A.; Johnson-Ansah, H.; Noel, M.P.; Rousselot, P.; Mahon, F.X. Discontinuation of dasatinib or nilotinib in chronic myeloid leukemia: interim analysis of the STOP 2G-TKI study. *Blood,* **2017**, *129*(7), 846-854.
[http://dx.doi.org/10.1182/blood-2016-09-742205] [PMID: 27932374]

[68] Imagawa, J.; Tanaka, H.; Okada, M.; Nakamae, H.; Hino, M.; Murai, K.; Ishida, Y.; Kumagai, T.; Sato, S.; Ohashi, K.; Sakamaki, H.; Wakita, H.; Uoshima, N.; Nakagawa, Y.; Minami, Y.; Ogasawara, M.; Takeoka, T.; Akasaka, H.; Utsumi, T.; Uike, N.; Sato, T.; Ando, S.; Usuki, K.; Morita, S.; Sakamoto, J.; Kimura, S. Discontinuation of dasatinib in patients with chronic myeloid leukaemia who have maintained deep molecular response for longer than 1 year (DADI trial): a multicentre phase 2 trial. *Lancet Haematol.,* **2015**, *2*(12), e528-e535.
[http://dx.doi.org/10.1016/S2352-3026(15)00196-9] [PMID: 26686407]

[69] Hochhaus, A.; Masszi, T.; Giles, F.J.; Radich, J.P.; Ross, D.M.; Gómez Casares, M.T.; Hellmann, A.; Stentoft, J.; Conneally, E.; García-Gutiérrez, V.; Gattermann, N.; Wiktor-Jedrzejczak, W.; le Coutre, P.D.; Martino, B.; Saussele, S.; Menssen, H.D.; Deng, W.; Krunic, N.; Bedoucha, V.; Saglio, G. Treatment-free remission following frontline nilotinib in patients with chronic myeloid leukemia in chronic phase: results from the ENESTfreedom study. *Leukemia,* **2017**, *31*(7), 1525-1531.
[http://dx.doi.org/10.1038/leu.2017.63] [PMID: 28218239]

[70] Ross, D.M.; Masszi, T.; Gómez Casares, M.T.; Hellmann, A.; Stentoft, J.; Conneally, E.; Garcia-Gutierrez, V.; Gattermann, N.; le Coutre, P.D.; Martino, B.; Saussele, S.; Giles, F.J.; Radich, J.P.; Saglio, G.; Deng, W.; Krunic, N.; Bédoucha, V.; Gopalakrishna, P.; Hochhaus, A. Durable treatment-free remission in patients with chronic myeloid leukemia in chronic phase following frontline nilotinib: 96-week update of the ENESTfreedom study. *J. Cancer Res. Clin. Oncol.,* **2018**, *144*(5), 945-954.
[http://dx.doi.org/10.1007/s00432-018-2604-x] [PMID: 29468438]

[71] Saglio, G.; Sharf, G.; Almeida, A.; Bogdanovic, A.; Bombaci, F.; Čugurović, J.; Deekes, N.; Garcia-Gutiérrez, V.; de Jong, J.; Narbutas, Š.; Westerweel, P.; Zackova, D. Considerations for treatment-free remission in patients with chronic myeloid leukemia: a joint patient-physician perspective. *Clin. Lymphoma Myeloma Leuk.,* **2018**, *18*(6), 375-379.
[http://dx.doi.org/10.1016/j.clml.2018.04.005] [PMID: 29753691]

[72] Hughes, T.P.; Ross, D.M. Moving treatment-free remission into mainstream clinical practice in CML. *Blood,* **2016**, *128*(1), 17-23.
[http://dx.doi.org/10.1182/blood-2016-01-694265] [PMID: 27013442]

[73] Barnes, D.J.; Palaiologou, D.; Panousopoulou, E.; Schultheis, B.; Yong, A.S.M.; Wong, A.; Pattacini, L.; Goldman, J.M.; Melo, J.V. Bcr-Abl expression levels determine the rate of development of resistance to imatinib mesylate in chronic myeloid leukemia. *Cancer Res.,* **2005**, *65*(19), 8912-8919.
[http://dx.doi.org/10.1158/0008-5472.CAN-05-0076] [PMID: 16204063]

Frontiers in Natural Product Chemistry, 2019, *Vol. 5*, 55-94

CHAPTER 3

Effects of Dietary Polyphenols on Chronic Diseases: Epidemiological Data and Molecular Mechanisms of Action

Kazuo Yamagata[*]

Laboratory of Molecular Health Science of Food, Department of Food Bioscience and Biotechnology, College of Bioresource Sciences, Nihon University (NUBS), Fujisawa, Japan

Abstract: Non-communicable diseases (NCDs) such as cardiovascular diseases (CVD), type 2 diabetes mellitus (T2DMM), cancers, and chronic respiratory diseases are usually chronic in nature, and the mortality rate associated with these NCDs is high. However, epidemiological evidence implies a relationship between dietary polyphenols and reduced risk of a number of NCDs, and indicated that dietary polyphenols inhibit NCD-related pathological changes and prophylactically prevent occurrence of NCDs. In this review, I described the role of dietary polyphenols in the prevention of NCDs, and discussed the possible utility of several polyphenols as prophylactic agents for obesity, CVD, T2DMM, and cancer. Polyphenols are classified based on structure; particularly, flavonoids, which is further divided into six major subclasses, are the most common dietary polyphenols, and help in the prevention of NCDs. In addition, consumption of polyphenols was associated with a reduced risk of T2DMM and obesity. The preventive effect on NCD by polyphenols such as epigallocatechin gallate and resveratrol was associated with potent anti-oxidative and anti-inflammatory effects. Furthermore, these polyphenols regulated the signaling pathway, associated with NCDs. Polyphenol contributed to NCD prevention, and the protective effects may have resulted from its anti-oxidative and anti-inflammatory effect. The intake of polyphenol-rich diets such as vegetable and fruit is important for prevention of NCDs. In future, the difference in polyphenol preventive effects and novel mechanism for preventing NCDs with polyphenol, need to be clarified.

Keywords: Non communicable diseases, Reactive oxygen species, Polyphenol, Cardiovascular diseases, Type 2 diabetes mellitus, Cancers and chronic respiratory diseases.

[*] **Corresponding author Kazuo Yamagata:** Laboratory of Molecular Health Science of Food, Department of Food Bioscience and Biotechnology, College of Bioresource Sciences (NUBS), 1866, Kameino, Fujisawa, Kanagawa 252-8510, Japan. Tel: +81-466-84-3986; Fax: +81-466-84-3986; E-mail:yamagata.kazuo@nihon-u.ac.jp

Atta-ur-Rahman (Ed.)

1. INTRODUCTION

Non-communicable diseases (NCDs) are usually chronic diseases and are not infective in nature. NCDs progress slowly and clinical disease is apparent after a long period of progression. Such diseases are usually preventable by lifestyle modification. Important NCDs include cardiovascular diseases (CVDs) (coronary heart disease and cerebrovascular disease) , cancers, chronic respiratory diseases (chronic obstructed pulmonary disease and asthma), and type 2 diabetes mellitus (T2DMM). Unhealthy dietary habits, lack of exercise, smoking, and excessive alcohol consumption have been defined as risk factors for NDCs by the World Health Organization [1]. In 2008, NDCs accounted for 63% of mortalities (of 57 million deaths) worldwide [2]. Furthermore, it has been predicted that the global mortality rate from chronic disease may rise by at least 15-20% by 2020, and four major noninfectious diseases may account for 75% of deaths globally by 2030 [1]. It is estimated that 36 million people die of NCDs every year.

In many high-income countries, NCDs are reported to be the major causes of mortality, and data on these cause-specific deaths are systematically reported. However, such monitoring systems are absent in low-income economies [3]. In addition, the precision of cause-specific mortality data, as reported in high-income countries, is known to be imprecise. Improving the precision of such data would contribute toward devising proper prevention strategies and lowering NCD-specific mortality rates. The global increase in the prevalence of NCDs is related to aging, rapid urbanization, and the globalization of unhealthy lifestyles. Furthermore, the increase in per capita income and urbanization have led to lower consumption of traditional diets, and has enhanced oil, meat, refined sugar, and fat intake [4]. Singh *et al.* reported that urbanization has led to higher obesity rates and to increased incidence of NCDs such as CVDs [5]. Higher incidence of obesity, has led to an increase in obesity-related metabolic disorders including hypertension, insulin resistance, impaired glucose tolerance, and dyslipidemia. These pathologic conditions are major risk factors for CVD [6]. Thus, obesity has been associated with chronic diseases such as T2DMM, CVDs, hypertension, and several forms of cancer [7]. Table **1** summarizes the adverse effects of increased obesity [8]. Thus, the prevention of obesity is imperative for preventing the onset of various NCDs. In contrast, a vegetarian diet is linked to lower mortality rates (related to ischemic heart disease, and circulatory and cerebrovascular diseases), than an omnivorous diet [9].

The Mediterranean diet is considered a healthy dietary pattern, and greater adherence to this diet may improve health status [10]. The Mediterranean diet reduces the risks related to NCD; and, variety of factors including dietary pattern and lifestyle contribute to the health benefit of the Mediterranean diet [11].

Mediterranean diet comprises of large fish and seafood, white meat, fruits, as well as vegetables and some amounts of red meat [10]. In general, vegetarian diet includes numerous vegetables and fruits which are thought to contain important components such as polyphenols, dietary fiber, magnesium, vitamin C, and vitamin E, which may aid in the prevention of onset of NCDs. Though the detailed mechanism is yet unclear, the Mediterranean diet has been strongly implicated in the prevention of NCDs [12]. For example, PREDIMED (PREvencion con DIeta MEDiterranea) trial indicated that a vegetable-based mix of Mediterranean diet, which is rich in unsaturated fat and polyphenols, can be an ideal model for CVD prevention [10]. Furthermore, evidence from epidemiological research has indicated that Mediterranean diet led to a 9% decrease in overall mortality, a 6% decrease in the incidence of cancer, and a 9% decrease in the incidence of CVD [13]. There are numerous polyphenolic compounds; and information about the various classes of polyphenols and the polyphenolic content of several foods is presented in Table **2** [14].

These foods are not comprehensive, but rather were selected based on quantity of polyphenols in the food item and common rate of consumption. Polyphenol content of foods was obtained from Phenol Explorer. 2. Polyphenol subclasses displayed are examples and are not comprehensive; individual foods are divided by polyphenol subclass for only the flavonoid class.

Previous reports have indicated the importance of dietary polyphenols in the prevention of obesity and obesity-related chronic diseases. For example, intake of polyphenols including green tea catechins, resveratrol, and curcumin inhibited obesity and obesity-related inflammation [15]. Furthermore, polyphenols may function in CVD risk-reduction. Biological effects of polyphenols have been correlated to antioxidant activities. In addition, recent studies have suggested that immunomodulatory and vasodilatory effects of polyphenols may also be associated with CVD risk-reduction [14]. Furthermore, polyphenol-rich diets have the ability to prevent T2DMM [16]. Other studies suggested that intake of anthocyanins may also decrease the risk of T2DMM [17, 18], and that diet rich in fruits and vegetables may reduce the risk of certain cancers [19]. The mechanism of anticancer activity of several polyphenolic compounds has been a subject of recent research [20, 21]. Table **3** summarizes the antioxidant effects, radical scavenging activities, anti-inflammatory effects, and several other mechanisms implicated in the activity of polyphenols [14]. The anti-inflammatory activity of polyphenolic compounds is thought to be important in its protective effects against various NCDs.

NADPH, nicotinamide adenine dinucleotide phosphate; NF-kB, nuclear factor-kappa B; TNF-α; tumor necrosis factor-α; IL-1B, interleukin-1 beta; IL-6, interleukin 6; VCAM, vascular cell adhesion molecule; ICAM, intercellular adhesion molecule; MCP-1; monocyte chemoattractant protein-1; MIP, macrophage inflammatory protein; 2Nrf2, nuclear transcription factor erythroid-2 related factor- 2; CD40, Cluster of differentiation 40; MMP1, metalloproteinase I. Modulates tyrosine and serine-threonine protein kinases (MAPKs [*i.e.*, p38, JNK]) involved in signal transduction and cell activation.

Though it is known that polyphenols exert protective effects against NCDs, there are numerous mechanisms which contribute to the onset of NCDs. In addition, there are many polyphenolic compounds with varied modes of action. The aim of this review was to summarize the preventive activities of polyphenols against various NCDs, and present evidence to show the possible utility of these compounds in preventing obesity, CVD, T2DMM, and cancer. The author hopes that this work would be a valuable reference resource to provide information about the beneficial effects of polyphenols for future studies.

2. CHARACTERISTICS OF DIETARY POLYPHENOLS

Polyphenols are secondary plant metabolites with potential to improve health [22]. Polyphenols are a diverse set of compounds with phenolic hydroxyl groups, and contain direct linkages of a sugar moiety (including polysaccharides or monosaccharides) to an aromatic carbon. More than 7,000 polyphenolic compounds have been identified in plants [22]. In food, polyphenols are responsible for the bitterness, color, flavor, and odor. Fig. **1** shows a summary of the beneficial effects of polyphenols [22 - 24] (Fig. **1**).

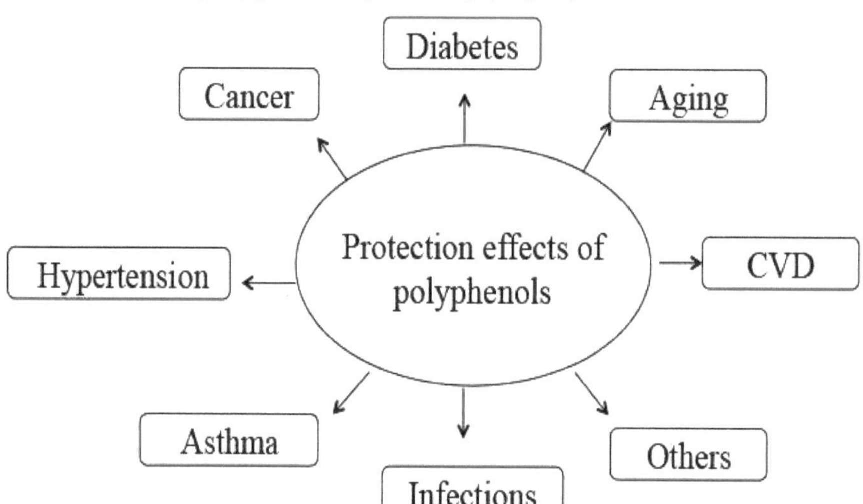

Fig. (1). Pleiotropic health benefits of dietary plant polyphenols.

Table 1. Adverse effects of obesity relate to cardiovascular diseases.

A.	**Increases in insulin resistance** (1) Glucose intolerance (2) Metabolic syndrome (3) Type 2 diabetes mellitus	E.	**Endothelial dysfunction**
		F.	**Increased systemic inflammation and prothrombotic state**
B.	**Hypertension**	G.	**Systolic and diastolic dysfunction**
C.	**Dyslipidemia** (1) Elevated total cholesterol (2) Elevated triglycerides (3) Elevated LDL cholesterol (4) Elevated non-HDL cholesterol (5) Elevated apolipoprotein-B (6) Elevated small, dense LDL particles (7) Decreased HDL cholesterol (8) Decreased apolipoprotein-A1	H.	**Heart failure**
		I.	**Coronary heart disease**
		J.	**Atrial fibrillation**
		K.	**Obstructive sleep apnea/sleep-disordered breathing**
		L.	**Albuminuria**
D.	**Abnormal left ventricular geometry** (1) Concentric remodeling (2) Left ventricular hypertrophy	M.	**Osteoarthritis**
		N.	**Cancers**

Adapted from reference [8].

Polyphenols are compounds found largely in fruits, vegetables, cereals, and beverages. Epidemiological studies have revealed that polyphenols provide significant protection against the development of several chronic diseases such as cardiovascular disease, cancer, diabetes, infections, aging, and asthma.

2.1. Classification of Polyphenol

Polyphenols are classified as phenolic acids, flavonoids, stilbenes, and lignans [22 [25], (Fig. **2**). Flavonoids are further divided into six major subclasses such as flavonols (such as quercetin and kaempferol), flavanones (such as naringenin and taxifolin), flavones (such as luteolin), flavanols (sometimes known as Flavan-3-ols, such as the catechins), anthocyanins (such as cyanidin), and isoflavones (such as genistein). Flavonoids are the most common dietary polyphenols, and help in the prevention of NCDs. Polyphenols are classified based on structure, and this classification helps in the elucidation of the biological effects of these compounds.

The flavonoids share a common structure consisting of 2 aromatic rings (A and B) bound together by 3 carbon atoms that form an oxygenated heterocycle (ring C). Polyphenols are classified as phenolic acids, flavonoids, stilbenes, and lignans (Fig. **2A**). Furthermore, flavonoids are categorized into 6 subclasses: flavonols, flavones, isoflavones, flavanones, anthocyanidins, and flavanols (catechins and proanthocyanidins) (Fig. **2B**).

Table 2. Polyphenol classes, compounds and content in common foods.

Polyphenol Class	Polyphenol Subclass	Example Compounds	Dietary Sources (mg/serving)			
			<25	25-50	50-100	>100
Flavonoids	Flavonols	Kaempferol, Myricetin, Quercetin	Black tea (22) Walnuts (19) Black Beans (10) Dark chocolate (7) Red wine (6) Almonds (1) White wine (1)	Spinach (36) Plum (31) Onion (29) Blueberry (29)	Capers (56)	
	Flavanones	Naringenin, Hesperetin	Red wine (1)		Grapefruit (67) Orange (63)	
	Flavan-3-ols	Catechin, Epigallocatechin Gallate, Procyanidin	Grape juice (5) Plum (4) White wine (2) Almonds (1) Blueberry (1)	Red wine (41) Cocoa (28)	Dark chocolate (60)	Black tea (176) Green tea (171)
	Flavones	Apigenin, Luteolin	Oregano (1)			
		Anthocyanidin, Anthocyanin	Red wine (20)	Black beans (35)	Blueberry (99)	
	Anthocyanins			Plum (32)		
	Isoflavones	Diadzein, Genistein		Tofu (35)		
Lignans	Lignans	Lariciresinol, Secoisolariciresinol			Flaxseed (61)	Sesame oil (217)

(Table 2) cont.....

Phenolic acids	Hydroxybenzoic acid; Hydroxycinnamic acids	Egallic Acid, Vanillic Acid, Caffeic Acid, Ferulic Acid	Grape juice (15)	Flaxseed (47)	Plum (59)	Coffee (509)
			Red wine (15)	Black tea (45)		Walnut (127)
			Rosemary (12)	Green olives (38)		Blueberry (101)
			Grapefruit (10)	Black beans (32)		
			Dark chocolate (7)			
			White wine (5)			
			Cocoa (2)			
			Oregano (2)			
			Rolled oats (1)			
Stilbenes	Stilbenes	Resveratrol,	Red wine (3)			
		Resveratrol 3-O-glycoside	White wine (1)			
Other polyphenols	Tyrosol, Curcuminoids	Hydroxytyrosol, Curcumin	Olive oil (8)		Green Olives (59)	
			Coffee (6)		Turmeric (54)	
			Red wine (4)			
			White wine (1)			
			White wine (1)			

Adapted from reference [14]

2.1.1. Phenolic Acids

Phenolic acids are categorized as derivatives of cinnamic acid and as derivatives of benzoic acid. Except in specific types of red fruit, black radish, and in onions, hydroxybenzoic acid content is generally minimal in most comestible plants [22]. P-coumaric, caffeic, ferulic, and sinapic acids are the most commonly encountered hydroxycinnamic acids and are more abundant than are hydroxybenzoic acids.

2.1.2. Flavonoids

Flavonoid is the generic designation of organic compounds which contain a basic flavan skeleton (a C6-C3-C6 structure with two benzene rings (C6) connected by three carbons (C3)). More than 4,000 species of flavonoids have been identified and have been categorized into six subclasses based on chemical structure: flavonols, flavones, flavanones, flavanols, anthocyanins, and isoflavones [22] (Fig. **2**). A flavonoid moiety is the main central polyphenolic group in polyphenolic compounds. Many biological effects pertaining to NCDs have been reported for flavonoids.

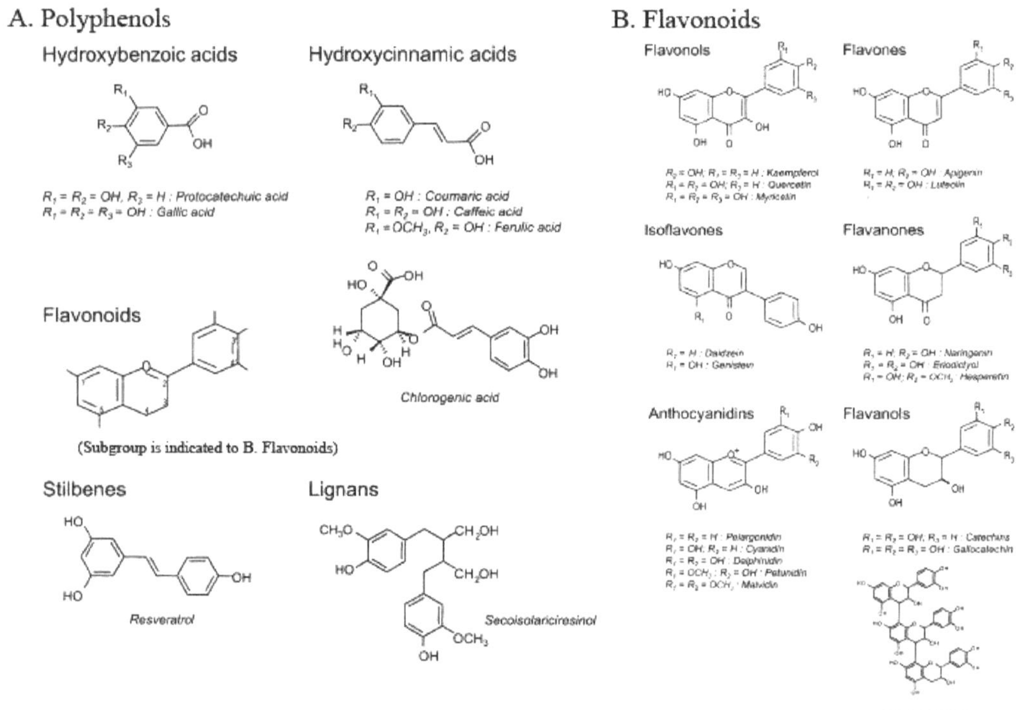

Fig. (2). Chemical structure of polyphenols.
Adapted from reference [25].

2.1.3. Stilbenes

Stilbenes contain two phenyl moieties flanked by a two-carbon methylene bridge. Historically, stilbenes were not recognized as food components, but as compounds synthesized by plants in response to infection or injury. However, when resveratrol was studied for its biological effects, it was recognized that resveratrol was a type of stilbene compound. Resveratrol is now considered as a typical stilbene, and is known as a wine polyphenol.

2.1.4. Lignans

Lignans are diphenolic compounds and are formed by the dimerization of two cinnamic acid residues [22]. Lignans are found abundantly in linseed [26]. Plant lignans such as secoisolariciresinol may function as phytoestrogens. Furthermore, reports of animal studies suggest that lignans may inhibit the development of cancer and atherosclerosis [27, 28].

Table 3. Major anti-inflammatory mechanisms and example phenolic compounds that elicit these effects.

A. Antioxidant Activity
Inhibition of reactive oxygen and nitrogen species • Direct scavenging of peroxynitrite, hydroxyl radicals, superoxide anion, nitric oxide
B. Modifies signaling cascades and transcriptional networks
Inhibition of pro-oxidant enzymes • Suppress activity and expression of endothelial NAPDH oxidase, lipoxygenase, myeloperoxidase, cyclooxygenase-2, phospholipase, inducible nitric oxide synthase (quercetin, apigenin, kaempferol) Blocks NFκB signaling and expression (resveratrol, quercetin) • Downregulates TNFα, IL1β, IL-6 synthesis (resveratrol, olive oil) • Reduces expression of VCAM-1 and ICAM-1 (resveratrol, olive oil) • Reduces MCP-1, MIP-1α expression (quercetin, resveratrol) Upregulation of NrF2 genes and thioredoxin to maintain redox state (epicatechin, tea)
C. Reduces adhesion of immune cells (T lymphocytes, monocytes) to endothelium
Suppression of adhesion markers on endothelium, vascular smooth muscle cells: CD40. • VCAM, ICAM, E-selectin, P-selectin (red wine, nuts, olive oil) • Inhibit expression of MMP1 (resveratrol)
D. Counters endothelial dysfunction
• Downregulates endothelial contractility factor, decreases endothelin-1 expression and release (resveratrol) • Increases nitric oxide availability because of increased activity of endothelial nitric oxide synthase (delphinidin, quercetin, resveratrol, red wine) • Upregulates endothelial derived hyperpolarizing factor (red wine, grapes)

Adapted from reference [14].

2.2. Protective Action of Polyphenols Against Reactive Oxygen Species (ROS)-Associated NCDs

Many chronic diseases are associated with high ROS production induced by oxidative stress and protein oxidation [29, 30]. Abundant evidence exists to suggest a role for oxidative stress in the development and pathogenesis of NCDs such as diabetes, chronic lung disease, and CVD [31]. In CVD, oxidative stress is reported to be associated with endothelial dysfunction, atherosclerosis evolution, and the onset of myocardial infarction [32 - 34]. Ameliorating early endothelial dysfunction has been shown to be critical for the prevention of atherosclerosis and CVD [35]. Reduction of nitric oxide (NO) production is known to augment the onset of myocardial infarction. In particular, a reduction in vasodilative capacity is reported to be caused by ROS and by the lowering of endothelial NO synthase (eNOS)-dependent NO production in the vascular endothelial cell (Fig. **3**) [35]. Mitochondrial nicotinamide adenine dinucleotide phosphate (NADPH) oxidase and xanthine oxidase enzymes are known to be associated with ROS production within the vascular system [36, 37]. Interestingly, the flavonoids apigenin and naringenin have been shown to prevent endothelial dysfunction by regulating ROS/caspase-3 and NO pathway in endothelial cells exposed to high glucose. These effects suggest that flavonoids such as apigenin and naringenin may help prevent endothelial dysfunction and atherosclerosis associated with diabetes [38]. Furthermore, rutin, a citrus flavonoid, is a known antioxidant which has been reported to enhance the nuclear factor erythroid 2–related factor 2 (Nrf2)-induced antioxidant response in endothelial cells [39]. These effects of rutin have been linked to a reduced risk of CVD.

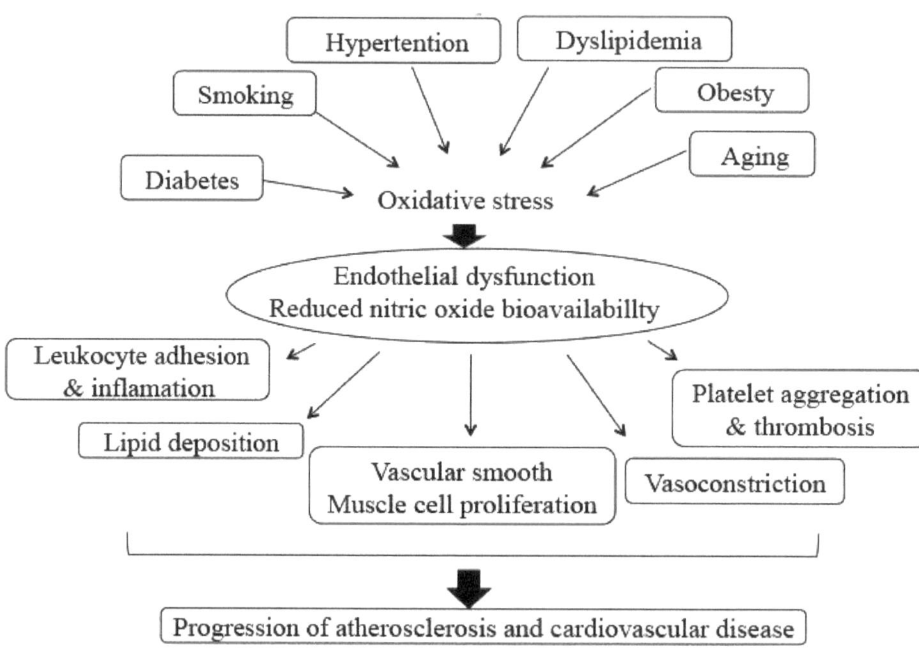

Fig. (3). Risk factors for atherosclerosis and cardiovascular disease caused by oxidative stress and endothelial dysfunction. Adapted from reference [35].

Early endothelial dysfunction is a critical point of intervention for the prevention of atherosclerosis and cardiovascular disease. This dysfunction could be an initial reversible step in the process of atherosclerosis.

ROS production occurs as a part of cellular metabolic processes, and antioxidant enzymes such as superoxide dismutase, glutathione reductase (GSR), glutathione peroxidase, and catalase protect the cell from ROS damage [40]. ROS bind to and oxidize DNA, lipid, and proteins, and cause pathological changes. These ROS-mediated effects have been implicated in the development of NCDs such as diabetes and CVDs [41, 42]. Recently, the inhibitory effect of curcumin on several enzymes associated with the ROS metabolic pathway has been implicated in its efficacy in blocking tumor cell proliferation [43]. In addition, in cervical cancer-derived cell lines, apigenin has been shown to induce apoptosis by enhanced mitochondrial redox impairment coupled with induction of ROS levels, and has also been shown to inhibit migration and invasion of cancer cells [44].

Furthermore, resveratrol enhances Nrf2 and superoxide dismutase (SOD) expression, and decreases intracellular superoxide anion in peripheral blood mononuclear cells (PBMCs) [45]. Oxidative stress plays an important role in T2DMM development. These results indicate that resveratrol has an antioxidant effect in the blood and in the PBMCs of patients with T2DMM. In addition, polyphenols in berries inhibited experimental nonalcoholic steatohepatitis by preventing lipid peroxidation and proinflammatory cytokines [46]. Therefore, polyphenolic antioxidation may inhibit several NCDs [47].

2.3. Protective Action of Polyphenols Against Inflammation

Inflammation is caused by the response of the immune system to infection. Inflammation causes many physiological and pathologic states, and affects numerous changes to signaling pathways connected to the expression of inflammatory markers, lipid peroxidation, and free radical generation [48]. Oxidative stress and oxidative tissue damage are known to be associated with chronic inflammatory and degenerative disorders [49]. For example, chronic diseases such as cancer, atherosclerosis, Alzheimer's disease, and metabolic disorders are known to involve oxidative stress [50, 51]. Many studies support the role of oxidative stress in inflammatory reactions in diabetic pathogenesis. The activation of the inflammatory transcription factor, nuclear factor (NF)-κB, induces the production of proinflammatory cytokines such as tumor necrosis factor (TNF) α and interleukin (IL)-6, and Meng *et al.* reported that inhibition of NF-κB is effective in the prevention of T2DMM [52].

In contrast, many polyphenols inhibit inflammation and are associated with a reduced risk of NCDs [53]. Resveratrol regulates glucose and lipid metabolism, and improves insulin resistance in arterial vessel walls of T2DMM rats. The protective effects of resveratrol are consistent with the reduction of NF-kappa B expression, and the reduction in interleukin (IL)-1β and IL-6 levels in the blood

[54]. Furthermore, resveratrol inhibits the expression of TNFα, intercellular adhesion molecule1 (ICAM-1), and monocyte chemotactic protein-1 (MCP-1) in the vascular wall, and effectively inhibits inflammation. In rhesus monkeys, resveratrol regulates adipose insulin signaling and prevents the inflammatory response in adipose tissue, on high-fat, high-sugar diet [55]. Anti-inflammatory effect in adipose tissues by resveratrol may improve glucose metabolism.

In a prior publication, we have demonstrated that a catechin from tea, epigallocatechin gallate (EGCG), prevents TNFα-enhanced vascular cell adhesion molecule (VCAM)-1 expression caused by inflammation, and apoptosis-induction related to microtubule-associated protein 1A/1B-light chain 3 (LC3) expression in endothelial cells [56]. In endothelial cells, changes in endoplasmic reticulum stress (ER stress)-related thioredoxin-interacting protein (TXNIP) and NOD-like receptor pyrin domain containing-3 (NLRP3) signaling, induce endothelial dysfunction [57]. This pathway induces IL-1β production and enhances inflammation and cell death. Quercetin, luteolin, and EGCG have been shown to confer protection from ER stress-associated inflammatory and apoptotic damage in endothelial cells [57].

3. BIOAVAILABILITY AND ABSORPTION OF POLYPHENOLS

Most native polyphenols occur as esters, glycosides, or as polymers in vegetables and fruits [58]. The ingested polyphenols are modified by intestinal membrane enzymes and colonic microflora before being absorbed into the body. Further, methylation, sulfation, and/or glucuronidation occur in the liver and in the small intestine [59]. As a result, the molecular composition of the polyphenols is significantly modified as they reach the systemic circulation. The methylation of polyphenols usually occurs at the C3 and C4 positions [60]. Furthermore, in the intestine and in the liver, glucuronic acid conjugation is observed mostly at the C3 position [61].

Accurate evaluation and identification of the polyphenols consumed is difficult, and therefore the estimation of the amount of polyphenols absorbed is also difficult. However, it is accepted that polyphenols are absorbed into the body from ingested food. For example, it has been reported that the glucoside derivative of polyphenols is transported into the enterocytes by the sodium-dependent glucose co-transporter 1 (SGLT1) and is hydrolyzed by beta-glucosidase within the enterocyte [25]. A previous report has indicated that oligomers larger than trimers may not be absorbed in the small intestine [62, 63], Table **4** [58].

These results indicate that the effects attributed to polyphenols may be mediated either by the polyphenols and/or by their metabolites. Thus, multiple molecules including polyphenols and their bioactive derivatives may be associated with the preventative effects on NCDs [64].

4. PROTECTIVE EFFECT OF POLYPHENOLS AGAINST NCDS - EPIDEMIOLOGIC STUDIES

Large amounts of polyphenols are present in fruits and vegetables. Polyphenols are plant products present in tea, coffee, cocoa, red wine, and herbal teas [25]. In this chapter, we describe epidemiologic studies about the protective efficacy for the polyphenolic NCDs.

Table 4. Bioavailability of polyphenols consumed alone or foods in humans.

Polyphenol	Source	Quantity of polyphenol ingested (mg)	Maximum concentration in plasma (μM)	Excretion in urine (%)
Phenolic acids				
Caffeic acid		1000		27
Flavonols				
Quercetin	Onion	68	0.74	1.39
Quercetin	Apple	98	0.30	0.44
Quercetin-4-*O*-	Pure compound	202	0.30	0.35
rhamnoglucoside	Pure compound	144	3.2	0.8
Quercetin-4-*O*-	Onion	139	1.34	0.5
glucoside				
Quercetin Quercetin	Mixed black currant and apple juice, *1000 ml/d for 7 d*	6.4		
Catechins				
Epigallocatechin gallate	Green tea infusion, *1.2 g*	88	0.33	ND
Epigallocatechin	Green tea infusion, *5 g*	82	0.67	3.6
	Green tea infusion, *6 g*			
	Green tea extract			
Epicatechin gallate	Red wine, *120 ml*	33	ND	ND
Epicatechin	Pure compound	32	0.27	6.2
Epigallocatechin gallate		105	0.13-0.31	0.45
Epigallocatechin gallate		525	5.0	
Epigallocatechin gallate		34	4.4	
Catechin		500	0.072	
Catechin			2.0	

(Table 4) cont.....

Polyphenol	Source	Quantity of polyphenol ingested (mg)	Maximum concentration in plasma (μM)	Excretion in urine (%)
Isoflavones				
Genistein	Soy milk	19	0.74	19.8
Daidzein	Soy proteins, *60 g/d for 1 month*	25	0.79	5.3
Genistein	Soy proteins, *60 g/d for 28 d*	20	0.50	9.2
Daidzein	Soy proteins, *20 g/d for 9 d*	25	0.91	2.5
Genistein		80		8.7
Daidzein		36		26
Genistein		23		
Daidzein		13		
Flavanones				
Naringin	Grapefruit juice, *120 ml*	43	<43	8.8
Naringin	Grapefruit and orange juice, *1250 ml each*	689		6.8
Hesperidin	Pure compounds	89		24.4
Naringin		500		4.9
Hesperidin		500		3.0
Anthocyanins				
Anthocyanins	Red wine, *300 ml*			1.0-6.7

Adapted from reference [62]

4.1. Cardiovascular Disease

In a cohort study conducted in women from the United Kingdom, the association between fruit intake and CVD-specific mortality was investigated [65]. In this study, total fruit consumption data from 30,458 women aged 35-69 years was acquired using a 217-item food frequency questionnaire. A high total fruit intake was associated with a lower risk of CVD and coronary heart disease mortality, with a 6-7% reduction in risk for each 80 g/day portion consumed. However, the type of fruit consumed affected the outcome, though the effect was not statistically significant. High intake of grapes and citrus fruits was associated with a decreased risk of CVD and stroke. In a study of 30 women and 26 men (average weight, 79 kg; average age, 50 years), the participants consumed 240 mL of cranberry juice or a placebo beverage twice daily. Results of the study showed that blood pressure, the levels of serum C-reactive protein, and triglycerides decreased in the cranberry juice group, compared to those in the placebo beverage group. The fasting plasma glucose was lower in the cranberry juice group than that in the placebo group. Furthermore, cranberry juice intake was reported to have reduced insulin resistance and lowered CVD risk as demonstrated by parameters such as blood pressure, C-reactive protein levels, triglyceride levels, and glucose levels [66]. In the PREDIMED study, the relationship between habitual polyphenolic intake and the incidence of CVD events was studied in 7,172 participants including 273 CVD subjects, using a 137-item questionnaire

[67]. Higher polyphenolic intake, particularly the intake of lignans, flavanols, and hydroxybenzoic acids, was associated with a decrease in CVD risk. Bilberries contain abundant quantities of polyphenols, and the association between bilberry intake and biomarkers of inflammation in participants with increased risk of CVD was studied by Karlsen *et al.* In the randomized controlled trial, the participants consumed bilberry juice (n = 31) or water (n = 31) for four weeks. Plasma quercetin and p-coumaric acid increased in the bilberry juice group. Using a monocytic cell line, the researchers also discovered that quercetin and p-coumaric acid inhibited NF-κB activation (leading to the expression of C-reactive protein, IL-6, IL-15, INF-γ and TNF-α). These results thus show that bilberry polyphenols may potentially lower inflammation [68]. Therefore, these effects of polyphenol indicate the potential to inhibit inflammation and prevent the progression of CVD.

4.2. Cancer

Mediterranean foods reduce the risk of cancer [69]. A mechanism for the cancer prevention activity of Mediterranean foods may involve the optimal balance between Omega 6 and Omega 3 fatty acids [70]. Furthermore, fruits, vegetables, olive oil, and wine, which form the cornerstones of the Mediterranean diet, contain high amounts of fiber, antioxidants, and polyphenols [69]. A recent report has indicated that the intake of nuts contributes to a decrease in the risk of colorectal, endometrial, lung, and pancreatic cancers. In the NIH-AARP diet study, 566,407 participants aged 50-71 years were followed for a median 15.5 years [71]. The study estimated the intake of peanut butter and other nuts using a questionnaire. In this previous study, 966 esophageal adenocarcinoma, 323 squamous cell carcinoma, 698 gastric cardiac gland cancers, and 732 stomach non-cardiac adenocarcinomas were incident. Compared with participants who did not consume nuts or peanut butter, the high nut consumption group had a lower risk of gastric non-cardiac adenocarcinoma. It is thought that polyphenols, fiber, vitamins, and minerals included in nuts confer protective anticancer properties from the nuts. Polyphenols may also contribute toward the anticancer activity of a variety of nuts. In addition, epidemiologic studies have revealed anticancer effects of polyphenolic EGCG against prostate cancer [72]. The study researched the association between habitual green tea and EGCG intake and prostate cancer (PCA) risk in Chinese men in Hong Kong. Habitual intake of green tea, black, oolong, and pu'er tea was evaluated by a questionnaire in 404 PCA cases and in 395 controls. Findings from this study revealed that increased EGCG intake decreased the risk of PCA.

4.3. Type 2 Diabetes Mellitus

Polyphenolic intake is also reported to be associated with a low risk of T2DMM [73]. Preliminary clinical trials indicated that resveratrol and anthocyanins had anti-diabetic effects in humans with improvement in blood glucose in T2DMM patients with insulin resistance [74]. In a study conducted in Eastern Europe, dietary polyphenol consumption and the risk of the T2DMM were studied in 5,806 participants who were non-diabetic at baseline. The participants were followed up for 2-4 years and the incidence of T2DMM was monitored. During the follow-up period, T2DMM occurred in 456 participants. In comparing extreme quartiles, polyphenolic intake was associated inversely with the risk of T2DMM. In a double-blinded, randomized, controlled, crossover study, the effect of polyphenol-rich chocolate on T2DMM was examined [75]. Ten study participants with T2DMM were asked to ingest 75 g of glucose 60 min after consuming high-polyphenol chocolate, and functional and serum biomarkers for endothelial function were assessed. The results of the study indicated that intake of polyphenols-rich chocolate may significantly improve endothelial function. The intake of polyphenol-rich chocolate reduces the endothelial dysfunction and risk of T2DMM. In addition, the study revealed that polyphenols may regulate the expression of endothelial adhesion molecules and the production of 15-F2t-isoprostane. These results indicate that intake of the chocolate containing polyphenol protects from endothelial dysfunction and oxidative stress in T2DMM. In a cohort study by Vitale *et al.* [76], the eating habits of 2,573 men and women aged 50-75 years were examined using a questionnaire. A total of 683.3±5.8 mg/day of polyphenol, obtained mainly from nonalcoholic beverages, was consumed by the participants. Additional sources of dietary polyphenols (accounting for 35% of the total polyphenol intake) included: fruits (23.0%), alcoholic beverages (14.0%), vegetables (12.4%), cereal products and tubers (4.6%), legumes (3.7%), and oils (2.1%). In this previous study, chocolate, cakes, and nuts were negligible sources of polyphenols. Flavonoids (47.5%) and phenolic acids (47.4%) were the main types of polyphenols consumed. Polyphenolic intake decreased body mass index and a differential pattern of polyphenolic intake was observed in subjects with T2DMM.

In a study by Sun *et al.*, evaluation of the effect of polyphenols on T2DMM was performed by analysis of diet-derived polyphenolic metabolites excreted in the urine of subjects [77]. Eight polyphenols such as naringenin, hesperetin, quercetin, isorhamnetin, catechin, epicatechin, caffeic acid, and ferulic acid were quantified by liquid chromatography/mass spectrometry, and the results showed that hesperetin levels in the urine were associated with T2DMM risk. In addition, naringenin and hesperetin (flavanons) and quercetin and isorhamnetin (flavonols) levels were associated with low T2DMM risk. These results indicate that intake of an as yet unidentified, specific flavonoid-containing flavanon and the flavonol components, may be associated with low T2DMM risk.

5. PROTECTIVE EFFECT OF POLYPHENOLS AGAINST OBESITY - EPIDEMIOLOGIC STUDIES

Obese or overweight individuals are at an increased risk of mortality [78], and obesity is an important risk factor for various chronic diseases [15, 79]. Previous randomized clinical trials showed that polyphenol reduces weight [80]. In addition, several reports have indicated that polyphenol-rich fruits and vegetables decrease body weight and increase energy expenditure [81 - 83]. Effects of dietary polyphenols such as EGCG, resveratrol, and curcumin have been tested in cells, animal, and human studies of obesity [15]. Weight reduction, with the use of EGCG, was reported in human participants [15]. However, in intervention clinical trials, polyphenol-rich food or polyphenolic extracts was shown not to affect weight or waist circumference [84].

In a recent cross-sectional study of 573 participants, total polyphenol levels, biomarker levels, and total urinary polyphenol excretion were evaluated in urine samples [85]. Polyphenol levels were reported to be inversely related to body weight and obesity in elderly study participants. Furthermore, it was also reported that high-polyphenol intake may be involved in decreasing the body weight of elderly participants at high CVD risk. On the other hand, consuming whole grains increased the levels of serum dihydroferulic acid and fecal ferulic acid in a study including 80 overweight/obese subjects [86]. Consumption of whole grains also reduced plasma TNF-α, enhanced plasma IL-10, and caused changes in the composition of enterobacterial communities. However, polyphenols derived from whole grains may not affect obesity and weight loss. Mielgo-Ayuso *et al.* reported that the consumption of EGCG did not improve weight-loss-induced changes in CVD risk factors in obese Caucasian women [87]. Thus, a review of existing studies showed that there is no consensus on the effect of dietary polyphenols on obesity. Though the reasons for the lack of agreement between studies are not clear, it is possible that differences in the type or quantity of dietary polyphenols may have led to the differences in outcomes.

6. MOLECULAR MECHANISMS OF ACTION OF EGCG AND RESVERATROL INVOLVED IN THE PREVENTION OF OBESITY AND NCDS

In previous section, evidence was presented to show that polyphenol intake may prevent the onset of NCDs such as obesity, CVD, cancer, and T2DMM.

Polyphenols are present in common plants such as tea, coffee, cocoa, red wine and herbal teas. EGCG [88] and resveratrol [89] are typical polyphenols, and are known to be beneficial to health. In this section, the prophylactic properties of EGCG and resveratrol in the prevention of various NCDs will be described. In animal and *in vitro.* experiments, we described a polyphenolic potential mechanism. However, direct extrapolation is not possible in humans, and the examination in humans is further necessary.

6.1. Obesity

6.1.1. EGCG

The catechin content of green tea is comparable to that of black tea and oolong tea [90]. A 2 g portion of green tea contains 500 mg of catechin. Green tea catechins commonly found are epigallocatechin gallate (EGCG, 68-69%), epigallocatechin (EGC, circa 15-18%), epicatechin gallate (ECG, 5-6%), and epicatechin (EC, 2-5%). EGCG accounts for the majority of catechin content in green tea [91].

The mechanism by which green tea prevents obesity has been analyzed in cell culture models. Such studies have shown that tea catechins may reduce body fat by inducing apoptosis of adipocytes. Catechin 3-gallate (CG), EGC, epicatechin 3-gallate, and epigallocatechin 3-gallatecatechin have been shown to inhibit intracellular lipid accumulation during the differentiation of 3T3-L1 adipocytes [92]. The inhibitory effects of CG and the EGC were stronger than that of the other catechins. Furthermore, EGCG (at 10 μM) arrested the cell cycle of mature 3T3-L1 adipocytes in the G2/M stage [93]. EGCG increased DNA fragmentation and caspase-3 activity in mature 3T3-L1 adipocytes [94]. These results indicate that EGCG induces apoptosis in adipocytes. Catechins also blocked the expression of peroxisome proliferator-activated receptor (PPAR)γ2 and CCAAT-enhancer-binding protein (C/EBP)α, suggesting that tea catechins prevent obesity through inhibition of adipocyte differentiation. Lin *et al.*, in a study of preadipocytes and adipocytes [95], using both laser scanning cytometry and dUTP nick-end labeling assays, showed that EGCG increased apoptosis of mature adipocytes. Taken together, the above evidence strongly suggests that EGCG inhibits the differentiation of preadipocytes and induces apoptosis of mature adipocytes. Furthermore, there is evidence to suggest that EGCG inhibits lipid accumulation in 3T3-L1 adipocytes [95, 96].

Peroxisome proliferator-activated receptor gamma (PPARγ) and C/EBPα play a critical role in lipogenesis and adipocyte differentiation [97]. These proteins control lipid synthesis and fatty acid oxidation by regulating the expression of acetyl-coenzyme A carboxylase (ACC) and sterol regulatory element-binding protein 1c (SREBP-1c) [97]. The effect of EGCG on adipocyte differentiation has been reported to be associated with the expression and 5' AMP-activated protein kinase (AMPK)-activation of PPARγ and C/EBPα in adipocytes [93]. Though AMPK modulation is reported to be involved in most pathways leading to anti-obesity effects, EGCG has not been reported to work through AMPK modulation; it is thought that EGCG relates its anti-obesity effects by blocking IGF-mediated mitogenesis of 3T3-L1 preadipocytes *via* the 67-kDa laminin receptor [98]. EGCG is also reported to induce 67LR/eNOS pathways and improve cardiovascular function while mediating anticancer effects (Fig **4**) [99]. Thus, the anti-obesity effects of EGCG may be achieved through multiple pathways.

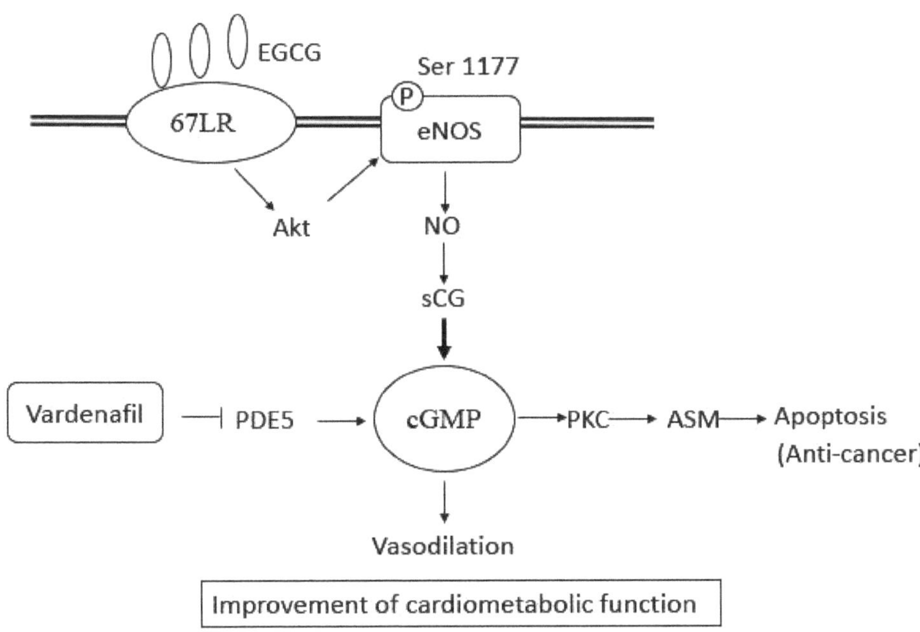

Fig. (4). Epigallocatechin gallate (EGCG)-activated endothelial nitric oxide synthase (eNOS) pathways that improve cardiovascular function and leads to anticancer effects in the presence of a phosphodiesterase 5 (PDE5) inhibitor. Adapted from reference [99].

EGCG induces an increase in cyclic guanosine monophosphate (cGMP) levels through a specific receptor (67LR) which stimulates the Akt/eNOS pathway. This pathway induces vasodilation which contributes to improvement in cardiovascular function. Inhibition of PDE5 following treatment with Vardenafil leads to elevations of cGMP levels in cancer cells. This enhanced cGMP activates protein kinase C (PKC)δ/acidic sphingomyelinase (ASM) that is associated with apoptosis.

6.1.2. Resveratrol

Resveratrol, a typical polyphenol, is found in grapes, wine, peanuts, and also in berries such as mulberries [100, 101]. It occurs as cis and trans isomers. Trans-resveratrol is present in red grape juice (3.38 mg/L) [102] and in the outer skin of the grape [103]. The unstable cis form is often converted into the trans form by ultraviolet irradiation and by fermentation [104]. Both trans and cis isomers of resveratrol are reported to have similar antioxidant and biological activities.

Several studies have shown that resveratrol inhibits the gene expression of fatty acid synthase, lipoprotein lipase (LPL), SREBP1c, and stearoyl-CoA desaturase-1 (SCD1), and reduces intracellular triglyceride accumulation in 3T3L1 adipocytes [93, 105, 106]. Furthermore, resveratrol is also reported to inhibit the differentiation of preadipocytes, reduce adipocyte proliferation, enhance adipocyte apoptosis, and regulate fatty acid β-oxidation [93, 107]. Resveratrol may effect lipogenesis and promote fatty acid β-oxidation by inducing the expression of AMPK, silent information regulator 2/sirtuin 1 (SIRT1), and peroxisome proliferator-activated receptor-γ co-activator 1α (PGC-1α) [108, 109]. At a concentration of 10-100 μM, resveratrol is reported to decrease the growth of and induce apoptosis of adipocytes [106]. At these concentrations, resveratrol is also known to inhibit the expression of fatty acid binding protein 4 (FABP4), PPARγ, and C/EBPα, and blocks preadipocyte differentiation. Treating adipocytes with an AMPK inhibitor reverses these effects of resveratrol [110]. These results indicate that resveratrol mediates anti-obesity effects through AMPK activation.

6.2. Cardiovascular Disease

Epidemiologic and clinical studies show that intake of fruit and vegetables is linked to a reduction in CVD-related mortality [111]). Polyphenols have been reported to lower CVD risk by reducing oxidative stress and activating several signaling pathways [112] (Fig. **5**).

A number of studies support the notion that a diet rich in fruits and vegetables is associated with reduced cardiovascular complications and mortality. Polyphenol-rich diets have been related to reduced CVD risks. The Fig. summarizes the possible mechanisms of action of polyphenols in reducing oxidative stress and in influencing signaling pathways to decrease CVD risk. eNOS: endothelial nitric oxide synthase; NO: nitric oxide; IL-6: interleukin-6; PPARγ: peroxisome proliferator-activated receptor gamma; HDL: high-density lipoprotein; PGC-1α: peroxisome proliferator-activated receptor-γ co-activator 1α; CYP7A1: cholesterol 7 alpha-hydroxylase; AMPK: AMP-activated protein kinase; HMGR: 3-hydroxy-3-methylglutaryl-coenzyme A reductase; LOX-1: oxidized low-density lipoprotein (LDL) receptor-1; VCAM-1: vascular cell adhesion molecule-1; ICAM-1:intercellular adhesion molecule-1; TNFα: tumor-necrotic factor alpha; SIRT-1: silent information regulator 2/sirtuin 1; ROS: reactive oxygen species.

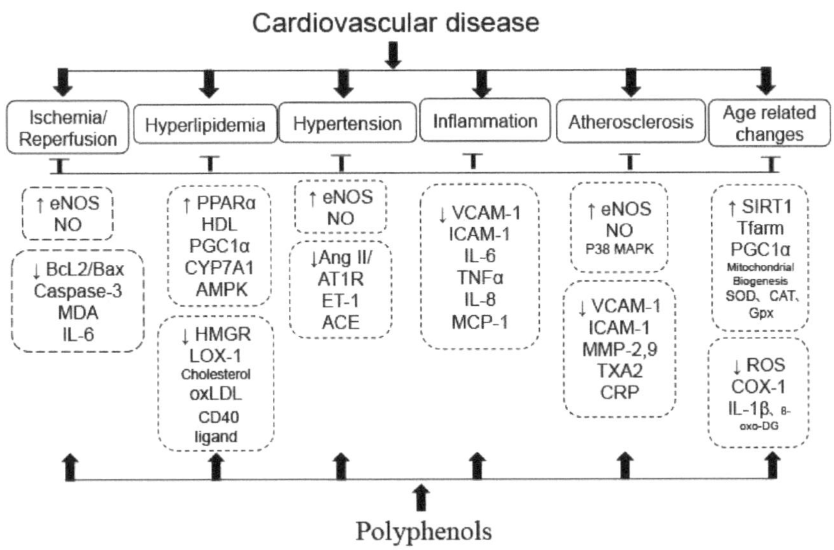

Fig. 5. Mechanisms of protection by polyphenols in cardiovascular disease. Adapted from reference [112].

6.2.1. EGCG

EGCG exerts beneficial and preventive effects with reference to CVD [88]. EGCG is reported to inhibit endothelial dysfunction and prevent cardiac cell damage, cardiac hypertrophy, and hypertension. In a study using the spontaneously hypertensive rat (SHR), green tea consumption was observed to induce eNOS, improve endothelial dysfunction, and cause vasodilatation [113]. EGCG also increased gene expression of eNOS in human vascular endothelial cells [114]. The stimulation of NO production by EGCG was associated with the regulation of p38 mitogen-activated protein kinase (MAPK) phosphorylation. The activation of phosphatidyl inositol-3 kinase (PI3 kinase) and p38 MAPK by EGCG caused upregulation of Nrf2 and the activation of extracellular signal–regulated kinase (ERK)1/2 [115]. EGCG thus increased heme oxygenase-1 (HO-1) production and inhibited the expression of enhanced VCAM-1 [56, 116]. On the other hand, in a different study, high dose green tea catechins improved plasma lipid profiles in healthy women [117]. Furthermore, intake of the tea including EGCG (58%) decreased fatty plaque development in the aortas of apolipoprotein E (ApoE)-deficient mice [118]. EGCG has been reported to inhibit the activity of the rate-limiting enzyme in cholesterol synthesis, hydroxyl-3-methyl-glutaryl-CoA reductase (HMGR), thus lowering cholesterol synthesis

[119]. The secretion and synthesis of endothelin-1 (ET-1) is regulated by the transcription factor forkhead box protein O1 (FOXO1). Studies proved that EGCG regulates FOXO1 by AMPkinase and Akt-mediated phosphorylation in endothelial cells [120]. Furthermore, EGCG inhibits NADPH oxidase and oxidized LDL receptor 1 (LOX-1) expression through activation of the NFκB pathway [121]. The above evidence, taken together, shows how EGCG may effectively prevent CVD.

6.2.2. Resveratrol

Resveratrol is a stilbene compound and is synthesized in response to stressful stimuli by plants [122]. The effect of resveratrol on cardiovascular risk has been studied widely [123, 124]. Intake of resveratrol has been shown to improve lipid profiles and cholesterol levels [125, 126]. Resveratrol induces eNOS activity and increases vasodilatation in vascular endothelial cells [127, 128]. In coronary arterial walls, resveratrol increases the expression of quinone reductase 1 (NQO1) and of HO-1 by modulating the Nrf-2 pathway, and enhances glutathione synthesis [129]. Furthermore, resveratrol inhibits the production and biosynthesis of thromboxane A2 (TXA2). These activities of resveratrol inhibit platelet adhesion and platelet aggregation, and thus resveratrol exhibits anti-thrombotic and ant-atheromatous properties. In addition, the protective effect of resveratrol against CVD is thought to be caused by inhibition of cardiac structural alteration [125]. Furthermore, resveratrol inhibits heart damage, induced in ischemia/reperfusion (I/R) injury. These effects of resveratrol explain its preventative effects on CVD. Several potential effects of resveratrol have been reported for atherogenesis and impaired metabolism [124] (Fig **6**).

Resveratrol has antioxidant and anti-inflammatory properties and induces endothelial nitric oxide synthase (eNOS). The Fig. summarizes possible mechanisms involved in disease prevention by resveratrol. AMPK:AMP-activated protein kinase; ARE: antioxidant response element; eNOS: endothelial NO synthase; HMG-CoA reductase: 3-hydroxy-3-methyl-glutaryl-CoA reductase; ICAM-1:intercellular adhesion molecule-1; LDL: low density lipoprotein; MCP-1: monocyte chemotactic protein-1; NF-κB: nuclear factor-kappa B; Nox1: NADPH oxidase 1; Nrf2: nuclear factor (erythroid-derived 2)-like 2; PAI-1: plasminogen activator inhibitor-1; PGC-1α: peroxisome proliferator-activated receptor-γ co-activator 1α; ROS: reactive oxygen species; SIRT-1: silent information regulator 2/sirtuin 1; SMC: smooth muscle cells; VCAM-1: vascular cell adhesion molecule-1.

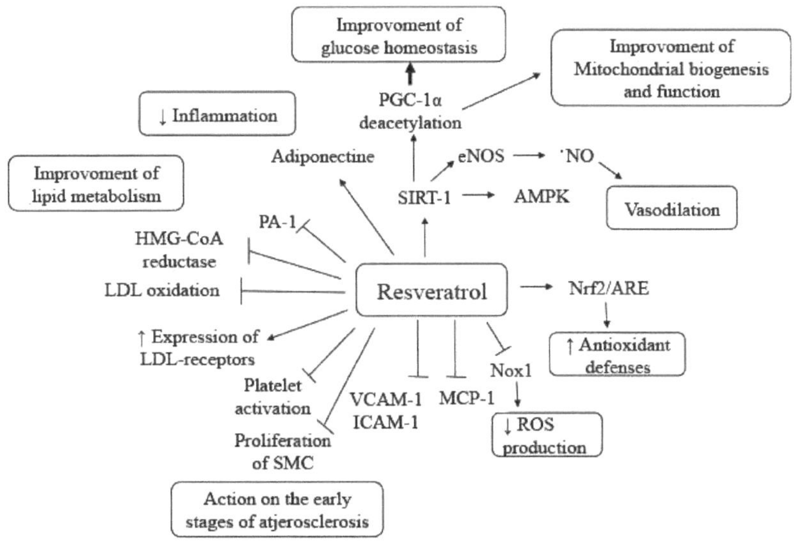

Fig. (6). Several potential effects of resveratrol on atherosclerosis and impaired. Adapted from reference [124].

6.3. Cancer

Epidemiological findings show that intake of a diet rich in vegetables reduces the risk of certain cancers [130]. One of the factors of such a diet leading to reduced cancer risks is the presence of natural polyphenols [131].

6.3.1. EGCG

Literature evidence shows that EGCG inhibits survivin, a potent anti-apoptotic protein, and increases Bax and TNF-related apoptosis-inducing ligand expression in several gastric cancer cells lines (MKN-1, MKN-28, MKN-45, NUGC-3, and TMK-1) [132], indicating that EGCG has potent apoptotic effects on cancer cells. It has also been reported that EGCG inhibits stem cell growth in colorectal cancer [133] and breast cancer [134]. EGCG is further known to inhibit estrogen-dependent breast cancer cell (MCF-7) proliferation [135], and downregulate estrogen receptor (ER)α expression in ER+/progesterone receptor (PR+) breast cancer cells [136]. Matrix metalloproteinase-2 (MMP-2) is closely related to metastatic potential in lung cancer. Deng *et al.* showed that EGCG inhibits invasion and migration, through the inhibition of MMP-2 expression and induces G2/M arrest *via* c-Jun N-terminal kinase (JNK) signaling in lung cancer cells [137]. The anticancer activity of EGCG involves the regulation of signal transduction in various cancer types. For example, EGCG regulates Akt, ERK1/2 and p38MAPK pathway in colon cancer [138], and the β-catenin pathway in human gastric cancer cells (AZ521) [139], to mediate anti-proliferative effects. Thus, EGCG may inhibit multiple cancer cells by modulating various pathways.

6.3.2. Resveratrol

Resveratrol is mainly found in red wine, grapes, and in berries [122]. Wang *et al.* showed that resveratrol inhibited invasion and metastasis in the human lung cancer cell line A549 [140]. In addition, resveratrol also inhibited the growth of gastric cancer cells and augmented cells senescence. In glioma cells, resveratrol prevented temozolomide-enhanced G2 inhibition leading to mitotic catastrophe, and reinforced temozolomide-induced senescence [141]. In a nude mouse xenograft model, resveratrol inhibited the proliferation of gastric cancer cells [142]. In addition, it has been reported that resveratrol augmented ROS production and induced DNA lesions and apoptosis in human gastric adenocarcinoma cells [143]. In lymphoma cell lines, resveratrol has been reported to inhibit the activation of Akt, lower ROS production, and enhance apoptosis [144]. Similarly, resveratrol has also been reported to induce apoptosis in colorectal cancer. It is thought that resveratrol upregulates ROS production, promotes autophagy, and induces caspase-dependent apoptosis in colorectal and gastric cancer cells. ROS production due to resveratrol is also known to cause DNA lesions in cancer cells [145]. There is also evidence to suggest that the anticancer activity of resveratrol may be associated with the modulation of topoisomerase II [146]. In contrast, in drug-resistant colorectal cancer cells, resveratrol inhibited the expression of multi-drug resistance protein 1 (MDR1) and decreased drug efflux [147]. Aires *et al.* reported that upon administration of oral resveratrol in colorectal cancer patients, high concentrations of conjugated resveratrol compounds such as RSV-3-O-sulfate were detected in the large intestine [148]. It is thus possible that these resveratrol conjugated compounds may be associated with the anticancer activity of resveratrol [148].

6.4. Type 2 Diabetes Mellitus

6.4.1. EGCG

Several studies have demonstrated the anti-diabetic effects of EGCG in animal and culture cell models [149, 150]. For example, EGCG is reported to inhibit glucose-induced cytotoxicity, and to improve viability and insulin secretory function in rat pancreatic β-cell line [151, 152]. These effects of EGCG have been shown to be mediated *via* the expression of insulin receptor substrate (IRS), Akt, and FoxO1 [152]. In addition, EGCG is known to improve mitochondrial function. IRS1 functions as an important signal for mediating insulin effects and regulates the survival and growth of the β-cell [153]. Akt is necessary for the activation of IRS, and FOXO1 phosphorylation by Akt ameliorates glucolipotoxicity. FOXO1 induces the expression of neurogenic differentiation factor and Maf A and regulates apoptotic inhibition and cell proliferation in β-cells [154, 155]. EGCG improves the function of the β-cell by modulating this insulin signaling cascade at various levels. Furthermore, EGCG inhibits cytokine-induced apoptosis through Bcl-2 and Bax expression in the β-cell [156]. EGCG inhibits free fatty acid (FFA)-induced insulin resistance in the C2C12 mouse myoblast cell through multiple signaling pathways. EGCG inhibits IRS1 serine phosphorylation, PKC potentiation, and the potentiation of the AMPK cascade. In addition, EGCG activates kinases (such as activated AMPK, ERK1/2, and p38 MAPK), stimulates glucose uptake [157, 158], and inhibits lipid accumulation through the AMPK/ACC signaling pathway [159]. ER stress is associated with insulin resistance and the dysfunction of the β-cell in dB/dB mice and in T2DMM subjects [160]. EGCG has also been shown to reduce the expression of the ER stress marker DNA-damage inducible transcript 3 (Ddit3) in dB/dB mice, preventing islet dysfunction. The mitochondrial fatty acid transporter L-Cpt-1 of the β-cell is associated with insulin secretion [160], and EGCG has been reported to decrease L-Cpt-1 expression and improve insulin secretion by the β-cell. Reports show that EGCG significantly reduces the expression of Beclin1 and dynamin-related protein 1 (DRP1) that participate in the autophagy pathway within the skeletal muscle [161]. EGCG is also reported to inhibit excessive mitochondrial autophagy and muscle autophagy by inhibiting the ROS/ERK/JNK-p53 pathway [161]. The above mentioned activities of EGCG contribute to the anti-diabetic effects of EGCG, and offer possible explanations for its efficacy in improving insulin secretion, glucose uptake, insulin resistance, glucose tolerance, and oxidative stress. EGCG thus seems to exert protective effects against diabetes through multiple signaling pathways.

6.4.2. Resveratrol

Resveratrol prevents diabetes and exerts anti-hyperglycemic effects, which are reported to be associated with glucose transport into the cell. A previous report has shown that resveratrol stimulates glucose uptake in streptozotocin-induced diabetic rats [162, 163], by stimulating increased localization of glucose transporters on the cytoplasmic membrane. In a streptozotocin-induced diabetes rat model, resveratrol intake increased the expression of glucose transporter 4 (GLUT4) [164, 165]. Resveratrol has been reported to mediate anti-diabetic effects by improving mitochondrial function and energy expenditure *via* modulation of Sirtuin1 [166, 167]. In addition, resveratrol increased the level of adiponectin, which inhibits inflammatory changes, leading to amelioration of insulin resistance in adipocytes [168]. FOXO1 and AMPK signaling pathway have been reported to be associated with resveratrol-induced production of adiponectin [169]. Similarly, resveratrol is reported to augment the expression of

FOXO1 and adiponectin in human visceral fat cells [170]. PPARγ is known to regulate adiponectin secretion. Resveratrol is reported to increase PPARγ activity and contribute to the increased expression of adiponectin, leading to anti-diabetic effects within the fat cell [171]. In addition, resveratrol enhances PPAR mediated uncoupling protein (UCP-) 1, 2, and 3 expressions in visceral white adipose [172]. Furthermore, a double-blind randomized clinical trial indicated that the green tea polyphenols consumption reduces albuminuria in diabetic patients [173]. These reports indicate that resveratrol contributes to diabetes prevention by modulating glucose uptake.

CONCLUSION

An abundance of epidemiological and *in vitro.* evidence supports the anti-NCD effects of several dietary polyphenols. The intake of vegetables and fruits enhances an internal polyphenolic level, and may be involved in health. Dietary polyphenols exert their anti-NCD effects by targeting various cellular signaling pathways. This review focused on the possible utility of several polyphenols in the prevention of NCDs such as obesity, CVD, T2DMM, and cancer. The possible signaling pathways involved in the effects of flavonoids on NCDs have also been discussed. Polyphenols exert their effects by antioxidant activity, and by influencing functional aspects such as energy metabolism and insulin sensitivity in peripheral tissues. Carefully designed human trials are required to further evaluate the potential of dietary polyphenols in preventing or treating NCDs. Consumption of polyphenol-rich foods such as vegetables and fruits are important for the prevention of NCDs. Future investigations will likely uncover novel mechanisms by which dietary polyphenols exert protective effects.

ABBREVIATIONS

AMPK	AMP-activated protein kinase
ARE, reductase	antioxidant response element
CVD	cardiovascular diseases
eNOS	endothelial NO synthase
HMG-CoA	3-hydroxy-3-methyl-glutaryl-CoA reductase
ICAM-1	intercellular adhesion molecule-1
LDL	low density lipoprotein
MCP-1	monocyte chemotactic protein-1
NCDs	Non-communicable diseases
NO	nitric oxide
NADPH	nicotinamide adenine dinucleotide phosphate

NF-κB	nuclear factor-kappa B
Nox1	NADPH oxidase 1
Nrf2	nuclear factor (erythroid-derived 2)-like 2
PAI-1	plasminogen activator inhibitor-1
PGC-1α	peroxisome proliferator-activated receptor-γ co-activator 1α
ROS	reactive oxygen species
SIRT-1	silent information regulator 2/sirtuin 1
SMC	smooth muscle cells
T2DMM	Type 2 diabetes mellitus
VCAM-1	vascular cell adhesion molecule-1

CONSENT FOR PUBLICATION

Not applicable.

CONFLICT OF INTEREST

The author confirms that this chapter contents have no conflict of interest.

ACKNOWLEDGMENTS

The authors received no specific funding for this work.

REFERENCES

[1] World Health Organization. Global Health Observatory 2011 . http://www.who.int/gho/ncd/en/index.html Accessed May, 2, 2011

[2] Alwan, A.; Maclean, D.R.; Riley, L.M.; d'Espaignet, E.T.; Mathers, C.D.; Stevens, G.A.; Bettcher, D. Monitoring and surveillance of chronic non-communicable diseases: progress and capacity in high-burden countries. *Lancet,* **2010**, *376*(9755), 1861-1868. [http://dx.doi.org/10.1016/S0140-6736(10)61853-3] [PMID: 21074258]

[3] Jaspers, L.; Colpani, V.; Chaker, L.; van der Lee, S.J.; Muka, T.; Imo, D.; Mendis, S.; Chowdhury, R.; Bramer, W.M.; Falla, A.; Pazoki, R.; Franco, O.H. The global impact of non-communicable diseases on households and impoverishment: a systematic review. *Eur. J. Epidemiol.,* **2015**, *30*(3), 163-188. [http://dx.doi.org/10.1007/s10654-014-9983-3] [PMID: 25527371]

[4] Tilman, D.; Clark, M. Global diets link environmental sustainability and human health. *Nature,* **2014**, *515*(7528), 518-522. [http://dx.doi.org/10.1038/nature13959] [PMID: 25383533]

[5] Singh, P.N.; Arthur, K.N.; Orlich, M.J.; James, W.; Purty, A.; Job, J.S.; Rajaram, S.; Sabaté, J. Global epidemiology of obesity, vegetarian dietary patterns, and noncommunicable disease in Asian Indians. *Am. J. Clin. Nutr.,* **2014**, *100* Suppl. 1, 359S-364S. [http://dx.doi.org/10.3945/ajcn.113.071571] [PMID: 24847857]

[6] Fuster, J.J.; Ouchi, N.; Gokce, N.; Walsh, K. Obesity-induced changes in adipose tissue microenvironment and their impact on cardiovascular disease. *Circ. Res.,* **2016**, *118*(11), 1786-1807. [http://dx.doi.org/10.1161/CIRCRESAHA.115.306885] [PMID: 27230642]

[7] Tsai, A.G.; Williamson, D.F.; Glick, H.A. Direct medical cost of overweight and obesity in the USA: a quantitative systematic review. *Obes. Rev.,* **2011**, *12*(1), 50-61.
[http://dx.doi.org/10.1111/j.1467-789X.2009.00708.x] [PMID: 20059703]

[8] Lavie, C.J.; Milani, R.V.; Ventura, H.O. Obesity and cardiovascular disease:risk factor, paradox, and impact of weight loss *J. Am. Coll. Cardiol,* **2009**, *53*(21), 1925-1932.

[9] Li, D. Effect of the vegetarian diet on non-communicable diseases. *J. Sci. Food Agric.,* **2014**, *94*(2), 169-173.
[http://dx.doi.org/10.1002/jsfa.6362] [PMID: 23965907]

[10] Martínez-González, M.A.; Salas-Salvadó, J.; Estruch, R.; Corella, D.; Fitó, M.; Ros, E. PREDIMED INVESTIGATORS. Benefits of the mediterranean diet: insights from the PREDIMED study. *Prog. Cardiovasc. Dis.,* **2015**, *58*(1), 50-60.
[http://dx.doi.org/10.1016/j.pcad.2015.04.003] [PMID: 25940230]

[11] Martinez-Lacoba, R.; Pardo-Garcia, I.; Amo-Saus, E.; Escribano-Sotos, F. Mediterranean diet and health outcomes: a systematic meta-review. *Eur. J. Public Health,* **2018**, *28*(5), 955-961.
[http://dx.doi.org/10.1093/eurpub/cky113] [PMID: 29992229]

[12] Caretto, A.; Lagattolla, V. Non-communicable diseases and adherence to Mediterranean diet. *Endocr. Metab. Immune Disord. Drug Targets,* **2015**, *15*(1), 10-17.
[http://dx.doi.org/10.2174/1871530314666141027095140] [PMID: 25612762]

[13] Sofi, F.; Cesari, F.; Abbate, R.; Gensini, G.F.; Casini, A. Adherence to Mediterranean diet and health status: meta-analysis. (), -.*BMJ,* **2008**, *337* a1344.
[http://dx.doi.org/10.1136/bmj.a1344] [PMID: 18786971]

[14] Tangney, C.C.; Rasmussen, H.E. Polyphenols, inflammation, and cardiovascular disease. *Curr. Atheroscler. Rep,* **2013**, *15*(5), 324.
[http://dx.doi.org/10.1007/s11883-013-0324-x]

[15] Wang, S.; Moustaid-Moussa, N.; Chen, L.; Mo, H.; Shastri, A.; Su, R.; Bapat, P.; Kwun, I.; Shen, C.L. Novel insights of dietary polyphenols and obesity. *J. Nutr. Biochem.,* **2014**, *25*(1), 1-18.
[http://dx.doi.org/10.1016/j.jnutbio.2013.09.001] [PMID: 24314860]

[16] Xiao, J.B.; Högger, P. Dietary polyphenols and type 2 diabetes: current insights and future perspectives. *Curr. Med. Chem.,* **2015**, *22*(1), 23-38.
[http://dx.doi.org/10.2174/0929867321666140706130807] [PMID: 25005188]

[17] Matsukawa, T.; Inaguma, T.; Han, J.; Villareal, M.O.; Isoda, H. Cyanidin-3-glucoside derived from black soybeans ameliorate type 2 diabetes through the induction of differentiation of preadipocytes into smaller and insulin-sensitive adipocytes. *J. Nutr. Biochem.,* **2015**, *26*(8), 860-867.
[http://dx.doi.org/10.1016/j.jnutbio.2015.03.006] [PMID: 25940979]

[18] Guo, X.; Yang, B.; Tan, J.; Jiang, J.; Li, D. Associations of dietary intakes of anthocyanins and berry fruits with risk of type 2 diabetes mellitus: a systematic review and meta-analysis of prospective cohort studies. *Eur. J. Clin. Nutr.,* **2016**, *70*(12), 1360-1367.
[http://dx.doi.org/10.1038/ejcn.2016.142] [PMID: 27530472]

[19] Zhou, Y.; Zheng, J.; Li, Y.; Xu, D.P.; Li, S.; Chen, Y.M.; Li, H.B. Natural polyphenols for prevention and treatment of cancer. *Nutrients,* **2016**, *8*(8)E515
[http://dx.doi.org/10.3390/nu8080515] [PMID: 27556486]

[20] Sur, S.; Pal, D.; Mandal, S.; Roy, A.; Panda, C.K. Tea polyphenols epigallocatechin gallete and theaflavin restrict mouse liver carcinogenesis through modulation of self-renewal Wnt and hedgehog pathways. *J. Nutr. Biochem.,* **2016**, *27*, 32-42.
[http://dx.doi.org/10.1016/j.jnutbio.2015.08.016] [PMID: 26386739]

[21] Nemec, M.J.; Kim, H.; Marciante, A.B.; Barnes, R.C.; Hendrick, E.D.; Bisson, W.H.; Talcott, S.T.; Mertens-Talcott, S.U. Polyphenolics from mango (Mangifera indica L.) suppress breast cancer ductal carcinoma in situ proliferation through activation of AMPK pathway and suppression of mTOR in

athymic nude mice. *J. Nutr. Biochem.,* **2017**, *41*, 12-19.
[http://dx.doi.org/10.1016/j.jnutbio.2016.11.005] [PMID: 27951515]

[22] Pandey, K.B.; Rizvi, S. Plant polyphenols as dietary antioxidants in human health and disease. *Oxid. Med. Cell Longev,* **2009**, *2*(5), 270-278.
[http://dx.doi.org/10.4161/oxim.2.5.9498]

[23] Graf, B.A.; Milbury, P.E.; Blumberg, J.B. Flavonols, flavones, flavanones, and human health: epidemiological evidence. *J. Med. Food,* **2005**, *8*(3), 281-290.
[http://dx.doi.org/10.1089/jmf.2005.8.281] [PMID: 16176136]

[24] Arts, I.C.; Hollman, P.C. Polyphenols and disease risk in epidemiologic studies. *Am. J. Clin. Nutr.,* **2005**, *81*(1) Suppl., 317S-325S.
[http://dx.doi.org/10.1093/ajcn/81.1.317S] [PMID: 15640497]

[25] Manach, C.; Scalbert, A.; Morand, C.; Remesy, C.; Jimenez, L. Polyphenols:food sources and bioavailability. *Am. J. Clin. Nutr,* **2004**, *79*(5), 727-747.

[26] Prasad, K.; Dhar, A. Flaxseed and Diabetes. *Curr. Pharm. Des.,* **2016**, *22*(2), 141-144.
[http://dx.doi.org/10.2174/1381612822666151112151230] [PMID: 26561065]

[27] Freise, C.; Querfeld, U. The lignan (+)-episesamin interferes with TNF-α-induced activation of VSMC *via* diminished activation of NF-κB, ERK1/2 and AKT and decreased activity of gelatinases. *Acta Physiol. (Oxf.),* **2015**, *213*(3), 642-652.
[http://dx.doi.org/10.1111/apha.12400] [PMID: 25267105]

[28] Grosso, G.; Godos, J.; Lamuela-Raventos, R.; Ray, S.; Micek, A.; Pajak, A.; Sciacca, S.; D'Orazio, N.; Del Rio, D.; Galvano, F. A comprehensive meta-analysis on dietary flavonoid and lignan intake and cancer risk: Level of evidence and limitations. *Mol. Nutr. Food Res.,* **2017a**, *61*(4)
[http://dx.doi.org/10.1002/mnfr.201600930] [PMID: 27943649]

[29] Berlett, B.S.; Stadtman, E.R. Protein oxidation in aging, disease, and oxidative stress. *J. Biol. Chem.,* **1997**, *272*(33), 20313-20316.
[http://dx.doi.org/10.1074/jbc.272.33.20313] [PMID: 9252331]

[30] Santilli, F.; D'Ardes, D.; Davì, G. Oxidative stress in chronic vascular disease: From prediction to prevention. *Vascul. Pharmacol.,* **2015**, *74*, 23-37.
[http://dx.doi.org/10.1016/j.vph.2015.09.003] [PMID: 26363473]

[31] Valenzuela, R.; Das, U.N.; Videla, L.A.; Llorente, C.G. Nutrients and diet: a relationship between oxidative stress, aging, obesity, and related noncommunicable diseases. *Oxid. Med. Cell. Longev.,* **2018**, *2018*7460453
[http://dx.doi.org/10.1155/2018/7460453] [PMID: 30116490]

[32] Sugamura, K.; Keaney, J.F., Jr Reactive oxygen species in cardiovascular disease. *Free Radic. Biol. Med.,* **2011**, *51*(5), 978-992.
[http://dx.doi.org/10.1016/j.freeradbiomed.2011.05.004] [PMID: 21627987]

[33] Raedschelders, K.; Ansley, D.M.; Chen, D.D.Y. The cellular and molecular origin of reactive oxygen species generation during myocardial ischemia and reperfusion. *Pharmacol. Ther.,* **2012**, *133*(2), 230-255.
[http://dx.doi.org/10.1016/j.pharmthera.2011.11.004] [PMID: 22138603]

[34] Hyderali, B.N.; Mala, K. Oxidative stress and cardiovascular complications in polycystic ovarian syndrome. *Eur. J. Obstet. Gynecol. Reprod. Biol.,* **2015**, *191*, 15-22.
[http://dx.doi.org/10.1016/j.ejogrb.2015.05.005] [PMID: 26066290]

[35] Park, K.H.; Park, W.J. Endothelial dysfunction: clinical implications in cardiovascular disease and therapeutic approaches *J. Korean Med. Sci, 30*(9), 1213-1225.**2015**,

[36] Cai, H.; Harrison, D.G. Endothelial dysfunction in cardiovascular diseases: the role of oxidant stress. *Circ. Res.,* **2000**, *87*(10), 840-844.
[http://dx.doi.org/10.1161/01.RES.87.10.840] [PMID: 11073878]

[37] Paravicini, T.M.; Touyz, R.M. NADPH oxidases, reactive oxygen species, and hypertension: clinical implications and therapeutic possibilities. *Diabetes Care,* **2008**, *31* Suppl. 2, S170-S180. [http://dx.doi.org/10.2337/dc08-s247] [PMID: 18227481]

[38] Qin, W.; Ren, B.; Wang, S.; Liang, S.; He, B.; Shi, X.; Wang, L.; Liang, J.; Wu, F. Apigenin and naringenin ameliorate PKCβII-associated endothelial dysfunction *via* regulating ROS/caspase-3 and NO pathway in endothelial cells exposed to high glucose. *Vascul. Pharmacol.,* **2016**, *85*, 39-49. [http://dx.doi.org/10.1016/j.vph.2016.07.006] [PMID: 27473516]

[39] Sthijns, M.M.J.P.E.; Schiffers, P.M.; Janssen, G.M.; Lemmens, K.J.A.; Ides, B.; Vangrieken, P.; Bouwman, F.G.; Mariman, E.C.; Pader, I.; Arner, E.S.J.; Johansson, K.; Bast, A. Haenen. G.R.M.M. Rutin protects against H2O2-triggered impaired relaxation of placental arterioles and induces Nrf2-mediated adaptation in human umbilical vein endothelial cells exposed to oxidative stress. *Biochim. Biophys. Acta,* **2017**, *1861* 5 Pt A, 1177-1189. [http://dx.doi.org/10.1016/j.bbagen.2017.03.004]

[40] Urso, M.L.; Clarkson, P.M. Oxidative stress, exercise, and antioxidant supplementation. *Toxicology,* **2003**, *189*(1-2), 41-54. [http://dx.doi.org/10.1016/S0300-483X(03)00151-3] [PMID: 12821281]

[41] Selvaraju, V.; Joshi, M.; Suresh, S.; Sanchez, J.A.; Maulik, N.; Maulik, G. Diabetes, oxidative stress, molecular mechanism, and cardiovascular disease--an overview. *Toxicol. Mech. Methods,* **2012**, *22*(5), 330-335. [http://dx.doi.org/10.3109/15376516.2012.666648] [PMID: 22394340]

[42] Venkataraman, K.; Khurana, S.; Tai, T.C. Oxidative stress in aging--matters of the heart and mind. *Int. J. Mol. Sci.,* **2013**, *14*(9), 17897-17925. [http://dx.doi.org/10.3390/ijms140917897] [PMID: 24002027]

[43] Larasati, Y.A.; Yoneda-Kato, N.; Nakamae, I.; Yokoyama, T.; Meiyanto, E.; Kato, J.Y. Curcumin targets multiple enzymes involved in the ROS metabolic pathway to suppress tumor cell growth. *Sci. Rep.,* **2018**, *8*(1), 2039. [http://dx.doi.org/10.1038/s41598-018-20179-6] [PMID: 29391517]

[44] Souza, R.P.; Bonfim-Mendonca, P.S.; Gimenes, F.; Ratti, B.A.; Kaplum, V.; Bruschi, M.L.; Souza, R.P.; Bonfim-Mendonça, P.S.; Gimenes, F.; Ratti, B.A.; Kaplum, V.; Bruschi, M.L.; Nakamura, C.V.; Silva, S.O.; Maria-Engler, S.S.; Consolaro, M.E. Oxidative stress triggered by apigenin induces apoptosis in a comprehensive panel of human cervical cancer-derived cell lines. *Oxid. Med. Cell. Longev.,* **2017**, *2017*1512745 [http://dx.doi.org/10.1155/2017/1512745] [PMID: 28191273]

[45] Seyyedebrahimi, S.; Khodabandehloo, H.; Nasli Esfahani, E.; Meshkani, R. The effects of resveratrol on markers of oxidative stress in patients with type 2 diabetes: a randomized, double-blind, placebo-controlled clinical trial. *Acta Diabetol.,* **2018**, *55*(4), 341-353. [http://dx.doi.org/10.1007/s00592-017-1098-3] [PMID: 29357033]

[46] Wu, S.; Yano, S.; Hisanaga, A.; He, X.; He, J.; Sakao, K.; Hou, D.X. Polyphenols from Lonicera caerulea L. berry attenuate experimental nonalcoholic steatohepatitis by inhibiting proinflammatory cytokines productions and lipid peroxidation. *Mol. Nutr. Food Res.,* **2017**, *61*(4) [http://dx.doi.org/10.1002/mnfr.201770044] [PMID: 27935258]

[47] Miranda, A.R.; Albrecht, C.; Cortez, M.V.; Soria, E.A. Pharmacology and toxicology of polyphenols with potential ss neurotropic agents in non-communicable diseases. *Curr. Drug Targets,* **2018**, *19*(2), 97-110. [http://dx.doi.org/10.2174/1389450117666161220152336] [PMID: 28000547]

[48] Haase, G.M.; Prasad, K.N. Oxidative damage and inflammation biomarkers: strategy in hearing disorders. *Otol. Neurotol.,* **2016**, *37*(8), e303-e308. [http://dx.doi.org/10.1097/MAO.0000000000001072] [PMID: 27518139]

[49] López-López, A.L.; Jaime, H.B.; Escobar Villanueva, M.D.C.; Padilla, M.B.; Palacios, G.V.; Aguilar,

F.J.A. Chronic unpredictable mild stress generates oxidative stress and systemic inflammation in rats. *Physiol. Behav.*, **2016**, *161*, 15-23.
[http://dx.doi.org/10.1016/j.physbeh.2016.03.017] [PMID: 27063246]

[50] Bonomini, F.; Rodella, L.F.; Rezzani, R. Metabolic syndrome, aging and involvement of oxidative stress. *Aging Dis.*, **2015**, *6*(2), 109-120.
[http://dx.doi.org/10.14336/AD.2014.0305] [PMID: 25821639]

[51] Cheignon, C.; Tomas, M.; Bonnefont-Rousselot, D.; Faller, P.; Hureau, C.; Collin, F. Oxidative stress and the amyloid beta peptide in Alzheimer's disease. *Redox Biol.*, **2018**, *14*, 450-464.
[http://dx.doi.org/10.1016/j.redox.2017.10.014] [PMID: 29080524]

[52] Meng, B.; Li, J.; Cao, H. Antioxidant and antiinflammatory activities of curcumin on diabetes mellitus and its complications. *Curr. Pharm. Des.*, **2013**, *19*(11), 2101-2113.
[PMID: 23116316]

[53] Cases, J.; Romain, C.; Dallas, C.; Gerbi, A.; Cloarec, M. Regular consumption of Fiit-ns, a polyphenol extract from fruit and vegetables frequently consumed within the Mediterranean diet, improves metabolic ageing of obese volunteers: a randomized, double-blind, parallel trial. *Int. J. Food Sci. Nutr.*, **2015**, *66*(1), 120-125.
[http://dx.doi.org/10.3109/09637486.2014.971229] [PMID: 25358490]

[54] Zheng, X.; Zhu, S.; Chang, S.; Cao, Y.; Dong, J.; Li, J.; Long, R.; Zhou, Y. Protective effects of chronic resveratrol treatment on vascular inflammatory injury in streptozotocin-induced type 2 diabetic rats:Role of NF-kappa B signaling *Eur. J. Pharmacol*, **2013**. pii: S0014-2999(13)00793-0.

[55] Jimenez-Gomez, Y.; Mattison, J.A.; Pearson, K.J.; Martin-Montalvo, A.; Palacios, H.H.; Sossong, A.M.; Ward, T.M.; Younts, C.M.; Lewis, K.; Allard, J.S.; Longo, D.L.; Belman, J.P.; Malagon, M.M.; Navas, P.; Sanghvi, M.; Moaddel, R.; Tilmont, E.M.; Herbert, R.L.; Morrell, C.H.; Egan, J.M.; Baur, J.A.; Ferrucci, L.; Bogan, J.S.; Bernier, M.; de Cabo, R. Resveratrol improves adipose insulin signaling and reduces the inflammatory response in adipose tissue of rhesus monkeys on high-fat, high-sugar diet. *Cell Metab.*, **2013**, *18*(4), 533-545.
[http://dx.doi.org/10.1016/j.cmet.2013.09.004] [PMID: 24093677]

[56] Yamagata, K.; Xie, Y.; Suzuki, S.; Tagami, M. Epigallocatechin-3-gallate inhibits VCAM-1 expression and apoptosis induction associated with LC3 expressions in TNFα-stimulated human endothelial cells. *Phytomedicine,* **2015**, *22*(4), 431-437.
[http://dx.doi.org/10.1016/j.phymed.2015.01.011] [PMID: 25925964]

[57] Wu, J.; Xu, X.; Li, Y.; Kou, J.; Huang, F.; Liu, B.; Liu, K. Quercetin, luteolin and epigallocatechin gallate alleviate TXNIP and NLRP3-mediated inflammation and apoptosis with regulation of AMPK in endothelial cells. *Eur. J. Pharmacol.*, **2014**, *745*, 59-68.
[http://dx.doi.org/10.1016/j.ejphar.2014.09.046] [PMID: 25446924]

[58] D'Archivio, M.; Filesi, C.; Di Benedetto, R.; Gargiulo, R.; Giovannini, C.; Masella, R. Polyphenols, dietary sources and bioavailability. *Ann. Ist. Super. Sanita,* **2007**, *43*(4), 348-361.
[PMID: 18209268]

[59] Day, A.J.; Williamson, G. Biomarkers for exposure to dietary flavonoids: a review of the current evidence for identification of quercetin glycosides in plasma. *Br. J. Nutr.*, **2001**, *86* Suppl. 1, S105-S110.
[http://dx.doi.org/10.1079/BJN2001342] [PMID: 11520427]

[60] Lee, M.J.; Maliakal, P.; Chen, L.; Meng, X.; Bondoc, F.Y.; Prabhu, S.; Lambert, G.; Mohr, S.; Yang, C.S. Pharmacokinetics of tea catechins after ingestion of green tea and (-)-epigallocatechin-3-gallate by humans: formation of different metabolites and individual variability. *Cancer Epidemiol. Biomarkers Prev.*, **2002**, *11*(10 Pt 1), 1025-1032.
[PMID: 12376503]

[61] Spencer, J.P.; Chowrimootoo, G.; Choudhury, R.; Debnam, E.S.; Srai, S.K.; Rice-Evans, C. The small intestine can both absorb and glucuronidate luminal flavonoids. *FEBS Lett.*, **1999**, *458*(2), 224-230.

[http://dx.doi.org/10.1016/S0014-5793(99)01160-6] [PMID: 10481070]

[62] Scalbert, A; Williamson, G Dietary intake and bioavailability of polyphenols. *J. Nutr,* **2000**, *130* 8S, 2073S-2085S.

[63] Scalbert, A.; Morand, C.; Manach, C.; Rémésy, C. Absorption and metabolism of polyphenols in the gut and impact on health. *Biomed. Pharmacother.,* **2002**, *56*(6), 276-282. [http://dx.doi.org/10.1016/S0753-3322(02)00205-6] [PMID: 12224598]

[64] Prasad, C.; Imrhan, V.; Juma, S.; Maziarz, M.; Prasad, A.; Tiernan, C.; Vijayagopal, P. Bioactive plant metabolites in the management of non-communicable metabolic diseases: looking at opportunities beyond the horizon. *Metabolites,* **2015**, *5*(4), 733-765. [http://dx.doi.org/10.3390/metabo5040733] [PMID: 26703752]

[65] Lai, H.T.; Threapleton, D.E.; Day, A.J.; Williamson, G.; Cade, J.E.; Burley, V.J. Fruit intake and cardiovascular disease mortality in the UK Women's Cohort Study. *Eur. J. Epidemiol.,* **2015**, *30*(9), 1035-1048. [http://dx.doi.org/10.1007/s10654-015-0050-5] [PMID: 26076918]

[66] Novotny, J.A.; Baer, D.J.; Khoo, C.; Gebauer, S.K.; Charron, C.S. Cranberry juice consumption lowers markers of cardiometabolic risk, including blood pressure and circulating C-reactive protein, triglyceride, and glucose concentrations in adults. *J. Nutr.,* **2015**, *145*(6), 1185-1193. [http://dx.doi.org/10.3945/jn.114.203190] [PMID: 25904733]

[67] Tresserra-Rimbau, A.; Rimm, E.B.; Medina-Remón, A.; Martínez-González, M.A.; de la Torre, R.; Corella, D.; Salas-Salvadó, J.; Gómez-Gracia, E.; Lapetra, J.; Arós, F.; Fiol, M.; Ros, E.; Serra-Majem, L.; Pintó, X.; Saez, G.T.; Basora, J.; Sorlí, J.V.; Martínez, J.A.; Vinyoles, E.; Ruiz-Gutiérrez, V.; Estruch, R.; Lamuela-Raventós, R.M. PREDIMED Study Investigators. Inverse association between habitual polyphenol intake and incidence of cardiovascular events in the PREDIMED study. *Nutr. Metab. Cardiovasc. Dis.,* **2014**, *24*(6), 639-647. [http://dx.doi.org/10.1016/j.numecd.2013.12.014] [PMID: 24552647]

[68] Karlsen, A.; Paur, I.; Bøhn, S.K.; Sakhi, A.K.; Borge, G.I.; Serafini, M.; Erlund, I.; Laake, P.; Tonstad, S.; Blomhoff, R. Bilberry juice modulates plasma concentration of NF-kappaB related inflammatory markers in subjects at increased risk of CVD. *Eur. J. Nutr.,* **2010**, *49*(6), 345-355. [http://dx.doi.org/10.1007/s00394-010-0092-0] [PMID: 20119859]

[69] Giacosa, A.; Barale, R.; Bavaresco, L.; Gatenby, P.; Gerbi, V.; Janssens, J.; Johnston, B.; Kas, K.; La Vecchia, C.; Mainguet, P.; Morazzoni, P.; Negri, E.; Pelucchi, C.; Pezzotti, M.; Rondanelli, M. Cancer prevention in Europe: the Mediterranean diet as a protective choice. *Eur. J. Cancer Prev.,* **2013**, *22*(1), 90-95. [http://dx.doi.org/10.1097/CEJ.0b013e328354d2d7] [PMID: 22644232]

[70] de Lorgeril, M.; Salen, P. Helping women to good health: breast cancer, omega-3/omega-6 lipids, and related lifestyle factors. *BMC Med.,* **2014**, *12*, 54. [http://dx.doi.org/10.1186/1741-7015-12-54] [PMID: 24669767]

[71] Hashemian, M.; Murphy, G.; Etemadi, A.; Dawsey, S.M.; Liao, L.M.; Abnet, C.C. Nut and peanut butter consumption and the risk of esophageal and gastric cancer subtypes. *Am. J. Clin. Nutr.,* **2017**, *106*(3), 858-864. [http://dx.doi.org/10.3945/ajcn.117.159467] [PMID: 28768652]

[72] Lee, P.M.Y.; Ng, C.F.; Liu, Z.M.; Ho, W.M.; Lee, M.K.; Wang, F.; Kan, H.D.; He, Y.H.; Ng, S.S.M.; Wong, S.Y.S.; Tse, L.A. Reduced prostate cancer risk with green tea and epigallocatechin 3-gallate intake among Hong Kong Chinese men. *Prostate Cancer Prostatic Dis.,* **2017**, *20*(3), 318-322. [http://dx.doi.org/10.1038/pcan.2017.18] [PMID: 28417981]

[73] Grosso, G.; Stepaniak, U.; Micek, A.; Kozela, M.; Stefler, D.; Bobak, M.; Pajak, A. Dietary polyphenol intake and risk of type 2 diabetes in the Polish arm of the Health, Alcohol and Psychosocial factors in Eastern Europe (HAPIEE) study. *Br. J. Nutr.,* **2017b**, *118*(1), 60-68. [http://dx.doi.org/10.1017/S0007114517001805] [PMID: 28799519]

[74] Mellor, D.D.; Madden, L.A.; Smith, K.A.; Kilpatrick, E.S.; Atkin, S.L. High-polyphenol chocolate reduces endothelial dysfunction and oxidative stress during acute transient hyperglycaemia in Type 2 diabetes: a pilot randomized controlled trial. *Diabet. Med.,* **2013**, *30*(4), 478-483. [http://dx.doi.org/10.1111/dme.12030] [PMID: 23039340]

[75] Mellor, D.D.; Madden, L.A.; Smith, K.A.; Kilpatrick, E.S.; Atkin, S.L. High-polyphenol chocolate reduces endothelial dysfunction and oxidative stress during acute transient hyperglycaemia in Type 2 diabetes: a pilot randomized controlled trial. *Diabet. Med.,* **2013**, *30*(4), 478-483. [http://dx.doi.org/10.1111/dme.12030] [PMID: 23039340]

[76] Vitale, M.; Masulli, M.; Rivellese, A.A.; Bonora, E.; Cappellini, F.; Nicolucci, A.; Squatrito, S.; Antenucci, D.; Barrea, A.; Bianchi, C.; Bianchini, F.; Fontana, L.; Fornengo, P.; Giorgino, F.; Gnasso, A.; Mannucci, E.; Mazzotti, A.; Nappo, R.; Palena, A.P.; Pata, P.; Perriello, G.; Potenziani, S.; Radin, R.; Ricci, L.; Romeo, F.; Santini, C.; Scarponi, M.; Serra, R.; Timi, A.; Turco, A.A.; Vedovato, M.; Zavaroni, D.; Grioni, S.; Riccardi, G.; Vaccaro, O. TOSCA.IT Study Group.Dietary intake and major food sources of polyphenols in people with type 2 diabetes: The TOSCA.IT Study. *Eur. J. Nutr.,* in press

[77] Sun, Q.; Wedick, N.M.; Tworoger, S.S.; Pan, A.; Townsend, M.K.; Cassidy, A.; Franke, A.A.; Rimm, E.B.; Hu, F.B.; van Dam, R.M. Urinary Excretion of select dietary polyphenol metabolites is associated with a lower risk of type 2 diabetes in proximate but not remote follow-up in a prospective investigation in 2 cohorts of US women. *J. Nutr.,* **2015**, *145*(6), 1280-1288. [http://dx.doi.org/10.3945/jn.114.208736] [PMID: 25904735]

[78] Borrell, L.N.; Samuel, L. Body mass index categories and mortality risk in US adults: the effect of overweight and obesity on advancing death. *Am. J. Public Health,* **2014**, *104*(3), 512-519. [http://dx.doi.org/10.2105/AJPH.2013.301597] [PMID: 24432921]

[79] Meydani, M.; Hasan, S.T. Dietary polyphenols and obesity. *Nutrients,* **2010**, *2*(7), 737-751. [http://dx.doi.org/10.3390/nu2070737] [PMID: 22254051]

[80] Farhat, G.; Drummond, S.; Al-Dujaili, E.A.S. Polyphenols and their role in obesity management: a systematic review of randomized clinical trials. *Phytother. Res.,* **2017**, *31*(7), 1005-1018. [http://dx.doi.org/10.1002/ptr.5830] [PMID: 28493374]

[81] Dallas, C.; Gerbi, A.; Elbez, Y.; Caillard, P.; Zamaria, N.; Cloarec, M. Clinical study to assess the efficacy and safety of a citrus polyphenolic extract of red orange, grapefruit, and orange (Sinetrol-XPur) on weight management and metabolic parameters in healthy overweight individuals. *Phytother. Res.,* **2014**, *28*(2), 212-218. [http://dx.doi.org/10.1002/ptr.4981] [PMID: 23554029]

[82] Most, J.; Goossens, G.H.; Jocken, J.W.; Blaak, E.E. Short-term supplementation with a specific combination of dietary polyphenols increases energy expenditure and alters substrate metabolism in overweight subjects. *Int. J. Obes.,* **2014**, *38*(5), 698-706. [http://dx.doi.org/10.1038/ijo.2013.231] [PMID: 24317366]

[83] Barth, S.W.; Koch, T.C.; Watzl, B.; Dietrich, H.; Will, F.; Bub, A. Moderate effects of apple juice consumption on obesity-related markers in obese men: impact of diet-gene interaction on body fat content. *Eur. J. Nutr.,* **2012**, *51*(7), 841-850. [http://dx.doi.org/10.1007/s00394-011-0264-6] [PMID: 22038464]

[84] Rangel-Huerta, O.D.; Aguilera, C.M.; Martin, M.V.; Soto, M.J.; Rico, M.C.; Vallejo, F.; Tomas-Barberan, F.; Perez-de-la-Cruz, A.J.; Gil, A.; Mesa, M.D. Normal or high polyphenol concentration in orange juice affects antioxidant activity, blood pressure, and body weight in obese or overweight adults. *J. Nutr.,* **2015**, *145*(8), 1808-1816. [http://dx.doi.org/10.3945/jn.115.213660] [PMID: 26136593]

[85] Guo, X.; Tresserra-Rimbau, A.; Estruch, R.; Martínez-González, M.A.; Medina-Remón, A.; Fitó, M.; Corella, D.; Salas-Salvadó, J.; Portillo, M.P.; Moreno, J.J.; Pi-Sunyer, X.; Lamuela-Raventós, R.M. Polyphenol levels are inversely correlated with body weight and obesity in an elderly population after

5 years of follow up (The Randomised PREDIMED Study). *Nutrients,* **2017**, *9*(5)E452 [http://dx.doi.org/10.3390/nu9050452] [PMID: 28467383]

[86] Vitaglione, P.; Mennella, I.; Ferracane, R.; Rivellese, A.A.; Giacco, R.; Ercolini, D.; Gibbons, S.M.; La Storia, A.; Gilbert, J.A.; Jonnalagadda, S.; Thielecke, F.; Gallo, M.A.; Scalfi, L.; Fogliano, V. Whole-grain wheat consumption reduces inflammation in a randomized controlled trial on overweight and obese subjects with unhealthy dietary and lifestyle behaviors: role of polyphenols bound to cereal dietary fiber. *Am. J. Clin. Nutr.,* **2015**, *101*(2), 251-261. [http://dx.doi.org/10.3945/ajcn.114.088120] [PMID: 25646321]

[87] Mielgo-Ayuso, J.; Barrenechea, L.; Alcorta, P.; Larrarte, E.; Margareto, J.; Labayen, I. Effects of dietary supplementation with epigallocatechin-3-gallate on weight loss, energy homeostasis, cardiometabolic risk factors and liver function in obese women: randomised, double-blind, placebo-controlled clinical trial. *Br. J. Nutr.,* **2014**, *111*(7), 1263-1271. [http://dx.doi.org/10.1017/S0007114513003784] [PMID: 24299662]

[88] Eng, Q.Y.; Thanikachalam, P.V.; Ramamurthy, S. Molecular understanding of Epigallocatechin gallate (EGCG) in cardiovascular and metabolic diseases. *J. Ethnopharmacol.,* **2018**, *210*, 296-310. [http://dx.doi.org/10.1016/j.jep.2017.08.035] [PMID: 28864169]

[89] Öztürk, E.; Arslan, A.K.K.; Yerer, M.B.; Bishayee, A. Resveratrol and diabetes: A critical review of clinical studies. *Biomed. Pharmacother.,* **2017**, *95*, 230-234. [http://dx.doi.org/10.1016/j.biopha.2017.08.070] [PMID: 28843911]

[90] Basu, A.; Lucas, E.A. Mechanisms and effects of green tea on cardiovascular health. *Nutr. Rev.,* **2007**, *65*(8 Pt 1), 361-375. [http://dx.doi.org/10.1111/j.1753-4887.2007.tb00314.x] [PMID: 17867370]

[91] Chen, Z.; Zhu, Q.Y.; Tsang, D.; Huang, Y. Degradation of green tea catechins in tea drinks. *J. Agric. Food Chem.,* **2001**, *49*(1), 477-482. [http://dx.doi.org/10.1021/jf000877h] [PMID: 11170614]

[92] Furuyashiki, T.; Nagayasu, H.; Aoki, Y.; Bessho, H.; Hashimoto, T.; Kanazawa, K.; Ashida, H. Tea catechin suppresses adipocyte differentiation accompanied by down-regulation of PPARgamma2 and C/EBPalpha in 3T3-L1 cells. *Biosci. Biotechnol. Biochem.,* **2004**, *68*(11), 2353-2359. [http://dx.doi.org/10.1271/bbb.68.2353] [PMID: 15564676]

[93] Chen, S.; Li, Z.; Li, W.; Shan, Z.; Zhu, W. Resveratrol inhibits cell differentiation in 3T3-L1 adipocytes *via* activation of AMPK. *Can. J. Physiol. Pharmacol.,* **2011**, *89*(11), 793-799. [PMID: 22017765]

[94] Wu, B.T.; Hung, P.F.; Chen, H.C.; Huang, R.N.; Chang, H.H.; Kao, Y.H. The apoptotic effect of green tea (-)-epigallocatechin gallate on 3T3-L1 preadipocytes depends on the Cdk2 pathway. *J. Agric. Food Chem.,* **2005**, *53*(14), 5695-5701. [http://dx.doi.org/10.1021/jf050045p] [PMID: 15998135]

[95] Lin, J.; Della-Fera, M.A.; Baile, C.A. Green tea polyphenol epigallocatechin gallate inhibits adipogenesis and induces apoptosis in 3T3-L1 adipocytes. *Obes. Res.,* **2005**, *13*(6), 982-990. [http://dx.doi.org/10.1038/oby.2005.115] [PMID: 15976140]

[96] Moon, H.S.; Chung, C.S.; Lee, H.G.; Kim, T.G.; Choi, Y.J.; Cho, C.S. Inhibitory effect of (---epigallocatechin-3-gallate on lipid accumulation of 3T3-L1 cells. *Obesity (Silver Spring),* **2007**, *15*(11), 2571-2582. [http://dx.doi.org/10.1038/oby.2007.309] [PMID: 18070748]

[97] Kim, H.; Hiraishi, A.; Tsuchiya, K.; Sakamoto, K. (-) Epigallocatechin gallate suppresses the differentiation of 3T3-L1 preadipocytes through transcription factors FoxO1 and SREBP1c. *Cytotechnology,* **2010**, *62*(3), 245-255. [http://dx.doi.org/10.1007/s10616-010-9285-x] [PMID: 20596890]

[98] Ku, H.C.; Liu, H.S.; Hung, P.F.; Chen, C.L.; Liu, H.C.; Chang, H.H.; Tsuei, Y.W.; Shih, L.J.; Lin, C.L.; Lin, C.M.; Kao, Y.H. Green tea (-)-epigallocatechin gallate inhibits IGF-I and IGF-II stimulation

of 3T3-L1 preadipocyte mitogenesis *via* the 67-kDa laminin receptor, but not AMP-activated protein kinase pathway. *Mol. Nutr. Food Res.*, **2012**, *56*(4), 580-592. [http://dx.doi.org/10.1002/mnfr.201100438] [PMID: 22495985]

[99] Kim, H.S.; Quon, M.J.; Kim, J.A. New insights into the mechanisms of polyphenols beyond antioxidant properties; lessons from the green tea polyphenol, epigallocatechin 3-gallate. *Redox Biol.*, **2014**, *2*, 187-195. [http://dx.doi.org/10.1016/j.redox.2013.12.022] [PMID: 24494192]

[100] Burns, J.; Yokota, T.; Ashihara, H.; Lean, M.E.; Crozier, A. Plant foods and herbal sources of resveratrol. *J. Agric. Food Chem.*, **2002**, *50*(11), 3337-3340. [http://dx.doi.org/10.1021/jf0112973] [PMID: 12010007]

[101] Hurst, W.J.; Glinski, J.A.; Miller, K.B.; Apgar, J.; Davey, M.H.; Stuart, D.A. Survey of the trans-resveratrol and trans-piceid content of cocoa-containing and chocolate products. *J. Agric. Food Chem.*, **2008**, *56*(18), 8374-8378. [http://dx.doi.org/10.1021/jf801297w] [PMID: 18759443]

[102] Romero-Pérez, A.I.; Ibern-Gómez, M.; Lamuela-Raventós, R.M.; de La Torre-Boronat, M.C. Piceid, the major resveratrol derivative in grape juices. *J. Agric. Food Chem.*, **1999**, *47*(4), 1533-1536. [http://dx.doi.org/10.1021/jf981024g] [PMID: 10564012]

[103] Frémont, L. Biological effects of resveratrol. *Life Sci.*, **2000**, *66*(8), 663-673. [http://dx.doi.org/10.1016/S0024-3205(99)00410-5] [PMID: 10680575]

[104] Soleas, G.J.; Diamandis, E.P.; Goldberg, D.M. Resveratrol: a molecule whose time has come? And gone? *Clin. Biochem.*, **1997**, *30*(2), 91-113. [http://dx.doi.org/10.1016/S0009-9120(96)00155-5] [PMID: 9127691]

[105] Kang, N.E.; Ha, A.W.; Kim, J.Y.; Kim, W.K. Resveratrol inhibits the protein expression of transcription factors related adipocyte differentiation and the activity of matrix metalloproteinase in mouse fibroblast 3T3-L1 preadipocytes. *Nutr. Res. Pract.*, **2012**, *6*(6), 499-504. [http://dx.doi.org/10.4162/nrp.2012.6.6.499] [PMID: 23346299]

[106] Kwon, J.Y.; Seo, S.G.; Yue, S.; Cheng, J.X.; Lee, K.W.; Kim, K.H. An inhibitory effect of resveratrol in the mitotic clonal expansion and insulin signaling pathway in the early phase of adipogenesis. *Nutr. Res.*, **2012**, *32*(8), 607-616. [http://dx.doi.org/10.1016/j.nutres.2012.06.014] [PMID: 22935344]

[107] Lasa, A.; Schweiger, M.; Kotzbeck, P.; Churruca, I.; Simón, E.; Zechner, R.; Portillo, M.P. Resveratrol regulates lipolysis *via* adipose triglyceride lipase. *J. Nutr. Biochem.*, **2012**, *23*(4), 379-384. [http://dx.doi.org/10.1016/j.jnutbio.2010.12.014] [PMID: 21543206]

[108] Pacholec, M.; Bleasdale, J.E.; Chrunyk, B.; Cunningham, D.; Flynn, D.; Garofalo, R.S.; Griffith, D.; Griffor, M.; Loulakis, P.; Pabst, B.; Qiu, X.; Stockman, B.; Thanabal, V.; Varghese, A.; Ward, J.; Withka, J.; Ahn, K. SRT1720, SRT2183, SRT1460, and resveratrol are not direct activators of SIRT1. *J. Biol. Chem.*, **2010**, *285*(11), 8340-8351. [http://dx.doi.org/10.1074/jbc.M109.088682] [PMID: 20061378]

[109] Beher, D.; Wu, J.; Cumine, S.; Kim, K.W.; Lu, S.C.; Atangan, L.; Wang, M. Resveratrol is not a direct activator of SIRT1 enzyme activity. *Chem. Biol. Drug Des.*, **2009**, *74*(6), 619-624. [http://dx.doi.org/10.1111/j.1747-0285.2009.00901.x] [PMID: 19843076]

[110] Chen, S.; Xiao, X.; Feng, X.; Li, W.; Zhou, N.; Zheng, L.; Sun, Y.; Zhang, Z.; Zhu, W. Resveratrol induces Sirt1-dependent apoptosis in 3T3-L1 preadipocytes by activating AMPK and suppressing AKT activity and survivin expression. *J. Nutr. Biochem.*, **2012**, *23*(9), 1100-1112. [http://dx.doi.org/10.1016/j.jnutbio.2011.06.003] [PMID: 22137261]

[111] Stefler, D.; Pikhart, H.; Kubinova, R.; Pajak, A.; Stepaniak, U.; Malyutina, S.; Simonova, G.; Peasey, A.; Marmot, M.G.; Bobak, M. Fruit and vegetable consumption and mortality in Eastern Europe: longitudinal results from the health, alcohol and psychosocial factors in Eastern Europe study. *Eur. J. Prev. Cardiol.*, **2016**, *23*(5), 493-501.

[http://dx.doi.org/10.1177/2047487315582320] [PMID: 25903971]

[112] Khurana, S.; Venkataraman, K.; Hollingsworth, A.; Piche, M.; Tai, T.C. Polyphenols:benefits to the cardiovascular system in health and in aging. *Nutrients,* **2013**, *5*(10), 3779-3827.

[113] Appeldoorn, M.M.; Venema, D.P.; Peters, T.H.; Koenen, M.E.; Arts, I.C.; Vincken, J.P.; Gruppen, H.; Keijer, J.; Hollman, P.C. Some phenolic compounds increase the nitric oxide level in endothelial cells *in vitro.. J. Agric. Food Chem.,* **2009**, *57*(17), 7693-7699. [http://dx.doi.org/10.1021/jf901381x] [PMID: 19722703]

[114] Appeldoorn, M.M.; Venema, D.P.; Peters, T.H.; Koenen, M.E.; Arts, I.C.; Vincken, J.P.; Gruppen, H.; Keijer, J.; Hollman, P.C. Some phenolic compounds increase the nitric oxide level in endothelial cells *in vitro.. J. Agric. Food Chem.,* **2009**, *57*(17), 7693-7699. [http://dx.doi.org/10.1021/jf901381x] [PMID: 19722703]

[115] Appeldoorn, M.M.; Venema, D.P.; Peters, T.H.; Koenen, M.E.; Arts, I.C.; Vincken, J.P.; Gruppen, H.; Keijer, J.; Hollman, P.C. Some phenolic compounds increase the nitric oxide level in endothelial cells *in vitro. J. Agric. Food Chem.,* **2009**, *57*(17), 7693-7699. [http://dx.doi.org/10.1021/jf901381x] [PMID: 19722703]

[116] Liu, P.L.; Liu, J.T.; Kuo, H.F.; Chong, I.W.; Hsieh, C.C. Epigallocatechin gallate attenuates proliferation and oxidative stress in human vascular smooth muscle cells induced by interleukin-1β *via* heme oxygenase-1. *Mediators Inflamm.,* **2014**, *2014*523684 [http://dx.doi.org/10.1155/2014/523684] [PMID: 25386047]

[117] Takechi, R.; Alfonso, H.; Hiramatsu, N.; Ishisaka, A.; Tanaka, A.; Tan, L.; Lee, A.H. Elevated plasma and urinary concentrations of green tea catechins associated with improved plasma lipid profile in healthy Japanese women. *Nutr. Res.,* **2016**, *36*(3), 220-226. [http://dx.doi.org/10.1016/j.nutres.2015.11.010] [PMID: 26923508]

[118] Miura, Y.; Chiba, T.; Tomita, I.; Koizumi, H.; Miura, S.; Umegaki, K.; Hara, Y.; Ikeda, M.; Tomita, T. Tea catechins prevent the development of atherosclerosis in apoprotein E-deficient mice. *J. Nutr.,* **2001**, *131*(1), 27-32. [http://dx.doi.org/10.1093/jn/131.1.27] [PMID: 11208934]

[119] Cuccioloni, M.; Mozzicafreddo, M.; Spina, M.; Tran, C.N.; Falconi, M.; Eleuteri, A.M.; Angeletti, M. Epigallocatechin-3-gallate potently inhibits the *in vitro* activity of hydroxy-3-methyl-glutaryl-CoA reductase. *J. Lipid Res.,* **2011**, *52*(5), 897-907. [http://dx.doi.org/10.1194/jlr.M011817] [PMID: 21357570]

[120] Reiter, C.E.; Kim, J.A.; Quon, M.J. Green tea polyphenol epigallocatechin gallate reduces endothelin-1 expression and secretion in vascular endothelial cells: roles for AMP-activated protein kinase, Akt, and FOXO1. *Endocrinology,* **2010**, *151*(1), 103-114. [http://dx.doi.org/10.1210/en.2009-0997] [PMID: 19887561]

[121] Ou, H.C.; Song, T.Y.; Yeh, Y.C.; Huang, C.Y.; Yang, S.F.; Chiu, T.H.; Tsai, K.L.; Chen, K.L.; Wu, Y.J.; Tsai, C.S.; Chang, L.Y.; Kuo, W.W.; Lee, S.D. EGCG protects against oxidized LDL-induced endothelial dysfunction by inhibiting LOX-1-mediated signaling. *J. Appl. Physiol.,* **2010**, *108*(6), 1745-1756. [http://dx.doi.org/10.1152/japplphysiol.00879.2009] [PMID: 20203069]

[122] Kuršvietienė, L.; Stanevičienė, I.; Mongirdienė, A.; Bernatonienė, J. Multiplicity of effects and health benefits of resveratrol. *Medicina (Kaunas),* **2016**, *52*(3), 148-155. [http://dx.doi.org/10.1016/j.medici.2016.03.003] [PMID: 27496184]

[123] Zordoky, B.N.; Robertson, I.M.; Dyck, J.R. Preclinical and clinical evidence for the role of resveratrol in the treatment of cardiovascular diseases. *Biochim. Biophys. Acta,* **2015**, *1852*(6), 1155-1177. [http://dx.doi.org/10.1016/j.bbadis.2014.10.016] [PMID: 25451966]

[124] Bonnefont-Rousselot, D. Resveratrol and Cardiovascular Diseases. *Nutrients,* **2016**, *8*(5)E250 [http://dx.doi.org/10.3390/nu8050250] [PMID: 27144581]

[125] Baur, J.A.; Sinclair, D.A. Therapeutic potential of resveratrol: the *in vivo* evidence. *Nat. Rev. Drug Discov.,* **2006**, *5*(6), 493-506.
[http://dx.doi.org/10.1038/nrd2060] [PMID: 16732220]

[126] Borriello, A.; Cucciolla, V.; Della Ragione, F.; Galletti, P. Dietary polyphenols: focus on resveratrol, a promising agent in the prevention of cardiovascular diseases and control of glucose homeostasis. *Nutr. Metab. Cardiovasc. Dis.,* **2010**, *20*(8), 618-625.
[http://dx.doi.org/10.1016/j.numecd.2010.07.004] [PMID: 20850033]

[127] Xia, N.; Förstermann, U.; Li, H. Resveratrol and endothelial nitric oxide. *Molecules,* **2014**, *19*(10), 16102-16121.
[http://dx.doi.org/10.3390/molecules191016102] [PMID: 25302702]

[128] Li, J.Y.; Huang, W.Q.; Tu, R.H.; Zhong, G.Q.; Luo, B.B.; He, Y. Resveratrol rescues hyperglycemia-induced endothelial dysfunction *via* activation of Akt. *Acta Pharmacol. Sin.,* **2017**, *38*(2), 182-191.
[http://dx.doi.org/10.1038/aps.2016.109] [PMID: 27941804]

[129] Ungvari, Z.; Bagi, Z.; Feher, A.; Recchia, F.A.; Sonntag, W.E.; Pearson, K.; de Cabo, R.; Csiszar, A. Resveratrol confers endothelial protection *via* activation of the antioxidant transcription factor Nrf2. *Am. J. Physiol. Heart Circ. Physiol.,* **2010**, *299*(1), H18-H24.
[http://dx.doi.org/10.1152/ajpheart.00260.2010] [PMID: 20418481]

[130] Peng, C.; Luo, W.P.; Zhang, C.X. Fruit and vegetable intake and breast cancer prognosis: a meta-analysis of prospective cohort studies. *Br. J. Nutr.,* **2017**, *117*(5), 737-749.
[http://dx.doi.org/10.1017/S0007114517000423] [PMID: 28366183]

[131] Zhou, Y.; Zheng, J.; Li, Y.; Xu, D.P.; Li, S.; Chen, Y.M.; Li, H.B. Natural polyphenols for prevention and treatment of cancer. *Nutrients,* **2016**, *8*(8)E515
[http://dx.doi.org/10.3390/nu8080515] [PMID: 27556486]

[132] Onoda, C.; Kuribayashi, K.; Nirasawa, S.; Tsuji, N.; Tanaka, M.; Kobayashi, D.; Watanabe, N. (---Epigallocatechin-3-gallate induces apoptosis in gastric cancer cell lines by down-regulating survivin expression. *Int. J. Oncol.,* **2011**, *38*(5), 1403-1408.
[PMID: 21344159]

[133] Toden, S.; Tran, H.M.; Tovar-Camargo, O.A.; Okugawa, Y.; Goel, A. Epigallocatechin-3-gallate targets cancer stem-like cells and enhances 5-fluorouracil chemosensitivity in colorectal cancer. *Oncotarget,* **2016**, *7*(13), 16158-16171.
[http://dx.doi.org/10.18632/oncotarget.7567] [PMID: 26930714]

[134] Mineva, N.D.; Paulson, K.E.; Naber, S.P.; Yee, A.S.; Sonenshein, G.E. Epigallocatechin-3-gallate inhibits stem-like inflammatory breast cancer cells. *PLoS One,* **2013**, *8*(9)e73464
[http://dx.doi.org/10.1371/journal.pone.0073464] [PMID: 24039951]

[135] Tu, S.H.; Ku, C.Y.; Ho, C.T.; Chen, C.S.; Huang, C.S.; Lee, C.H.; Chen, L.C.; Pan, M.H.; Chang, H.W.; Chang, C.H.; Chang, Y.J.; Wei, P.L.; Wu, C.H.; Ho, Y.S. Tea polyphenol (-)-epigallocatech-n-3-gallate inhibits nicotine- and estrogen-induced α9-nicotinic acetylcholine receptor upregulation in human breast cancer cells. *Mol. Nutr. Food Res.,* **2011**, *55*(3), 455-466.
[http://dx.doi.org/10.1002/mnfr.201000254] [PMID: 21370452]

[136] De Amicis, F.; Russo, A.; Avena, P.; Santoro, M.; Vivacqua, A.; Bonofiglio, D.; Mauro, L.; Aquila, S.; Tramontano, D.; Fuqua, S.A.; Andò, S. *in vitro* mechanism for downregulation of ER-α expression by epigallocatechin gallate in ER+/PR+ human breast cancer cells. *Mol. Nutr. Food Res.,* **2013**, *57*(5), 840-853.
[http://dx.doi.org/10.1002/mnfr.201200560] [PMID: 23322423]

[137] Deng, Y.T.; Lin, J.K. EGCG inhibits the invasion of highly invasive CL1-5 lung cancer cells through suppressing MMP-2 expression *via* JNK signaling and induces G2/M arrest. *J. Agric. Food Chem.,* **2011**, *59*(24), 13318-13327.
[http://dx.doi.org/10.1021/jf204149c] [PMID: 22082235]

[138] Cerezo-Guisado, M.I.; Zur, R.; Lorenzo, M.J.; Risco, A.; Martín-Serrano, M.A.; Alvarez-Barrientos, A.; Cuenda, A.; Centeno, F. Implication of Akt, ERK1/2 and alternative p38MAPK signalling pathways in human colon cancer cell apoptosis induced by green tea EGCG. *Food Chem. Toxicol.,* **2015**, *84*, 125-132.
[http://dx.doi.org/10.1016/j.fct.2015.08.017] [PMID: 26303273]

[139] Tanaka, T.; Ishii, T.; Mizuno, D.; Mori, T.; Yamaji, R.; Nakamura, Y.; Kumazawa, S.; Nakayama, T.; Akagawa, M. (-)-Epigallocatechin-3-gallate suppresses growth of AZ521 human gastric cancer cells by targeting the DEAD-box RNA helicase p68. *Free Radic. Biol. Med.,* **2011**, *50*(10), 1324-1335.
[http://dx.doi.org/10.1016/j.freeradbiomed.2011.01.024] [PMID: 21277973]

[140] Wang, H.; Zhang, H.; Tang, L.; Chen, H.; Wu, C.; Zhao, M.; Yang, Y.; Chen, X.; Liu, G. Resveratrol inhibits TGF-β1-induced epithelial-to-mesenchymal transition and suppresses lung cancer invasion and metastasis. *Toxicology,* **2013**, *303*, 139-146.
[http://dx.doi.org/10.1016/j.tox.2012.09.017] [PMID: 23146760]

[141] Filippi-Chiela, E.C.; Thomé, M.P.; Bueno e Silva, M.M.; Pelegrini, A.L.; Ledur, P.F.; Garicochea, B.; Zamin, L.L.; Lenz, G. Resveratrol abrogates the temozolomide-induced G2 arrest leading to mitotic catastrophe and reinforces the temozolomide-induced senescence in glioma cells. *BMC Cancer,* **2013**, *13*, 147.
[http://dx.doi.org/10.1186/1471-2407-13-147] [PMID: 23522185]

[142] Yang, Q.; Wang, B.; Zang, W.; Wang, X.; Liu, Z.; Li, W.; Jia, J. Resveratrol inhibits the growth of gastric cancer by inducing G1 phase arrest and senescence in a Sirt1-dependent manner. *PLoS One,* **2013**, *8*(11)e70627
[http://dx.doi.org/10.1371/journal.pone.0070627] [PMID: 24278101]

[143] Wang, Z.; Li, W.; Meng, X.; Jia, B. Resveratrol induces gastric cancer cell apoptosis *via* reactive oxygen species, but independent of sirtuin1. *Clin. Exp. Pharmacol. Physiol.,* **2012**, *39*(3), 227-232.
[http://dx.doi.org/10.1111/j.1440-1681.2011.05660.x] [PMID: 22211760]

[144] Hussain, A.R.; Uddin, S.; Bu, R.; Khan, O.S.; Ahmed, S.O.; Ahmed, M.; Al-Kuraya, K.S. Resveratrol suppresses constitutive activation of AKT *via* generation of ROS and induces apoptosis in diffuse large B cell lymphoma cell lines. *PLoS One,* **2011**, *6*(9)e24703
[http://dx.doi.org/10.1371/journal.pone.0024703] [PMID: 21931821]

[145] Colin, D.J.; Limagne, E.; Ragot, K.; Lizard, G.; Ghiringhelli, F.; Solary, É.; Chauffert, B.; Latruffe, N.; Delmas, D. The role of reactive oxygen species and subsequent DNA-damage response in the emergence of resistance towards resveratrol in colon cancer models. *Cell Death Dis.,* **2014**, *5*e1533
[http://dx.doi.org/10.1038/cddis.2014.486] [PMID: 25412311]

[146] Demoulin, B.; Hermant, M.; Castrogiovanni, C.; Staudt, C.; Dumont, P. Resveratrol induces DNA damage in colon cancer cells by poisoning topoisomerase II and activates the ATM kinase to trigger p53-dependent apoptosis. *Toxicol. in vitro,* **2015**, *29*(5), 1156-1165.
[http://dx.doi.org/10.1016/j.tiv.2015.04.015] [PMID: 25952326]

[147] Wang, Z.; Zhang, L.; Ni, Z.; Sun, J.; Gao, H.; Cheng, Z.; Xu, J.; Yin, P. Resveratrol induces AMPK-dependent MDR1 inhibition in colorectal cancer HCT116/L-OHP cells by preventing activation of NF-κB signaling and suppressing cAMP-responsive element transcriptional activity. *Tumour Biol.,* **2015**, *36*(12), 9499-9510.
[http://dx.doi.org/10.1007/s13277-015-3636-3] [PMID: 26124005]

[148] Aires, V.; Limagne, E.; Cotte, A.K.; Latruffe, N.; Ghiringhelli, F.; Delmas, D. Resveratrol metabolites inhibit human metastatic colon cancer cells progression and synergize with chemotherapeutic drugs to induce cell death. *Mol. Nutr. Food Res.,* **2013**, *57*(7), 1170-1181.
[http://dx.doi.org/10.1002/mnfr.201200766] [PMID: 23495229]

[149] Li, X.; Li, S.; Chen, M.; Wang, J.; Xie, B.; Sun, Z. (-)-Epigallocatechin-3-gallate (EGCG) inhibits starch digestion and improves glucose homeostasis through direct or indirect activation of PXR/CAR-mediated phase II metabolism in diabetic mice. *Food Funct.,* **2018**, *9*(9), 4651-4663.

[http://dx.doi.org/10.1039/C8FO01293H] [PMID: 30183039]

[150] Sampath, C.; Sang, S.; Ahmedna, M. *in vitro* and *in vivo* inhibition of aldose reductase and advanced glycation end products by phloretin, epigallocatechin 3-gallate and [6]-gingerol. *Biomed. Pharmacother.*, **2016**, *84*, 502-513. [http://dx.doi.org/10.1016/j.biopha.2016.09.073] [PMID: 27685794]

[151] Han, M.K. Epigallocatechin gallate, a constituent of green tea, suppresses cytokine-induced pancreatic beta-cell damage. *Exp. Mol. Med.*, **2003**, *35*(2), 136-139. [http://dx.doi.org/10.1038/emm.2003.19] [PMID: 12754418]

[152] Cai, E.P.; Lin, J.K. Epigallocatechin gallate (EGCG) and rutin suppress the glucotoxicity through activating IRS2 and AMPK signaling in rat pancreatic beta cells. *J. Agric. Food Chem.*, **2009**, *57*(20), 9817-9827. [http://dx.doi.org/10.1021/jf902618v] [PMID: 19803520]

[153] Withers, D.J.; Gutierrez, J.S.; Towery, H.; Burks, D.J.; Ren, J.M.; Previs, S.; Zhang, Y.; Bernal, D.; Pons, S.; Shulman, G.I.; Bonner-Weir, S.; White, M.F. Disruption of IRS-2 causes type 2 diabetes in mice. *Nature,* **1998**, *391*(6670), 900-904. [http://dx.doi.org/10.1038/36116] [PMID: 9495343]

[154] Buteau, J.; Accili, D. Regulation of pancreatic beta-cell function by the forkhead protein FoxO1. *Diabetes Obes. Metab.*, **2007**, *9* Suppl. 2, 140-146. [http://dx.doi.org/10.1111/j.1463-1326.2007.00782.x] [PMID: 17919188]

[155] Kluth, O.; Mirhashemi, F.; Scherneck, S.; Kaiser, D.; Kluge, R.; Neschen, S.; Joost, H.G.; Schürmann, A. Dissociation of lipotoxicity and glucotoxicity in a mouse model of obesity associated diabetes: role of forkhead box O1 (FOXO1) in glucose-induced beta cell failure. *Diabetologia,* **2011**, *54*(3), 605-616. [http://dx.doi.org/10.1007/s00125-010-1973-8] [PMID: 21107520]

[156] Low, I.C.; Chen, Z.X.; Pervaiz, S. Bcl-2 modulates resveratrol-induced ROS production by regulating mitochondrial respiration in tumor cells. *Antioxid. Redox Signal.*, **2010**, *13*(6), 807-819. [http://dx.doi.org/10.1089/ars.2009.3050] [PMID: 20367277]

[157] Lemieux, K.; Konrad, D.; Klip, A.; Marette, A. The AMP-activated protein kinase activator AICAR does not induce GLUT4 translocation to transverse tubules but stimulates glucose uptake and p38 mitogen-activated protein kinases alpha and beta in skeletal muscle. *FASEB J.*, **2003**, *17*(12), 1658-1665. [http://dx.doi.org/10.1096/fj.02-1125com] [PMID: 12958172]

[158] Pournourmohammadi, S.; Grimaldi, M.; Stridh, M.H.; Lavallard, V.; Waagepetersen, H.S.; Wollheim, C.B.; Maechler, P. Epigallocatechin-3-gallate (EGCG) activates AMPK through the inhibition of glutamate dehydrogenase in muscle and pancreatic ß-cells: A potential beneficial effect in the pre-diabetic state? *Int. J. Biochem. Cell Biol.*, **2017**, *88*, 220-225. [http://dx.doi.org/10.1016/j.biocel.2017.01.012] [PMID: 28137482]

[159] Deng, Y.T.; Chang, T.W.; Lee, M.S.; Lin, J.K. Suppression of free fatty acid-induced insulin resistance by phytopolyphenols in C2C12 mouse skeletal muscle cells. *J. Agric. Food Chem.*, **2012**, *60*(4), 1059-1066. [http://dx.doi.org/10.1021/jf204496f] [PMID: 22191431]

[160] Laybutt, D.R.; Preston, A.M.; Akerfeldt, M.C.; Kench, J.G.; Busch, A.K.; Biankin, A.V.; Biden, T.J. Endoplasmic reticulum stress contributes to beta cell apoptosis in type 2 diabetes. *Diabetologia,* **2007**, *50*(4), 752-763. [http://dx.doi.org/10.1007/s00125-006-0590-z] [PMID: 17268797]

[161] Yan, J.; Feng, Z.; Liu, J.; Shen, W.; Wang, Y.; Wertz, K.; Weber, P.; Long, J.; Liu, J. Enhanced autophagy plays a cardinal role in mitochondrial dysfunction in type 2 diabetic Goto-Kakizaki (GK) rats: ameliorating effects of (-)-epigallocatechin-3-gallate. *J. Nutr. Biochem.*, **2012**, *23*(7), 716-724. [http://dx.doi.org/10.1016/j.jnutbio.2011.03.014] [PMID: 21820301]

[162] Palsamy, P.; Subramanian, S. Resveratrol, a natural phytoalexin, normalizes hyperglycemia in streptozotocin-nicotinamide induced experimental diabetic rats. *Biomed. Pharmacother.*, **2008**, *62*(9), 598-605.
[http://dx.doi.org/10.1016/j.biopha.2008.06.037] [PMID: 18675532]

[163] Soufi, F.G.; Sheervalilou, R.; Vardiani, M.; Khalili, M.; Alipour, M.R. Chronic resveratrol administration has beneficial effects in experimental model of type 2 diabetic rats. *Endocr. Regul.*, **2012**, *46*(2), 83-90.
[http://dx.doi.org/10.4149/endo_2012_02_83] [PMID: 22540856]

[164] Gencoglu, H.; Tuzcu, M.; Hayirli, A.; Sahin, K. Protective effects of resveratrol against streptozotocin-induced diabetes in rats by modulation of visfatin/sirtuin-1 pathway and glucose transporters. *Int. J. Food Sci. Nutr.*, **2015**, *66*(3), 314-320.
[http://dx.doi.org/10.3109/09637486.2014.1003534] [PMID: 25666415]

[165] Tan, Z.; Zhou, L.J.; Mu, P.W.; Liu, S.P.; Chen, S.J.; Fu, X.D.; Wang, T.H. Caveolin-3 is involved in the protection of resveratrol against high-fat-diet-induced insulin resistance by promoting GLUT4 translocation to the plasma membrane in skeletal muscle of ovariectomized rats. *J. Nutr. Biochem.*, **2012**, *23*(12), 1716-1724.
[http://dx.doi.org/10.1016/j.jnutbio.2011.12.003] [PMID: 22569348]

[166] Higashida, K.; Kim, S.H.; Jung, S.R.; Asaka, M.; Holloszy, J.O.; Han, D.H. Effects of resveratrol and SIRT1 on PGC-1α activity and mitochondrial biogenesis: a reevaluation. *PLoS Biol.*, **2013**, *11*(7)e1001603
[http://dx.doi.org/10.1371/journal.pbio.1001603] [PMID: 23874150]

[167] Strycharz, J.; Rygielska, Z.; Swiderska, E.; Drzewoski, J.; Szemraj, J.; Szmigiero, L.; Sliwinska, A. SIRT1 as a Therapeutic Target in Diabetic Complications. *Curr. Med. Chem.*, **2018**, *25*(9), 1002-1035.
[http://dx.doi.org/10.2174/0929867324666171107103114] [PMID: 29110598]

[168] Lee, H.J.; Lim, Y.; Yang, S.J. Involvement of resveratrol in crosstalk between adipokine adiponectin and hepatokine fetuin-A *in vivo* and *in vitro*. *J. Nutr. Biochem.*, **2015**, *26*(11), 1254-1260.
[http://dx.doi.org/10.1016/j.jnutbio.2015.06.001] [PMID: 26282595]

[169] Wang, A.; Liu, M.; Liu, X.; Dong, L.Q.; Glickman, R.D.; Slaga, T.J.; Zhou, Z.; Liu, F. Up-regulation of adiponectin by resveratrol: the essential roles of the Akt/FOXO1 and AMP-activated protein kinase signaling pathways and DsbA-L. *J. Biol. Chem.*, **2011**, *286*(1), 60-66.
[http://dx.doi.org/10.1074/jbc.M110.188144] [PMID: 20980258]

[170] Wang, A.; Liu, M.; Liu, X.; Dong, L.Q.; Glickman, R.D.; Slaga, T.J.; Zhou, Z.; Liu, F. Up-regulation of adiponectin by resveratrol: the essential roles of the Akt/FOXO1 and AMP-activated protein kinase signaling pathways and DsbA-L. *J. Biol. Chem.*, **2011**, *286*(1), 60-66.
[http://dx.doi.org/10.1074/jbc.M110.188144] [PMID: 20980258]

[171] Kennedy, A.; Overman, A.; Lapoint, K.; Hopkins, R.; West, T.; Chuang, C.C.; Martinez, K.; Bell, D.; McIntosh, M. Conjugated linoleic acid-mediated inflammation and insulin resistance in human adipocytes are attenuated by resveratrol. *J. Lipid Res.*, **2009**, *50*(2), 225-232.
[http://dx.doi.org/10.1194/jlr.M800258-JLR200] [PMID: 18776171]

[172] Castrejón-Tellez, V.; Rodríguez-Pérez, J.M.; Pérez-Torres, I.; Pérez-Hernández, N.; Cruz-Lagunas, A.; Guarner-Lans, V.; Vargas-Alarcón, G.; Rubio-Ruiz, M.E. The effect of resveratrol and quercetin treatment on PPAR mediated uncoupling protein (UCP-) 1, 2, and 3 expression in visceral white adipose tissue from metabolic syndrome rats. *Int. J. Mol. Sci.*, **2016**, *17*(7)E1069
[http://dx.doi.org/10.3390/ijms17071069] [PMID: 27399675]

[173] Borges, C.M.; Papadimitriou, A.; Duarte, D.A.; Lopes de Faria, J.M.; Lopes de Faria, J.B. The use of green tea polyphenols for treating residual albuminuria in diabetic nephropathy: A double-blind randomised clinical trial. *Sci. Rep.*, **2016**, *6*, 28282.
[http://dx.doi.org/10.1038/srep28282] [PMID: 27320846]

CHAPTER 4

Overview of Past and Present Developments Towards Biotechnological and Molecular Approaches to Improve Taxol Production

Samavia Mubeen[1], Chun-Tao He[1], Bilal Ahmad Asad[2] and Zhong-Yi Yang[1,*]

[1] *State Key Laboratory for Biocontrol, School of Life Sciences, Sun Yat-Sen University, Xingang Xi Road 135, Guangzhou, 510275, China*

[2] *State Key Laboratory for Biology of Plant Diseases and Insect Pests, Institute of Plant Protection, Chinese Academy of Agricultural Sciences, Beijing, 100081, China*

Abstract: Taxol (paclitaxel) is one of the most used chemotherapeutic drugs, first isolated from Pacific yew tree *T. brevifolia*. It is used for several cancer treatments due to its unique mechanism of action. The demand for taxol supply was exceeded significantly due to its low accumulation in *Taxus sp.*, slow growth of the tree and high cost of extraction. Due to these reasons, considerable efforts have been carried out to explore the alternative sources, including plants other than *Taxus sp.*, total and semi-synthesis of taxol, plant cell culture technology, and endophytic fungi. The biosynthesis of taxol is a complex pathway and several genes associated with taxol biosynthesis are identified and cloned. Transcriptomic studies of the critical genes involved in taxol biosynthesis pathway provided valuable insight in gene regulation patterns about metabolite synthesis. Also, recent advances in metabolic engineering have demonstrated the potential of genes regulation to increase taxol production. This chapter provides a more in-depth insight into basic and applied research to increase taxol production.

Keywords: Biosynthetic pathway, Cancer treatment, Metabolic engineering, Natural products, Secondary metabolites, Taxol, *Taxus*, Taxol production, Taxanes, Taxol toxicity.

1. INTRODUCTION

“Natural products” also called “secondary metabolites” are organic molecules of low molecular weight (often less than 3,000 Daltons) with particular and exceptionally complex structures. The significant number of these substances

* **Corresponding author Zhong-Yi Yang:** State Key Laboratory for Biocontrol, School of Life Sciences, Sun Yat-Sen University, Xingang Xi Road 135, Guangzhou, 510275, China; Tel: +86 (20) 84112008; E-mail: adsyzy@mail.sysu.edu.cn

don't take part in the development and growth of the plant [1]. These substances assist the plants in survival by providing a defense mechanism against predators, and it also helps the plants to adapt their surrounding environment. Nevertheless, despite their importance for the plant itself, various secondary metabolites are also of great incentive to the human on account of their attractive natural and therapeutic activities [2 - 4]. From the beginning of human civilization, these vital organic substances of different plants have been used to treat diverse types of diseases. Indeed, at present plants are considered as the most significant source of natural drug compounds, and these substances constitute around 25% of the prescribed medication [5].

Natural products also used as chemotherapeutic agents either in natural and synthetic modified forms [6]. One-third of the anti-cancer agents used in medicine are natural products or their derivatives and produced on information that picked up from micro and macromolecules that exist in nature. Since 1940, food and drug administration (FDA) approved more than 140 anti-cancer agents for cancer treatment, among them, 60% are derived from natural products [7]. Natural product based cancer drugs that are involved in war against cancer include taxanes (paclitaxel, docetaxel), vinca alkaloids (vindesine, vincristine, vinorelbine, vinblastine), camptothecin and its derivatives (irinotecan, topotecan), anthracyclines (idarubicin, doxorubicin, epirubicin, daunorubicin), podophyllotoxin and its derivative (teniposide, etoposide) and others [8, 9]. 'Taxol' (generic name paclitaxel) is a most promising complex diterpene, alongside baccatin III (BAC III) and 10-deacetylbaccatin III (10-DAB III), widely used for cancer treatment. It is used to treat different types of cancer including breast cancer [10, 11], ovarian carcinomas [12, 13], skin cancer [14], and non-small cell lung cancer [15]. It is also used to treat neurodegenerative diseases such as Alzheimer's [16, 17] and also a useful compound for the drug-eluting coronary artery stents [18], and polycystic kidney disease [19]. Moreover, taxol was found effective against restenosis [20], psoriasis [21], and tauopathies [22] that require microtubules stabilization.

This chapter aims to summarize the current information available regarding the taxol development as drug and how it works to kill the cancer cells. We considered the recent progress in taxol production and also focused on optimizing strategies to improve taxol and related taxane obtained from the different sources for cheaper commercial production of taxol. Besides, we also cover the metabolic engineering strategies related to the microorganisms, heterologous plants, and *Taxus* cell cultures, to improve taxoids production. We also described the advances in molecular biology and genomics, which were made to overcome the gap in our knowledge of the taxol and other related taxoids biosynthesis. However, this chapter does not summarize the complete range of such published research studies.

2. TAXOL AND ITS SUCCESS STORY TO DRUG DEVELOPMENT

An open screening center named National cancer institute (NCI) was established by Cancer chemotherapy national service center (CCNSC) in 1955 to check the anti-cancer activities in chemical compounds collected by different external organizations and institutions. Even though the higher number of the compounds screened were of synthetic origin. Jonathan Hartwell, who was working in CCNSC, had an understanding of compounds derived from natural sources and started a screening program for natural products derived compounds [23]. Almost 115,000 plant extracts tested from 15,000 plant species in a joint screening program of NCI and the U.S. division of agriculture (USDA) [24]. As a result, taxol was isolated from the bark of *T. brevifolia* and identified as cytotoxic against KB cells obtained from a nasopharyngeal tumor [24]. It also tested against other preclinical models being used at that time [25]. The successive stages in the development of taxol as an anticancer drug presented in Fig. (**1**).

Taxol is a white to off-white color crystalline powder with the molecular formula of $C_{47}H_{51}NO_{14}$ [5]. According to the International union of pure and applied chemistry (IUPAC) nomenclature of organic chemistry the taxol chemical name is (2α,4α,5β,7β,10β,13α)-4,10-bis(acetyloxy)-13-{[(2*R*,3*S*)-3-(benzoylamino)-2-hydroxy-3-phenylpropanoyl]oxy}-1,7-dihydroxy-9-oxo-5,20-epoxytax-11-en-2-yl benzoate [26]. The molecular weight of the taxol is 853.9 Dalton (Da), and its melting temperature is 216 - 217 °C [5]. It is soluble in dimethyl sulfoxide (DMSO), ethanol and methanol but insoluble in water [26]. Taxol core consists of A, B, C ring system with numerous attached functional groups such as two acetyl groups, two OH groups, one benzoyl group, and an oxetane ring. A side chain or C13 (2′R,3′S)-N-benzoyl-3′-phenylisoserine bound at the C13 position of the taxol core with a benzoyl and hydroxyl group [27].

The high demand for taxol because of its unique mechanism of action against cancer cell peaked the global market of taxol at billion dollars in 2001. At present, Phyton Biotech is the leading taxol provider worldwide, which is now a subsidiary of DFB Pharmaceuticals Inc [28]. In recent years, extensive studies have been accomplished to develop second-generation taxoids to boost their viability and reduce toxicity. As a minimum, nine novel taxane analogs were undergone clinical trials in the last few years. Among new taxanes, nab-paclitaxel or Abraxane was approved by the FDA in 2005 for breast cancer treatment. More recently, in 2010, cabazitaxel was also approved by the FDA for prostate cancer treatment [29, 30]. Regardless of its low yield limit and complex nature of biosynthesis, low efficacy, high toxicity, taxol is the most significant drug for cancer treatment from the last four decades.

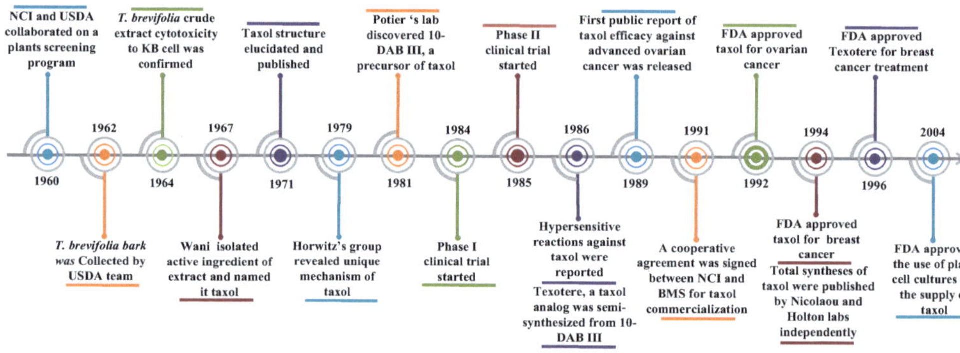

Fig. (1). Timeline highlight the pivotal discoveries and development stages of taxol as an anticancer drug.

3. CELL AND TAXOL FIGHT

Microtubules are long, hollow cylinders with approximately 25 nm in outer diameter, made up of a particular type of protein dimers called α- and β- tubulin. These α/β tubulin subunits are almost similar polypeptides with a molecular weight of approximately 55 kD. These tubulin dimers polymerize head-to-tail arrays into 13 linear proto-filaments which laterally associate to form a single microtubule. Microtubules are polar structures with two particular ends, and their polarity is critical to determine the direction of microtubules movement. The β subunit exposed end designated as a fast-growing (+) end while α subunit exposed end is slow-growing (-) end [31]. Microtubules are dynamic structures and alternate between the cycle of growth and cycle of shrinkage due to the rapid round of assembly and disassembly of tubulin dimers. This non-equilibrium behavior of microtubules is termed as dynamic instability [32]. In particular, the GTP molecule bound to both α and β tubulin subunits. The GTP bound to α tubulin subunit is stable while β-tubulin bound GTP is hydrolyzed to GDP shortly after polymerization and becomes non-exchangeable [33]. As long as the addition of GTP bound β tubulin is more rapid to the elongating microtubule than the hydrolysis of GTP, the microtubule holds a GTP cap at its (+) end, and the microtubule enlargement continues. However, if the rate of polymerization slows, the β tubulin bound GTP hydrolyzed to GDP at the (+) end and dissociated GDP bound tubulin. Eventually, this dissociation results in depolymerization and shrinkage of microtubule [31]. Taxol with the unique mechanism of action is a potential chemotherapeutic agent Fig. (**2**). Taxol binds to β-subunit of tubulin at N-terminal 31 amino acids position in the microtubule [34]. By stabilizing polymerization of microtubules and inhibiting from disassembly, taxol arrests the cell cycle at G_0/G_1 and G_2/M stages and induces the cell death in the cancer cell [35, 36]. It helps to polymerize tubulin dimers to form microtubules by inhibiting tubulin depolymerization even in the absence of factors such as GTP, microtubule-related proteins (MAPs), and ethylene glycol-bis-β-aminoethyl ether N,N' tetra-acetic acid (EGTA) are generally required for assembly of microtubules [37, 38].

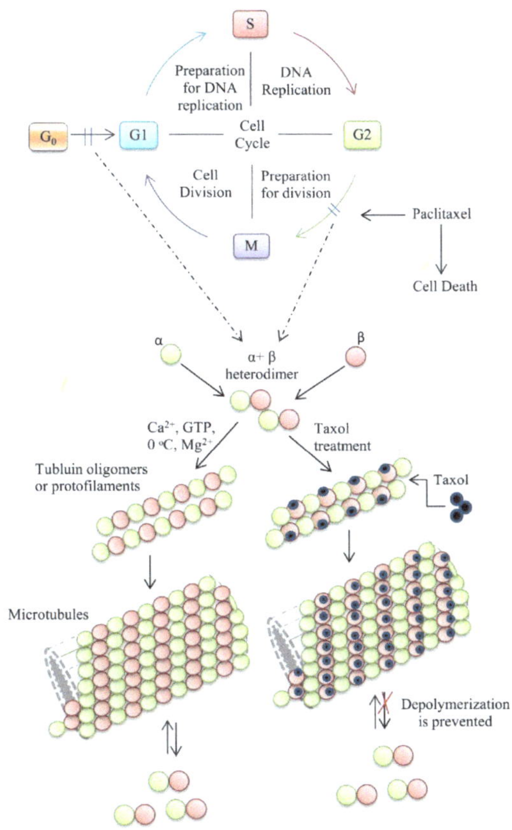

Fig. (2). General taxol mechanism of action.

Taxol also has mechanisms of action other than microtubule targeting. Mullins, *et al.* [39] described that the taxol restores the production of interleukin (IL)-12 in tumor-bearing hosts which drastically reduced the growth of the tumor by selective regulatory impairment of IL-12 p40 expression. It also reduced the tumor necrosis factor alpha (TNFα) receptors surface expression, which adds significance to its anti-cancer activity [40]. Likewise, It promotes the release of IL-1, IFN-α (interferon alpha) and IFN-β (interferon beta) to kill or inhibit cancer cells [41]. Taxol induces apoptosis through various mechanisms or transduction pathways which emerge to be independent of stabilization of microtubule. For a broader understanding of how transduction pathways involved in taxol-based cell killing; readers are referred to [42 - 44]. Moreover, taxol generates reactive oxygen species (ROS) by enhancing the activity of plasma membrane-associated nicotinamide adenine dinucleotide phosphate (NADPH) and increases hydroperoxide production, which participates to the efficient anticancer usage of taxol [45, 46]. Gan, *et al.* [47] found that taxol hindered the androgen receptor by initiating nuclear accumulation of forkhead box protein O1 (FOXO1) as one of the anticancer mechanisms. The non-chemotherapeutic utilization of taxol identifies the antineoplastic mechanisms. For instance, Sevko, *et al.* [48, 49] announced that taxol improved the adequacy of chemotherapy by obstructing the immune-suppressive potential of myeloid-derived suppressor cells. In addition to its utility in cancer treatment, taxol is likewise broadly utilized as a part of cell science.

4. TOXICITY OF TAXOL

4.1. Hypersensitivity

Hypersensitive reactions are often associated with chemotherapeutic agent taxol. These reactions usually occur during or shortly after taxol infusion. 78% of hyper-sensitive symptoms generally develop within the first 10-15 mints after infusion [50]. Hypersensitive reactions reported in 95% of cases during the first and second infusion [51]. In 3% of cases, reactions can develop in subsequent infusions. The taxol and docetaxel frequency of hypersensitivity differs between 8% and 50% [52].

4.2. Extravasation Reactions

The leakage of intravenously infused taxol into the soft tissue of the infusion region can occur in 0.1-6% cases [53]. The reactions due to intravenous leakage are generally mild; however, acute extravasation may happen with taxol [54], nab-paclitaxel [53] or docetaxel [10]. Taxanes are usually considered irritants. The leakage of high concentration of taxane into the soft tissues may also cause blistering reaction [55, 56]. Besides severe reactions such as chronic ulceration or necrosis can also develop in some cases [54, 57].

4.3. Cutaneous Toxicities

Warm sites of the body such as contact areas, folds, under dressings and pads, are more inclined to the taxane-induced rash. The development of bilateral, painful, and inflammatory intertriginous patches on the axillary and inguinal regions or neck folds is the most significant representation of taxane-induced toxicity [58]. The extensor muscles of the arm and lateral surfaces of the thighs and knees also reported with taxol toxicity. These toxicity reactions are dose-dependent and may develop several days after the first infusion [59]. Tropical steroids are typically used to manage these skin lesions. On the other hand, sometimes temporary taxanes interruption and dose reduction are required.

4.4. Neurotoxicity

As a therapeutic agent, taxol also affects neurons. It specifically affects the peripheral brain system and leads to a primarily sensory axonal neuropathy [60]. The higher single and cumulative doses increase the occurrence and severity of the neuropathy. The acute seriousness of neurological symptoms requires the termination or reduction of treatment. These symptoms can endure for months or years, even though side effects as a rule resolve after ceasing treatment [61]. The distal sensory axons start to degenerate as the neurotoxic dose reaches, and sensory symptom begins to appear in the hands and feet [62]. In case of severe neuropathy fiber loss, secondary demyelination, and axonal degeneration is revealed by peripheral nerve biopsy [63]. The primary symptoms of taxol-induced toxicity in patients include pain, numbness, and tingling [61]. Numerous studies on cultured neurons and rodents model have reported different agents that protect taxol-induced axonal degeneration [64 - 66]. The clinical trials of these agents have yielded mixed results, and there are right now no endorsed mediations.

4.5. Cardiac Arrhythmias

Taxol-induced electrocardiogram (ECG) changes include right and left bundle branch block, prolongation of QTc interval, and T-wave changes [67]. Sinus bradycardia is one of the most well-known arrhythmias associated with taxol. It is usually mild and temporary, with no symptoms. 29% of the cases reported sinus bradycardia when taxol is infused alone or combined with cisplatin. Momentary atrioventricular (AV) block have also been reported in rare cases [68]. Before the start of anticancer therapy with taxol, ECG, and clinical cardiovascular evaluation are useful to screen the signs of cardiomyopathy, conduction disturbances, and QTc intervals.

4.6. Gastrointestinal Effects

Typhlitis (cecal inflammation) has examined in phase I trial due to combining the infusion of taxol and doxorubicin within 72 hours [69]. The pathophysiological relationship has shown taxol-induced microtubular aster development in harmed epithelial cells, proposing mitotic arrest of mucosal cells proliferation [70]. Moreover, taxol administration is irregularly associated with nausea, vomiting, and esophagitis. Diarrhea has also associated with taxol-induced reactions, although these reactions are rare.

4.7. Taxol-induced Alopecia

Taxol rank among the top chemotherapy agents that induced alopecia. Taxol induces alopecia by dystrophic anagen effluvium mechanism [71, 72]. Alopecia may happen after the first treatment cycle. Taxol affects the scalp in a diffuse pattern in at least 60% of the treated patient [73]. The prolong treatments with higher doses, and multiple exposures may also affect other hair-bearing areas such as eyebrows, eyelashes, axillae, beard, and body [74]. Typically, the re-growth of the lost hair starts within three to six months after the last cycle treatment. However, more than one-third of cases observe the change in re-growing hair texture (more curly) and color (more grey) [72]. Total/near total hair loss universally examined in taxol-treated patients. Moreover, permanent/irreversible hair loss has also emerged recently [75].

The investigations on taxol are still progressing, and scientists are endeavoring to make it more efficient. Several studies centered on figuring out how to decrease taxol associated adverse effects, for example, the utilization of adjuvant for targeted drug delivery. One such study includes the utilization of a lectin, maackia amurensis agglutinin (MAA), as an adjuvant and demonstrated its adequacy in various cancers [76].

5. SOURCES AND PRODUCTION OF TAXOL

5.1. *Taxus* and Other Plant Sources of Taxol

The natural producer of the taxol is gymnosperm family *Taxaceae*, which includes *T. baccata* L. (English yew), *T. cuspidata* Sieb. and Zucc. (Japanese yew), *T. Canadensis* Marshall (Canadian yew), *T. brevifolia* Nutt. (Pacific yew or Western yew), *T. floridana* Champ. (Florida yew), *T. globosa* Schltdl. (Mexican yew), *T. wallichiana* Zucc. (Himalayan yew), *T. fuana* Nan Li and R.R. Mill, and *T. chinensis* (Pilger) Rehder (Chinese yew). Besides, two hybrids species *T. media* = *T. baccata* X *T. cuspidate* and *T. hunnewelliana* = *T. cuspidate* and *T. Canadensis* are also recognized [77, 78]. All the *Taxus* species are phylogenetically similar to each other. It is postulated that all the cultivars have the same common origin from *T. baccata*. Originally taxol was isolated from *T.*

brevifolia bark where it is present in a concentration of 0.01 – 0.05% [79]. After the noteworthy finding of anticancer activities, the search for taxol extended to cultivars, varieties, different organs and tissues of the species, which led to the discovery of taxol in all *Taxus* species. The most noteworthy average highest yield of taxol is present in bark followed by roots, leaves, wood, seedlings, and then twigs [80]. Other than *Taxus*, the four genera of this family are *Autotaxus*, *Pseudotaxus*, *Amenotaxus*, and *Torreya* [77]. Among these genera, a few simpler taxanes were obtained from *Pseudotaxus* [81] and *Autotaxus* [82]. Among gymnosperm, *Podocarpus gracilior* was the prime species outside family *Taxaceae* documented for taxol production, with 0.54 mg/Kg yield [83]. The claim for taxol production was insufficient in evidence due to the high-performance liquid chromatography (HPLC) and mass spectroscopy (MS) technique used for the experimental investigation [84]. Moreover, 10-DAB III precursor of taxol was also detected in needles of *P. massoniana* and *C. sinensis* [85].

After adequately exploring the taxol and other taxoids in gymnosperm, the search for taxol extended to angiosperm. The taxol production in angiosperm dates back to 1998 when Hoffman group was investigating some varieties of hazelnut (*C. avellana* cv. *Gasaway)*, observing why some varieties are resistant than others against eastern filberts blight. By analyzing purified extract, these scientists found traces of taxol in hazelnut by HPLC and MS analysis [86]. Initially, it was thought that the endophytic fungi reside in this tree are responsible for the production of taxol rather than hazel itself. Later, Bestoso, *et al.* [87] *in vitro* cell culture investigations on *C. avellana* revealed that hazel species possess metabolic pathway for taxane biosynthesis. Taxol and other taxanes including BAC-III, 10-DAB III, 10-deacetylpaclitaxel, 10-diacetyl-7-xylosyl-paclitaxel, 7-xylosy--paclitaxel, 7-epi-paclitaxel, Cephalomanine, paclitaxel C, have been obtained from shell, leaf, and kernel of *C. avellana* [88 - 90].

Moreover, few other angiosperm species like *Magujreothamnus speciosus*, *Justicia gendarussa*, and *Morinda citrifolia* also reported in the literature for taxol production [91, 92]. Throughout screening of chemical constituents, novel taxanes were identified in *Y. longistaminata* (tender burgeon), an angiosperm utilized as a consumable wild vegetable in China. The structures were distinguished as taxayunnansin B, L-iditol, and taxumairol E on the premise of NMR and MS [92]. Other than these compounds, the probability of taxol production from the angiosperm species exists yet so far continued.

5.2. Total Synthesis of Taxol

Two research groups independently reported the total synthesis of taxol in 1994.

They used comparatively simple and commercially accessible starting material [93, 94]. Holton synthesis started with the AB rings formation, followed by C-and D-rings. This linear synthesis initiated from a natural compound patchoulene oxide and consisted of 42 steps with the ultimate yield of 0.6% [95]. On the other hand, in Nicolaou's synthesis of taxol, A and C ring were constructed first by convergent approach then formed the B ring by a ring closure reaction. This synthesis consisted of 35 steps and yielded taxol of 0.06% [94]. Moreover, a racemic mixture also produced by Nicolau's strategy, which required an extra step of purification.

A year later, in 1995, Danishefsky used heck cyclization to synthesize taxol [96, 97]. This strategy was similar to Nicolau's convergent synthesis and involved 24 steps with a final yield of 0.02%. The starting material for this synthesis was Wieland-Miescher ketone. This material changed into complex enol triflate that contains an olefin at C-ring, which allows taxol synthesis through an intra-molecular heck reaction. Wender, *et al.* [98] reported the total chemical synthesis of taxol by fragmentation strategy of an epoxy-alcohol. α-pinene was the starting material of this strategy. Mukaiyama reported another method of taxol total synthesis [99]. This technique generated B ring first followed by A and C rings. In this technique, the starting material was industrially accessible neopentyl glycol or L-serines. Kuwajima and coworkers have published another procedure for Enantio-selective total synthesis of taxol. This method started from the construction of A and C ring and cyclization of Lewis acid mediated B-ring, which generate the required ABC configuration. The addition of the D ring gave the complete functional skeleton of taxol [100, 101].

Recently, researchers described another method of total synthesis of taxol from geraniol, and it was found different from the other six published techniques. This synthesis involved 36 steps and carried out in a mechanized synthesizer which produced a synthetic taxol intermediate. The prime reaction of this synthesis involved a microwave-assisted alkylation in generating the ABC ring system. The addition of the D ring leads to BAC III formation, a renowned taxol precursor [102, 103]. Other synthetic researchers have also made possible the total chemical synthesis by using Takahashi intermediate [104 - 106]. Although total chemical synthesis of taxol was an incredible success, its commercial application is not possible shortly due to lengthy steps of chemical synthesis and low yield. It makes taxol synthesis too complicated and too expensive. However, this does not mean that synthetic approaches towards taxol production should be abandoned.

5.3. Semi-synthesis of Taxol

One of the significant leaps forward intending to the taxol supply issue was the discovery of 10-DAB III, a precursor of taxol from the needle of *T. baccata.* A year later in 1982, it was isolated abundantly from *T. brevifolia* bark. This discovery provoked scientific community to develop semi-synthetic approaches to produce taxol. The complicated four ring tetracycline structure is already present in 10-DAB III. An acetyl group on the tenth carbon is the only missing component apart from the taxol-side chain. When 10-DAB III contains the acetyl group, the compound is known as BAC-III [107]. The formation of the C-13 side chain and its emergence with 10-DAB III is the prime condition of semi-synthesis of taxol which has been brilliantly reviewed by Wuts [108] and Barua, *et al.* [109]. Several semi-synthetic strategies reported in the literature, among these three distinct procedures are more efficient for semi-synthesis of taxol. The two of these procedures starts with 7-O-TES-baccatin-III. To obtained 7-O-T-S-baccatin-III, 10-DAB III first silylated and then acetylated as depicted by Denis, *et al.* [110]. The first synthetic procedure developed by Prof. Holton was revealed in U.S patent (No. 5,274,124) [111]. In this method, lithium ions of 7-O-T-S-baccatin-III react with the β-lactam to initiate the required amino acid chain of taxol at the position of C_{13}. The second synthetic procedure is based on combing of 7-O- TES-baccatin-III with oxazoline carboxylic acid by utilizing dicyclohexylcarbodiimide (DCC) or other related dehydrating agents. This procedure evolved by BMS was published in U.S. patent application (No. 07/995,443) and by Kingston, *et al.* [112]. The third synthetic procedure was developed by Commerçon, *et al.* [113], in which 7-O-TROC-baccatin- III coupled with a protected β-phenylisoserine side chain in the presences of DCC.

The 7-b-xylosyl-10-deacetylTaxol (XDT) is an analog of taxol, present in the dry bark of the yew plant with a yield of 0.5% [114]. The XDT compound has a 7-β-xylosyl moiety at the C_7 position. The removal of xylosyl group by biological and chemical hydrolysis converts XDT to 10-deacetylTaxol (DT) which can also be utilized to chemically semi-synthesize taxol through acetylation at position C_{10} (U.S. Patent 6,028,206) [115, 116]. The synthesis of taxol from DT is simple as compared to 10-DAB III due to the presence of a C_{13} side chain. To boost the commercial production of taxol from DT, efficient mechanism of XDT conversion to DT is needed. The chemical reactions that use periodate or other oxidizing agent and a hydrazine substitute to remove the sugar are costly and tedious. As opposed, the biological path by utilizing an enzyme β-xylosidase to remove D-xylose sugar from XDT is regarded as environmental friendly. Some bacterial strains, for example, *Cellulosimicrobium cellulans* XZ-5, *Enterobacter sp.* and *Moraxella sp.* have been accounted for XDT to DT conversion. However, bacterial strain converts the small amount of DT ranged from 0.23 – 0.76 mg/mL, which is most likely because of low levels of the enzyme in the native organisms [117, 118]. Recently a new β-xylosidase gene was cloned from *Lentinula edodes* and introduced into a yeast host *Pichia pastoris*. The conversions by recombinant yeast increased DT yield by 10.58 g/L, which is much higher than the earlier reports [114].

5.4. Production by Plant Cell Culture

The plant cell culture technology is the most promising methodology for sufficient production of taxol and related taxoids so far and has been extensively reviewed [27, 119 - 129]. The general outline of taxol and related taxane production at a commercial level is given in Fig. (**3**). Taxol and its derivatives initially investigated in callus, and cell suspension dedifferentiated culture (DDC) [130 - 135]. Different *Taxus* species were used to obtain taxol producing dedifferentiated cell culture including *T. brevifolia* [136], *T. media* [137], *T. chinensis* [138], *T. canadensis* [139], *T. cuspidata* [140, 141], and *T. globosa* [142].

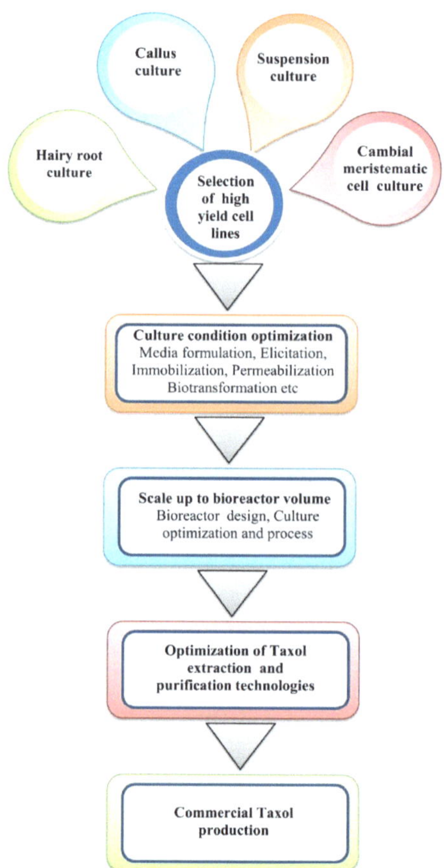

Fig. (3). Outline of taxol and related taxane production at the commercial level by cell culture technology.

Nevertheless, the productivity of the cell lines of the callus and cell suspension cultures are difficult to maintain over successive culture generations. Recently, attention has been rapidly moving towards the application of hairy root cultures which remain stable over consecutive generations for the production of taxol [143 - 145]. The use of hairy root culture for commercial production is still limited due to the cultivation of hairy culture on a large scale, and additional investigations are needed to produce taxol at commercial level. Besides, Lee and co-worker used multi-potent undifferentiated cambial meristematic cells (CMCs) with stem-cell-like properties to initiate cell cultures. These cells have smaller aggregate size, low growth variability, and more resistance to shear stresses. The high taxol yield of 102 mg/Kg (fresh cell weight) detected in CMCs generated from *T. cuspidate* as compared to needle and embryo-derived DDC with the final yield of 23 mg/Kg and 39 mg/Kg respectively [146]. Utilizing CMCs as a framework for subsequent metabolic engineering strategies may further increase the biosynthesis of taxol in these cells.

When the *Taxus* cell culture venture started, the production of the desired compound was limited. The simultaneous application of multiple approaches brings taxol yields up to a useful level in cell culture. Biosynthetic activities of the cultured cell were optimized to enhance the production of taxol, and related taxanes in cell culture for commercial development includes the selection of cell lines for high yield, culture conditions, media optimization, elicitation, usage of two-phase/two-stage cell culture and immobilization method [27]. Genetic difference or heterogeneity of cell in suspension culture demonstrates significant variation in their ability to produce secondary metabolites. To obtain stable production of taxol in *Taxus* cell culture, once high yielding cell line has been chosen, that must be screened further *via* repeated sub-culturing and stability analysis because cell line gradually decreases taxol production or lose the capacity altogether [27, 147 - 149]. Different basal media including Gamborg (B5), Murashige and Skoog (MS), Woody Plant Medium (WPM), Driver and Kuniyuki (DKW), and Schenk and Hildebrandt (SH) were studied to enhance and maintain biomass production in *Taxus* cell culture. DKW basal media was best for 10-DAB III and Baccatin III production. The maximum taxol yield was recorded in WPM basal media when the effect of different basal media was studied on *T. baccata* cell suspension culture [150].

Moreover, inducing agents such as temperature, light, time, pH, cultivation stage and concentration of oxygen also play a significant role in taxol production [151, 152]. Among the manipulative techniques used to increase metabolite production, elicitation is the most potent approach for the remarkable increase in the yield. Jasmonic acid (JA) is one of the most extensively used elicitors in cell cultures studies with a significant increase in taxol production [128, 153 - 155]. Among other elicitors that are commonly used to increase taxol production, alone or in combination include vanadyl (IV) sulfate, phenylalanine, arachidonic corrosive, salicylic corrosive, chlorocholine chloride, fungal culture and fungal extract, as well as osmotic regulators such as sucrose, mannitol, sorbitol, and polyethylene glycol [127, 131, 156 - 158]. After optimization of different parameters, successful large-scale cultivation of *Taxus* cells for taxol production was conducted in different types of bioreactors. In the study of Bentebibel, *et al.* [159], the maximum production of taxol (43.43 mg/L) and baccatin III (5.06 mg/L) was observed in the turbine stirred bioreactor, followed by Airlift and Wave bioreactors.

The cell acquired taxol inside the cell wall [160], and 7-10% of the total taxol discharged to the extracellular environment [161]. The taxol accumulation inside the cell causes feedback inhibition and degradation of the product. The use of cell-wall digesting enzymes increase 90% of the recovery rate of taxol in the extracellular medium [162]. The use of these enzymes cause the rupturing of the cell wall that leads to complete biomass destruction. Permeabilization of the cell by utilizing pH shock or chemical treatment is one of the methods that help to maintain cell viability and the further utilization of biomass [161]. The addition of low concentration of the permeabilizing agent, *i.e.*, hexadecane, decanol, and dibutyl phthalate increased total taxol content in the extracellular environment [163]. Cusido, *et al.* [164] demonstrated that taxol and related taxanes production does not depend on the growth of the cell culture and taxol accumulate during the stationary phase of the culture. These investigations led to the development of a two-phase cell culture system and the increase in taxol and baccatin III production in *Taxus* cell suspension culture is reported in different studies [132, 165]. Furthermore, Immobilisation by beads of calcium alginate in a bioreactor of *T. baccata* cells resulted in 43.43 mg/L taxol production at day 16, presenting 2.71 mg/L production rate per day [159]. The ultimate objective of all these investigations is to establish an environmental friendly and supportable biotechnological platform to produce a high amount of taxol from *Taxus* cell culture and to protect yew species in their natural environment.

5.5. Taxol Producing Endophytic Fungi

A fermentation process involving microorganisms is another most attractive approach for the supply of taxol. Firstly, *Taxus* species were screened for taxol producing endophytes before extended to other plant species. Up to the early 1990s, there was not any report of endophytes from *Taxus* species that produced taxol. After a few years of research, in 1994, *Taxomyces andreanae* was isolated from the earliest known source of the alkaloid *T. brevifolia* [166]. Despite the low the yield of taxol (24-50 ng/L) from fungi, this discovery induced a huge interest in scientists. Two years later, another taxol-producing endophytic fungus *Pestalotiopsis microspore* isolated from *T. wallichiana* inner bark, with the yield of 50 ng/L on semi-synthetic medium [167]. After the success of taxol-producing fungus isolation from *Taxus* species, search for taxol producing endophytes was extended to non-*Taxus* species. The surprising primary finding was the isolation of *P. microspore* from *Taxodium distichum* [168]. Since then, several reports have been published on the production of taxol in endophytes, and few of them isolated in the last decade are mentioned in Table 1. The host range of taxol-producing fungi contains the species of *Taxus* and non-*Taxus* species, including *Torreya grandifolia* [169], *Terminalia arjuna* [170], *Cypress* [171], and *Podocarpus* [172]. The fungus *Pestalotiopsis malicola* isolated as a saprophyte (from debris) has been reported to produce taxol, with the final yield of 186 mg/L in the liquid culture medium. Similarly, epiphytes (fungus from plant surfaces) have also been accounted as taxol producer, and the yield of epiphytic fungus is relatively similar to the most of isolated endophytes [173]. Presently, around 200 endophytes, representing more than 40 genera including; *Sporormia*, *Alternaria*, *Pestalotia*, *Pithomyces*, *Penicillium*, *Pestalotiopsis*, *Truncatella*, *Monochaetia*, and *Fusarium*, belonging to different order such as Ascomycota, Deuteromycota, Zygomycota, and few Basidiomycota were also reported to produce taxol [174, 175]. Numerous endophytic fungi are added to the list consistently, emphasize that merely a small portion of an expected one million (or more) endophytes species has been cultured and screened [176]. Unquestionably, none of these revelations has been effectively converted into industrial bioprocesses up until now.

However, Numerous techniques are used to improve the commercial production of taxol from endophytes includes strain improvement, fermentation condition optimization such as temperature, pH, and rotation speed as well as genetic engineering including mutagenesis and breeding of protoplasts [177 - 180]. The micro- and macroelement manipulation in culture medium influence the yields of taxol, such as the increase of sodium benzoate and the decrease of phosphate in *P. microspora* culture medium, a fungus isolated from *T. wallichiana* stimulate the production of taxol [181]. Besides mineral elements, the addition of chemical elicitors in culture medium also enhances the production of taxol. Yang, *et al.* [182] reported 0.07 to 0.35 mg/L increase in *P. aurantiogriseum* culture medium by addition of methyl jasmonate (MJ) and phenylalanine. In addition to chemical elicitors, the modification of culture medium of taxol-producing fungi with host plant crude extract boosts the production of taxol. When the *Periconia* sp. with the yield of 118 ng/L placed together with 100 mg/L of *Torreya taxifolia* extract in the MID culture medium, taxol production almost increased to 350 ng/L [169]. Similarly, co-culturing of *T. chinensis var. mairei* suspension cells with *F. mairei* resulted in a 38-fold increase in production of taxol in contrast to *Fusarium* alone [183]. More recently, co-culturing of one or more taxane producing endophytic fungi with non-taxane producing fungi from the same host plant also reported increasing taxol production [175].

Transformation and protoplast fusion are frequently used methods for strain improvement. A high taxol producing strain *F. mairei* K178 was obtained by protoplast mutation using diethyl sulfate (DES) and UV radiation. The production of taxol in improved strain *F. maire* K178 was increased from 20 to 225.2 mg/L after optimization of nutrients such as NaOAc, $MgSO_4$, and NH_4NO_3 in culture medium [179]. Besides, Zhao, *et al.* [184] completely inactivated the protoplast of strains UV40-19 and UL50-6 before fusion via 85 sec of radiation treatment and 5 min heating at 54 °C to obtain an improved strain of *Nodulisporium sylviforme.* The final yield of taxol was 468.62 ± 37.49 mg/L in the mutant strain HDF-68, which were 19.35% and 24.51% higher compared to the parental strains UL50-6 and UV40-19, respectively. Moreover, the four independent rounds of random shuffling of the genome via protoplast fusion increased taxol yield from 314 to 516 mg/L of NCEU-1 [185, 186].

In summary, none of these methods of taxol production are viable on large scale. Summary of all the methods of the taxol production is given in Table 2. Currently taxol production by semi-synthesis and cell culture method is the main source of clinical supply which is not enough to meet the increasing demand of taxol. To boost the production and reduce the price of the taxol and its analogs, collaborative research between different research groups should be encouraged and different research approaches should be adopted.

Table 1. List of taxol-producing fungi.

Host Plant	Endophytic Fungi	Area of Collection	Host Tissue	Taxol Yield (ug/L)	Detection Technique	Growth Medium	References
Ervatamia divaricata	*Pestalotiopsis breviseta*	india	Leaf	64 µg/L	UV spectroscopy, IR, HPLC, NMR, LC–MS	MID medium	[187]
Citrus medica	*Phyllosticta citricarpa*	India	Leaf	137-265 µg/L	TLC, HPLC, LC-MS	M1D medium	[188]
T. cuspidata	*Pestalotiopsis versicolor*	South Korea	Leaf and bark	478 µg/L	HPLC, ^{1}H-NMR, LC-MS	MID medium	[189]
T. cuspidata	*Pestalotiopsis neglecta*	South Korea	Leaf and bark	375 µg/L	HPLC, ^{1}H-NMR, LC-MS	MID medium	[189]

(Table 1) cont.....

Host Plant	Endophytic Fungi	Area of Collection	Host Tissue	Taxol Yield (ug/L)	Detection Technique	Growth Medium	References
T. baccata	*Gliocladium sp.*	India	-	10 µg/L	UV-spectroscopy, TLC, HPLC, ESI-MS, MS/MS, H-NMR	S7 medium	[190]
T. chinensis var. mairei	*Didymostilbe sp.*	China	Inner bark	8 - 15 µg/L	HPLC, LC–MS, CIEIA	PDA medium	[191]
T. baccata	*Paraconiothyrium variabile*	UK	Twig	1.75 ug/L	TLC, HPLC-DAD, LC-MS/MS	M1D medium	[192]
T. baccata	*Epicoccum nigrum*	UK	Twig	1.32 µg/L	TLC, HPLC-DAD, LC-MS/MS	M1D medium	[192]
T. wallichiana var. *mairei*	*Diaporthe phaseolorum*	China	Branch	219 µg/L BAC-III	HPLC, LC-MS	PDA medium	[193]
T. baccata sub sp.*wallichiana*	*Fusarium redolens*	India	Bark	70 µg/L	HPLC, LC-MS	S-7 medium	[194]
T. baccata	*Cladosporium sp.*	Iran	Leaf and stem	129 µg/L	HPLC	-	[194]
Catharanthus roseus	*Pestalotiopsis funerea*	Chennai	Leaf	92 µg/L	HPLC	MID medium	[195]
Taxus sp.	*Cladosporium cladosporioides*	Pakistan	Inner bark	140 µg/L	TLC, HPLC, UV spectroscopy	-	[196]
T. media	*Guignardia mangiferae*	China	Bark and leaf	0.72 µg/L	HPLC-MS	PDB medium	[197]
T. media	*Fusarium proliferatum*	China	Bark and leaf	0.24 µg/L	HPLC-MS	PDB medium	[197]
T. media	*Colletotrichum gloeosporioides*	China	Bark and leaf	0.12 µg/L	HPLC-MS	PDB medium	[197]
Corylus avellana	*Penicillium aurantiogriseum*	USA	Nuts	120 µg/L	HPLC-MS, NMR	PDB medium	[182]
T. cuspidata	*Aspergillus niger var. taxi*	China	Branch and trunk	273·46 µg/L	HPLC, MS	PDA medium	[198]
Tectona grandis	*Colletotrichum gleospoiroides*	India	Leaf	-	UV spectroscopy, TLC, HPLC	PDB medium	[199]
Ficus infectoria	*Pestalotiopsis stellata*	India	Leaf	0.044 µg/L	UV spectroscopy, IR, HPLC; MTT assay	M1D medium	[200]

(Table 1) cont.....

Host Plant	Endophytic Fungi	Area of Collection	Host Tissue	Taxol Yield (ug/L)	Detection Technique	Growth Medium	References
T. media	*Paraconiothyrium sp.*	Canada	Branch	20 μg/L	TLC, LC-MS, EIA	YPD medium	[201]
Rhizophora annamalayana	*Fusarium oxysporum*	-	Leaf	172.3 μg/L	IR, HPLC, TLC	PDA medium	[202]
Axus celebica	*Fusarium solani*	UK	Stem	1.6 μg/L	TLC, HPLC, MALDI, LC-ES--MS	PDA medium	[203]
T. chinensis	*M. anisopliae*	China	Stem	846.1 μg/L	HPLC, LC-MS	PDA medium	[204]
T. media	*Cladosporium cladosporioides*	China	Inner bark	800 μg/L	HPLC, LC-MS, NMR	PDA medium	[205]
Ginkgo biloba	*Phoma betae*	South Korea	Leaf	795 μg/L	UV, IR, NMR, LC-MS, TLC, HPLC	M1D medium	[206]
Justicia gendarussa	*Colletotrichum gloeosporioides*	India	Leaf	163.4 μg/L	HPLC	MID medium	[207]
Cupressus sp.	*Phyllosticta spinarum*	India	Leaf	235 μg/L	HPLC	M1D medium	[208]
Citrus medica,	*Phyllosticta citricarpa*	India	Leaf	265 μg/L	TLC, HPLC, LC-MS, H-NMR	M1D medium	[188]
Hibiscus rosasinensis	*Phyllosticta dioscoreae*	India	Leaf	298 μg/L	HPLC	M1D medium	[209]
Morinda citrifolia	*Lasiodiplodia theobromae*	-	Leaf	245 μg/L	TLC, HPTLC, HPLC, UV, IR, ^{1}H-NMR, FAB-MS	MID medium	[210]
Terminalia arjuna	*Chaetomella raphigera*	India	Leaf	79.6 μg/L	TLC, HPTLC, HPLC, UV, IR, ^{1}H-NMR, FAB-MS	MID Broth	[170]
T. wallichiana var. mairei	*Phoma medicaginis*	China	Bark	1215 μg/L	LC-MS	PDA medium	[211]
Phoma moricola	*Bauhinia tomentosa*	India	infected leaf	302 μg/L	HPLC	MID medium	[212]
Grammothele lineata	*Corchorus olitorius*	Bangladesh	-	382.2 μg/L	TLC, HPLC, FTIR, LC-ES--MS/MS	PDB medium	[213]
T. baccata	*Stemphylium sedicola*	Iran	Stem	6.9 ug/L	HPLC	PDB medium	[214]

*This table summarises the taxol-producing fungi that were isolated in last decades. Abbreviations indicate HPLC: High-performance liquid chromatography; TLC: Thin layer chromatography; LC-MS: Liquid chromatography-mass spectrometry; NMR: Nuclear magnetic resonance; H-NMR: Proton nuclear magnetic resonance. IR: Infrared radiations; MALDI: Matrix-assisted laser desorption ionisation; ESI-MS: electrospray ionization mass spectrometry; CIEIA: Comprtitive inhibition enzyme immunoassay; EIA: Enzyme immunoassay; FTIR: Fourier-transform infrared spectroscopy. FAB-MS: Fast-atom bombardment mass spectrometry.

Table 2. Summary of various methods of taxol production.

Source of Production	Advantages	Disadvantages	Potential at industrial scale
Isolation from *Taxus* sources	Simplest isolation route	Fully grown tree only able to provide 0.5 g of taxol and two to three fully grown trees are required to treat one patient effectively. The extraction process is destructive to the tree source, and mature yew tree required 200 years to develop fully. This form of direct plant isolation is clearly inefficient and non-sustainable.	Direct Isolation from the *Taxus* sp. bark was the only method for taxol production at the commercial level before the 90s. Extraction from natural sources led to its destruction. Now there are not enough trees to treat patients.
Total synthesis of taxol	The method starts with relatively simple and commercially available starting materials. The end product can be used directly. Don't have to perform laborious purifications.	The chemical synthesis involves lengthy processing steps with low final yield. The cost of the method is very high due to the use of different solvent and organic reagent. Some of these reagents are hazardous and toxic. The waste streams from the process also raise environmental concerns.	Total synthesis could not be implemented for large-scale industrial production. Lengthy steps and the environmental impacts for such a method are unacceptable.
Semi-synthesis of taxol	10-DAB III is the precursor molecule for semi-synthesis of taxol and present in the leaves and twigs in good yield. It is a renewable source that does not adversely impact on the ecosystem. It can also be obtained from nursery cultivated yew trees. Most of the structural complexity of the taxol molecule is already present in the 10-DAB III .	The semi-synthetic process is very complex with 7 isolation and 11 transformation steps. Several different solvents, organic reagents, and other material also present environmental concerns. The semi-synthesis is not very productive and subject to genetic and biological variables.	Indeed this method proved useful for industrial-scale production. BMS pharmaceutical owns a form with 30 billion yews which supply leaves for 10-DAB III extraction. BSM led to this method for commercialization by signing a cooperative research and development agreement with the Robert Holton, who invented the semi-synthetic route.

(Table 2) cont.....

Source of Production	Advantages	Disadvantages	Potential at industrial scale
Tissue culture technology	This method is a renewable source for taxol production. It is environmental friendly and not being subjected to pollution, climate, and season. Cell culture can grow independently from its unique and remote location. Moreover, fewer purification steps are required because of low interfering substances.	Taxol accumulation in cell culture negatively affects the cell culture resulting in growth inhibition and instability of taxol production. At the cellular level, such phenotypic pressure led to the formation and heterogeneity of the aggregate that causes production variability.	Plant cell culture contributed to the world taxol supply since the 1990s. Currently, taxol production is carried out in plant-cell fermentation technology developed by the Ithaca, New York biotechnology company Phyton Biotech, Inc. It uses up to 75,000 L bioreactors for industrial-scale production of taxol.
Isolation from endophytes	The process of taxol isolation from endophytic fungi is simple, and the downstream processing is secure.	There is a lack of comprehensive understanding of endophytes physiology, biology, genetic, etc with relation to taxol production. The method of fungi fermentation produces an unstable and meager yield. These problems are associated with other factors such as lengthy culture duration and sensitivity to shear stress. Moreover, fungi lost taxol production after repeated sub-culturing.	Undeniably, the taxol production from endophytes is not converted into the industrial process so far. The discovery of new taxol producing fungi continues today, but sustainability and yield are still not up to the desired levels.

6. TAXOL BIOSYNTHESIS AND METABOLIC ENGINEERING FOR TAXOL PRODUCTION

The precursor's dimethylallyl diphosphate (DMAPP) and isopentenyl diphosphate (IPP) is used to synthesize taxol. Two biosynthetic pathways have characterized DMAPP and IPP synthesis; 1) the mevalonate pathway (MVA), 2) the non-mevalonate pathway [215]. The non-mevalonate pathway is also known as the 2C-methyl-D-erythritol-4-phosphate pathway (MEP) and 1-deoxy-D-xylulose- 5-phosphate (DXP) [216]. The mevalonate pathway comprised of six enzymatic steps and produce precursor IPP from acetyl coenzyme-A for the synthesis of triterpenes and sesquiterpenes. The non-mevalonate pathway comprises seven enzymatic steps (Fig. **4**) and produces IPP from glyceraldehyde-3-phosphate and pyruvate [217]. The pathway leads to the synthesis of monoterpenes, diterpenes, and tetraterpenes. Eisenreich, *et al.* [218] demonstrate that the ring system of taxoid does not synthesize via the MVA pathway in taxol biosynthesis, which is the quality of diterpenes. On the other hand, in two different experiments, the *Taxus* cell culture supplemented with radioactively labeled mevalonate produced a high concentration of labeled taxol [219, 220]. Cusido group supplemented the *T. media* cell suspension culture with mevalonate and revealed that both pathways could be involved in taxol biosynthesis under their experiment condition [132]. It is at present acknowledged that the primary source for the biosynthesis of geranylgeranyl pyrophosphate (GGPP) and, therefore, of taxol, is the MEP pathway [221]. Moreover, some degree *Taxus* cells could utilize the MVA pathway as a source of IPP to yield taxol.

The biosynthesis of taxol requires the implementation of as many as 19 enzymes to produce the desired molecule. Numerous review articles have been published on the subject [222, 223]. IPP and DMAPP are the precursor molecules for the synthesis of GGPP by using the enzyme geranylgeranyl pyrophosphate synthase (GGPPS). GGPP converted to taxa 4(5), 11(12)-diene by the enzyme taxadiene synthase (TXS). After that, taxadiene 5α hydroxylase (T5αH) activity converted it into taxa 4(20),11(12)-dien-5α-ol. At this point, the taxol metabolic pathway is divided into two branches. One branch synthesized taxa 4(20), 11(12)-diene 5α, 13αdiol from taxa 4(20), 11(12)-dien-5α-ol by taxadiene 13α -hydroxylase (T13αH). The other branch of the pathway produces taxa 4(20), 11(12)-diene--α-yl acetate from taxa 4(20), 11(12)-dien-5α-ol by using enzyme taxadiene 5α-ol O-acetyltransferase (TDAT) which is then further converted to taxa 4(20), 11(12) diene 5α-acetoxy-10β-ol by taxane 10β-hydroxylase (T10βH) [224]. The taxa 4(20), 11(12) diene 5α-acetoxy-10β-ol used as a substrate of the taxoid 14β-hydroxylase (T14βH) and produce taxa-4(20),11(12)-dien-5α-acetoxy-1-β-14β-diol. This enzyme causes the diversion of the pathway and does not involve in the biosynthesis of the taxol [27]. These intermediates then undergo four further hydroxylations, an oxidation, and an epoxidation step. The hydroxylation steps are characterized by CYP450's, but these and other enzymes yet have not been fully revealed. These pathway steps produce a theoretical precursor 2-debenzoyltaxane which produce 10-DAB III by the activity of enzyme taxane 2α-O-benzoyltransferase (TBT). Then 10-DAB III converted to baccatin III by 10-deacetylbaccatin III-10-O-acetyltransferase (DBAT). The α-phenylalanine is the precursor of the taxane side chain, and enzyme phenylalanine aminomutase (PAM) converts it into β-phenylalanine. The esterification of the β-phenylalanine by an unknown enzyme produces β-phenylalanine CoA. The taxane side chain is then attached to the taxane body to yield 3′-N-debenzoyl-2-deoxyTaxol by the activity of enzyme baccatin III-13-O-phenylpropanoyl transferase (BAPT). An indefinite enzyme CYP450 then hydroxylates this transitional compound, and the final compound taxol is obtained by the enzyme 3′-N-debenzoyl-20-deoxyT-xol-N-benzoyltransferase (DBTNBT) (Fig. **4**) [223].

Recent advancements in synthetic biology and metabolic engineering describe the potential of the technically improved microbial host to produce a higher amount of desired natural complex compounds [225, 226]. A few steps of taxol biosynthesis have been introduced into different heterologous hosts such as *Saccharomyces cerevisiae, Escherichia coli,* and other higher plants. There is, by all accounts, an undeniable obstruction in constructing an extensive and complex pathway entirely in the heterologous expression system. The alteration of the entire pathway genes in the heterologous hosts is challenging, and significantly taxol biosynthesis genes regulation involving crosstalk signaling and epigenetic modulation itself remains an inadequately comprehended topic. Till date, except a few genes, there is no study available on getting the taxol using metabolic engineering and synthetic biology.

6.1. Taxol Production by Transgenic *Saccharomyces Cerevisiae*

S. cerevisiae has been chosen as heterologous host due to extensive available genetic information and molecular tools such as promoters, selection markers, and integrative and episomal vectors [227]. Recently, many enzymes that encode taxol biosynthesis gene have been isolated and practically expressed in *S. cerevisiae*. At first, Wang, *et al.* [228] transformed and introduced genes encoding the 3-hydroxyl-3- methylglutaryl-coenzyme A (HMG-CoA), GGPPS, and TXS to reconstruct a metabolic pathway in *S. cerevisiae* to produce taxadiene. The successful taxadiene production reported in *S. cerevisiae* by gas chromatography-mass spectrometry (GC-MS). Furthermore, Croteau and coworkers redesigned the primary steps of the biosynthetic pathway of taxol and introduced eight truncated genes encoding GGPPS, TXS, the cytochrome P450's (Cyt-450) taxoid 5α, 13α and 10β hydroxylases, TBT, TDAT, and DBAT acyltransferases into a single yeast host by utilizing three plasmid vectors that bearing different promoters. The Taxadiene-5α-ol was present in a little amount of ~25 mg/L of culture. The yield of taxadiene-5α-yl acetate and taxadiene-5α acetoxy-10β-ol was not recorded during this work. The taxadiene production was readily measurable with the final yield of 0.5 mg/g dry weight (DW) of the cells. However, a limitation in the pathway was experienced at the first Cyt-P450 hydroxylation step [227]. In order to increase the hydroxylation activity, *Taxus* Cyt-P450 reductase and Cyt-P450 oxygenase, which are involved in taxol biosynthesis, were co-expressed in yeast. The transgenic co-expression of these two enzymes in yeast demonstrated a significant primary step in redesigning the pathway of taxol biosynthesis in microbial expression system [229].

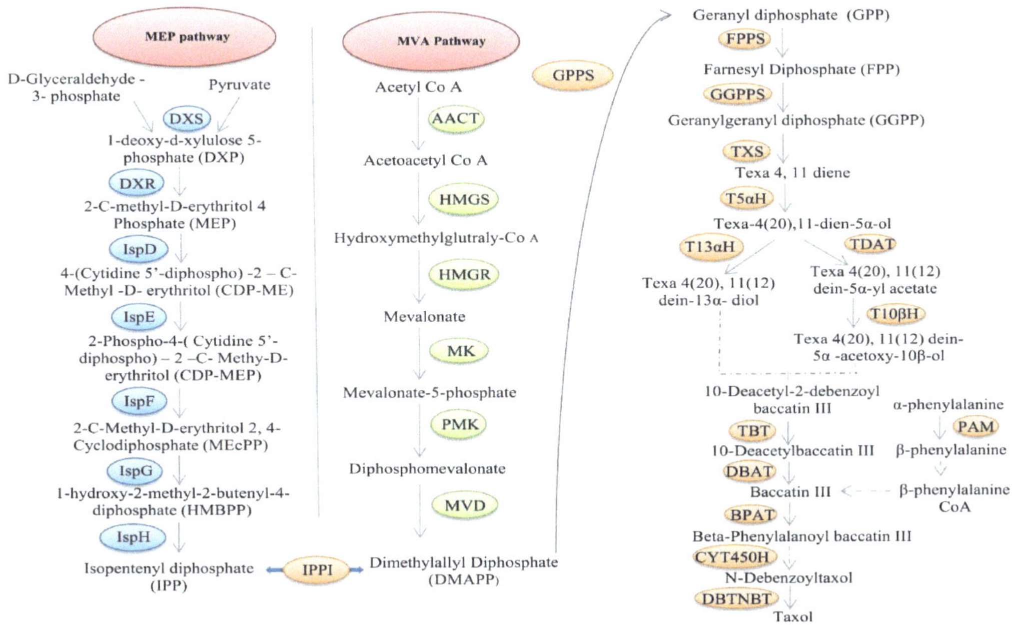

Fig. (4). Biosynthesis pathway of taxol. Abbreviations indicate enzymes: DXS: 1-deoxy-d-xylulo-e-5-phosphate synthase; DXR: deoxy-d-xylulose-5-phosphate reductoisomerase; IspD: 2-C-methy--d-erythritol 4-phosphate cytidylyltransferase; IspE: 4-(cytidine 5′-diphospho)-2-C-methyl-d-erythritol kinase; IspF: 2-C-methyl-d-erythritol 2,4-cyclodiphosphate synthase; IspG: 4-hydroxy-3-methylbut-2-enyl diphosphate synthase; IspH: 4-hydroxy-3-methylbut-2-enyl diphosphate reductase; AACT: acetoacetyl-CoA thiolase; HMGS: 3-hydroxy-3- methyl-glutaryl-CoA synthase; HMGR: 3-hydroxy-3- methyl-glutaryl-CoA reductase; MK: Mevalonate-5-kinase; PMK: Phosphomevalonate kinase; MVD: Mevalonate diphosphate decarboxylase; IPPI: Isopentenyl diphosphate isomerase; GGPPS: geranylgeranyl diphosphate synthase; TXS: taxadiene synthase; T5αH: taxadiene 5α hydroxylase; TDAT: taxadiene 5α-ol O-acetyltransferase; T10βH: taxane 10β-hydroxylase; T14βH: taxane 14β-hydroxylase; T13αH taxadiene 13α-hydroxylase; TBT: taxane 2α-O-benzoyltransferase; DBAT: 10-deacetylbaccatin III-10-O-acetyltransferase; PAM: phenylalanine aminomutase; BAPT: baccatin III-13- O-phenylpropanoyl transferase; CytP450H, cytochrome P450 hydroxylase; DBTNBT: 3′-N-debenzoyl-2′-deoxytaxol-N-benzoyltransferase.

Towards the successful genes expression of taxol biosynthesis, Engels and co-workers in 2008, introduced the early steps genes of taxol biosynthesis in *S. cerevisiae.* Moreover, they also introduced regulatory factors to restrain other undesirable pathways and to increase taxadiene production in genetically modified *S. cerevisiae*. The expression of *T. chinensis* TXS alone and co-expression of TXS and GGPP did not increment the levels of taxadiene. They made use of a truncated HMG-CoA reductase, the rate-controlling enzyme of the MVA pathway and UPC2-1, a mutated regulatory protein which plays a crucial role in cell to uptake steroid aerobically, which induced 50% increase in taxadiene production. Ultimately they used a truncated GGPP from *T. chinensis* with its counterpart from *Sulfolobus acidocaldarius*. The codon optimization of the TXS gene from *T. chinensis* resulted in 8.7 ± 0.85 mg/L high taxadiene production, which was 40-fold high as compared to control [230]. Recently, catalytic capabilities of six different GGPPSs enzymes from *Rana catesbeiana* (GGPPSrc), *Ginkgo biloba* (GGPPSgb), *Erwinia herbicola* (GGPPSeh) *Chlamydomonas reinhardtii* (GGPPScr), *Taxus baccata* x *Taxus cuspidate* (GGPPSbc), and *S. cerevisiae* (GGPPSsc) were analysed with famesyl diphosphate (FPP) substrate by enzyme substrate docking approach. Then, the taxadiene biosynthesis pathway redesigned and constructed in yeast by the TXS transformation and overexpression of erg20 and HMG-CoA reductase genes. The experimental results and computer predictions were similar. The engineered yeast with the GGPPSbc gene yield the highest taxadiene (72.8 mg/L) [231]. Despite these endeavors, tragically taxadiene production has not met the desired demand, and additional efforts are needed to reconstruct the taxol biosynthesis pathway in yeast metabolically.

6.2. Taxol and its Precursor's Production by *E.Coli*

E.coli is a single cell micro-organism and is considered a better expression system as compared to the yeast due to the simple central metabolic pathway and robust regulatory mechanism. The pathway of taxol metabolism comprises of an upstream isoprenoid pathway (native to *E. coli*) and heterologous downstream terpenoid pathway. In *E. coli* native upstream isoprenoid pathway, IPP and DMAPP synthesize low amount of GGPP due to the limited amount of its precursors. Huang and coworkers published the first reports on the construction of the taxol metabolic pathway in *E. coli* in 1998 and 2001. In 1998, during their first attempt, they encountered a limitation due to the formation of insoluble TXS in inclusion bodies. In 2001, they advanced their research and over-expressed three genes encoding isopentenyl diphosphate isomerase (IPPI), GGPPs, and TXS in a single *E. coli* strain. The transgenic strain produced a soluble form of taxadiene with the final yield of 1.3 mg/L under un-optimized conditions [232]. Unluckily, further development of the pathway was halted because of Cyt-P450 expression difficulties in the microbial system. It is assumed that Cyt-P450's lose their function due to insertion, inaccurate folding, and translation into the cell membrane.

Ajikumar, *et al.* [233] group adopted a combinatorial strategy to optimize taxadiene and taxadien-5α -ol, the initial two intermediates of taxol biosynthesis pathway. Analysts named this combinatorial strategy "multivariate-modular pathway engineering". In this strategy, the taxadiene biosynthesis pathway was divided into two modules; the first module was mainly a native upstream isoprenoid (MEP) module, comprises of eight-genes. In this module, only four genes (DXS, IPPI, IspD, and IspF) were carefully optimized by considering them as rate limiting. The second module was a downstream heterologous pathway to taxadiene, which comprises of only two-genes. A total of 32 constructs were prepared with different genotype, promoter strengths, and plasmid copy number. Among them, strain 26 produced the maximum taxadiene yield of 1020 ± 80 mg/L. To convert taxadiene to taxadiene-5α-ol, they also engineered the Cyt-P450 based oxidation in *E.coli.* The transgenic strain yielded 58 mg/L of taxadiene-5α-ol, which was 24,000 fold higher compared to that previously reported in *S. cerevisiae* [227]. In order to maximize the biosynthesis of taxadiene in *E. coli*, an in-silico comparison approach was adopted between maximum anticipated IPP yields and the thermodynamic properties of the DXP and MVA pathways by utilizing different sources of carbon and hosts [234]. The high potential of IPP production was found in *E. coli* and its DXP pathway. They further performed the optimization of taxadiene biosynthesis in various strains via the redesign of codon usage and combinatorial chromosomal engineering in endogenic DXP pathway. Consequently, a high taxadiene producing strain was successfully obtained with 876 ± 60 mg/L yield by merging the upstream DXP pathway (chromosomal engineered) and the downstream taxadiene biosynthesis pathway.

Boghigian, *et al.* [235] used B, and K derived strains of *E. coli* as host for heterologous production of taxadiene. In this experiment, the genes responsible for taxadiene precursors IPP and DMAPP of upstream MEP pathway introduced in *E. coli* using an inducible T7 promoter system. The genes encoding plasmid-borne GGPPS and TXS of the downstream taxadiene pathway were tested with T5, T7, and Trc inducible promoters. The K- derivative strain of *E. coli* yielded 2.5-fold higher taxadiene than the B-derivative strain of *E.coli.* Besides, transcriptome analysis revealed the significant differential expressions of genes in pyruvate metabolism between B and K strains, which explain the differences of taxadiene biosynthesis in these two strains.

The high concentration of oxygenated taxanes with a yield of 570 mg/L was obtained in *E.coli* by optimizing the expression of Cyt-P450, reductase partner interactions, and altering N-terminal modifications [236]. However, the presence of high titers of byproducts catalyzed by T5αH significantly restricted the production of taxadiene-5α-ol and the resulting taxanes [237]. To resolve this problem, many studies have been carried out to illustrate the specific mechanisms involved [237, 238]. Recently, Bian, *et al.* [239] established taxadiene production in mutant *E. coli* T2 and T4 by the engineering of the MVA pathway. The titers of taxadiene produced by mutants T2 and T4 were 11.3 ± 0.5 mg/L (13.2 mg/g DCW) and 5.0 ± 0.7 mg/L (5.9 mg/g DCW), respectively. They next used *A. alternata* TPF6 fungus to engineered MVA pathway with plant taxadiene forming gene introduction. Notably, the over-expressions of the IPPI, HMG-CoA reductase, and TXS were responsible for 61.9 ± 6.3 μg/L taxadiene in the engineered strain GB127. However, there are seven additional steps catalyzed by Cyt-P450 in taxol biosynthesis, which hinders the further study of taxol production in *E. coli.*

6.3. Transformation of *Taxus* Cell Culture

The genetic engineering of *Taxus* cell culture to increase taxol and other related taxoids production is remarkably challenging because of complexity in genetically transforming higher plants like *Taxus* and its slow growth capacity. The initial report about successful genetic transformation was published in 1994 [240]. To develop transgenic culture, *T. brevifolia* and *T. baccata* were genetically transformed using two wild-type *Agrobacterium tumefaciens*. Two years later, Luan, *et al.* [241] reported the transitory GUS gene expression in the embryo of *T. brevifolia.* Albeit none of these studies has given unambiguous affirmation of stable transformation.

Ho, *et al.* [242] carried out the first serious attempt for biotechnological production of taxanes through direct metabolic engineering approach. The transgenic cell culture of *T. mairei* by over-expressing TXS and DBAT genes produced the high yield of taxol. They also observed that the over-expression of TXS and DBAT gene in *T. mairei* is MJ dependent. Ketchum, *et al.* [243] depicted the long-term and stable transformation of the transgenic cell suspension culture of *Taxus*. They used *A. rhizogenes* with binary vector pCAMBIA1301 and *A. tumefaciens* with binary vector pCAMBIA1305.2 separately for the successful transformation of *T. cuspidata* cell lines. Besides, *A. rhizogenes* containing pCAMBIA1301 binary vector was also used to transform a cell line of *T. chinensis.* The two engineered cell lines of *T. cuspidata* were sustained for over 20 months. The transgenic cell line of *T. chinensis* was maintained for over 9 months with no discernable effect on growth or taxol production.

Hairy root cultures were established by transforming seedlings of *T. cuspidata* using *A. rhizogenes* [144]. Initially, 107 lines of hairy root were induced. However, only three lines were stably maintained over 10 months period. Among these hairy root lines, RC11106 root line accumulated 52.5 mg/L of taxol. Unfortunately, taxol production was deficient and inappropriate for commercial scale production. Highest taxol production of 221.8 μg/L was observed in hairy root culture of *T. media* var. Hicksii, when the culture medium of these cell lines supplemented with 100 μM of the precursors p-amino benzoic acid and L-phenylalanine along with MJ [244].

Transgenic cell culture of *T. media* with the same genetic traits as of parent culture was developed by dedifferentiation of the transformed roots. In this experiment, T-DNA of *A. rhizogenes* was induced in Rol C transformed cell line. Besides T-DNA of *A. rhizogenes* and TXS transgene of *T. baccata* under the control of 35S CaMV promoter were tested in TXS transformed cell line. The taxane production in TXS transformed cell line was 265% greater than the untransformed cell line (control) and 170% higher than the Rol C transformed cell line with MJ elicitation [245]. Over-expression of 9-cis-epoxycarotenoid dioxygenase (NCED) gene from *T. chinensis* in transformed *T. chinensis* cell line yielded 48% more abscisic acid (ABA) and 2.7-fold high taxol than the untransformed cell line. The TcNCED1 gene expression in transgenic *T. chinensis* cell line described its significant role in ABA biosynthesis, whereas TcNCED1 gene genetic engineering can also elevate the production of taxol [246]. Sykłowska-Baranek, *et al.* [247] developed hairy root cultures of *T. media* var. Hicksii from *in vitro* cultivated ten-year-old *Taxus* plantlets by using *A. tumefaciens* C58C1 strain that harboring TXS gene of *T. baccata.* Elicitors and Precursor's such as sodium nitroprusside, L-phenylalanine, MJ, and sucrose were used in different combinations to treat transgenic cell lines. The taxol yield of 10.78 mg/L was obtained when transgenic cell lines elicited with MJ + L-phenylalanine. In another study, the same *T. media* var. Hicksii hairy root cell lines carrying TXS transgene were supported with perfluorodecalin (PFD) in aerated and degassed form. The culture medium was treated with coronatine and MJ elicitor and fed with L-phenylalanine and sucrose precursor. The increase in taxanes production was 1,440.8 and 1,432.5 μg/g of DW at 0 and 14 day respectively when the transgenic hairy root cell lines were treated with MJ and supplemented with degassed PFD [145].

6.4. Taxol and its Precursor Production in Heterologous Plants

Plant systems are more favorable for metabolic engineering compared to the microbial system due to the presence of Cty-P450-related biosynthesis genes. These Cyt-P450s are challenging to express in the microbial system. Efforts of utilizing plant cells as heterologous host are not very common, mainly due to sophisticated transformation techniques; require more time to recover transgenic plant and slow growth rate as compared to the microbial system. The initial report on taxanes metabolic engineering in angiosperm was published in 2004 [248]. The accumulation of taxadiene was observed when a recombinant *T. baccata* TXS gene that lacks putative plastid-targeting protein and fusion of a C-terminal histidine (His) tag, constitutively expressed in *Arabidopsis thaliana.* These transgenic plants showed a decrease in hypocotyls length and flowering, growth retardation, and pale-bleached phenotype due to carotenoids and chlorophyll reduction. The lower production of endogenous carotenoids and chlorophylls suggests that the constitutive accumulation of TXS enzyme in the transgenic plant might cause alteration of the GGPP pool. The redirection of GGDP pools was further established by adopting a glucocorticoid-mediated system that drove to 30-fold higher more proficient GGPP recruitment for taxadiene production than the plants that were constitutively expressing the transgene. In 2008 Rontein and colleagues used *Nicotiana sylvestris* plant to introduce genes encoding T5αH and TXS under the control of a trichome specific promoter to produce an initial component of taxol biosynthesis pathway. The co-expression of these genes did not prompt the anticipated production of 5α-hydroxytaxa-4(20), 11(12)-diene in GC-MS profile, and taxadiene-5α-ol was not detected either. Instead, a novel taxane named 5(12)-oxa-3(11)-cyclotaxane (OCT), was characterized by NMR analysis and quantified as 2g/g fresh weight (FW) of leaf [249].

The TXS was also over-expressed in yellow-fruited tomato lines that cannot use GGPP for the biosynthesis of carotenoid. Kovacs, *et al.* [250] reported the redirection of the large available pool of GGPP toward taxadiene production in transgenic tomato plants leading to the yield of 160 mg/Kg taxadiene of dried-freeze fruit. The growth rate of transgenic tomato lines was slower than the controls and produced parthenocarpic fruits or fruits with less than ten viable seeds. It was assumed that the redirection of GGPP for the production of taxadiene might have reduced the level of available GGPP for the biosynthesis of phytohormones involved in growth and fruit development. Similarly, in bryophytes, TXS gene from *T. brevifolia* was constitutively expressed in the moss *Physcomitrella patens* using a ubiquitin promoter. In moss transformants, taxa-4(5),11(12)-diene was produced up to 0.05% FW of tissue. Unlike higher plants, transgenic *P. patens* did not exhibit growth inhibition due to alteration of diterpenoid metabolic pools [251]. A TXS gene from *T. brevifolia* was used to transform the roots of cultured ginseng (*Panax ginseng* C.A. Meyer) to produce taxadiene. The TXS gene was successfully introduced into the ginseng genome, without any change in phenotypes or growth difference. In the transgenic TSS3-2 line taxadiene accumulation was recorded 9.1 μg/g of DW. Elicitation with methyl jasmonate for 3 or 6 days resulted in increase taxadiene accumulation of 14.6 and 15.9 μg/g of DW, respectively [252].

Recently, Hasan, *et al.* [253] constitutively overexpressed the TbTXS gene under the control of CaMV 35S promoter in *Nicotiana benthamiana.*In the transgenic line, the taxadiene production was 11–27 μg/g of DW. Further treatment of the transgenic plant with MJ and the terpenoid pathway shunting with the suppression of the phytoene synthase gene resulted in increased accumulation of taxadiene up to 35 mg/g of DW. The metabolic engineering of taxol biosynthetic pathway in *Artemisia annua*, a Chinese medicinal herb plant, was also successfully performed [254]. The *A. tumefaciens*-mediated transformation of TXS gene within pCAMBIA1304 promoter ensued in the accumulation of taxadiene up to 129.7 μg/g DW of the stem. However, the high expression of TXS did not affect plant growth or photosynthesis in transgenic *A. annua*.

In summary, the functional expression of these enzymes and supporting complexes in the taxol pathway represent a significant challenge that requires scalable methods for enzymes expression and optimization *in vivo*. To date, no technologies can be deployed to engineer the pathway in its entirety, and further step-by-step optimization will be required to complete the taxol pathway.

7. MOLECULAR BASIS OF TAXOL BIOSYNTHESIS

7.1. Transcriptomic Studies for Genes Involved in Taxane Biosynthesis

Next-generation sequencing (NGS) technologies have been established for the evaluation of genome and transcriptome in non-model species that is independent to prior sequence depiction of a genome in the target species [255]. Illumina/Solexa, ABI/SOLiD, 454/Roche, and Helicos are the most commonly used high-throughput sequencing platform for the genomic research of non-model plant species [256]. The bibliometric investigation of *Taxus* species uncovered that information of taxane metabolomics, genomics, transcriptomics, and bioinformatics is as yet constrained and a lot is unknown on the process of epigenetic systems managing taxane biosynthesis [91]. In a primary study of transcriptome sequencing, Jennewein, *et al.* [257] performed the arbitrary sequencing of a cDNA library from MJ elicited *T. cuspidata* cells and revealed all biosynthesis genes of taxol identified at the time. As the first report on the transcriptomic study came out, using Illumina deep sequencing and 454 deep sequencings, many researchers reported transcriptomic study on different organs of *Taxus* species [146, 258 - 260]. Moreover, transcriptome sequencing of *T. chinensis*, *T. cuspidata*, *T. baccata* and *T. media* cultured cells grown under optimized conditions, and MJ elicitation was performed to identify genes and transcription factors (TFs) involved in taxol metabolic pathway [261 - 263]. Such studies confirmed the transcriptional reprogramming under MJ elicitation in taxol biosynthesis pathway. It also led to the recognition of numerous transcripts corresponding to genes involved in taxane biosynthesis, but it could not lead to the discovery of new genes.

In addition, different studies were also conducted to determine the correlation between plant transcriptome and taxane biosynthesis in terms of *Taxus* tissue type. The tag-based digital system of gene expression was used in a study conducted by Hao *et al.* [259]. He *de novo* assembled transcriptome sequence of three *T.mairie* tissues, including root, stem, and leaves. The root has a significant higher expression of taxane biosynthesis genes as compared to leaf and stem. Moreover, many novel and antisense transcripts were also identified. Similar tissues specific studies were also conducted in our lab by transcriptome profiling of *T. yunnanensis* WT and its hybrid cultivar Zd1 with high taxol content and Zd2 with high 10-DAB III contents in their needles. The higher transcript abundance was identified in needles than stem and root in Zd1 and Zd2 cultivar as compared to WT. Different from Zd1, it was identified that Zd2 and WT shared the same gene regulation pattern between tissues [264, 265]. In addition MicroRNAs (miRNAs) identification and MJ effect on their expression were also investigated by Illumina sequencing platform [266].

Since the initial study of Jennewein, *et al.* [257], numerous deep sequencing of *Taxus* transcriptomes have been attempted. These studies cover diverse *Taxus* species, different types of tissues (needles, bark, roots, cambial meristematic cells etc), and different kind of RNAs (mRNAs and microRNAs). A few of these studies have prompted the revelation of novel enzymes involved in the biosynthesis of taxol and undoubtedly will reveal more genes in the coming years.

7.2. TFs Involved in Taxanes Biosynthesis

Currently, not enough is known about molecular mechanisms responsible for the regulation of gene expression associated with taxol biosynthesis. Previously, a few investigations uncovered that TFs such as MYC2, WRKY, MYB, ERF, and BHLH play a positive regulatory role under MJ induction. The higher expression of the genes encoding these TFs assigned increase in taxol biosynthesis [261, 263, 267]. Li, *et al.* [267] identified a WRKY TF, TcWRKY1 as DBAT regulator from *T. chinensis* cells with the yeast one-hybrid system. JA specifically triggered the TcWRKY1 gene expression in *T. chinensis*. Amongst the vital regulatory elements, the biochemical analysis of TcWRKY1 revealed that it specifically interacted with the two W-box (TGAC) cis-elements. Over-expression of TcWRKY1 enhances DBAT expression in suspension cells of *T. chinensis* and the reduction in transcript levels of DBAT were observed by RNA interference (RNAi). Such observations implied that TF WRKY target DBAT gene and involved in the regulation of taxol biosynthesis. Similarly, an investigation was conducted by Lenka, *et al.* [268] on three JA-inducible bHLH TFs in *T. cuspidata*. Based on their high congruence to *Arabidopsis* MYC2, the bHLH TFs were named JAMYC (TcJAMYC1, TcJAMYC2, and TcJAMYC4). The congruence in sequence and expression between AtMYC2 and TcJAMYC referred a preserved feedback to JAs regardless of notable deviation between the lineage of angiosperm and gymnosperm. The results suggest that the TcJAMYC(s) are responsible for JA-mediated gene expression in taxol biosynthesis pathway, yet that they worked as negative regulator instead of a positive regulator. Moreover, 5'-flanking sequence of 550-bp was acquired by Zhang, *et al.* [269] and was verified as TXS promoter. The result of the deletion analysis revealed that GCC-box cis-elements from 150 to 131 were responsive to MJ. Then they distinguished two MJ responsive AP2/ERF TFs, TcERF15 and TcERF12 by binding with the key elements. The TXS gene expression reduced by 2.1 times in TcERF12-overexpressing cells, although increased by 2.5 times in TcERF15-overexpressing cells as a result of over-expression of TcERF12 and TcERF15 in suspension cells of *Taxus*. The above outcomes implied that TcERF12 and TcERF15 are the two efficient regulators transducing MJ signal to the biosynthesis of taxol. Further investigations of more TFs will help to figure out the patterns of regulation by elicitation of MJs and mechanisms at the molecular level of MJ-mediated biosynthesis of taxanes in species of *Taxus*.

SUMMARY

Researches on taxol are directed comprehensively since 1967, but the sustainable commercial supply is still a gigantic problem. Extensive search has been conducted to replace the natural *Taxus* sources, but the phytochemical examinations have demonstrated that taxoids are entirely constrained to the *Taxus* genus except for few angiosperm species and some endophytic fungi. Presently, semi-synthesis and plant cell technology are using as the main source of commercial taxol production. To boost the industrial production, different strategies related to plant cell culture and fermentation by endophytic fungi were combined, but the bottleneck of low and unstable yield still need to be resolved. The biosynthetic pathway of taxol involves numerous enzymatic steps from various enzyme classes, and the evolutionary basis of this pathway is still unsolved. Many of the pathway enzymes are presently known, and the corresponding genes have been cloned and characterised. This primary research led to the metabolic engineering for improvement in taxol production, and it was found that the transgene produced the significantly low amount of taxadiene. Such outcome demonstrates the requirement to restored endeavours related to metabolic engineering to boost yields. An additional difficulty is that not all of the taxol biosynthesis pathway enzymes have been recognized. Accordingly, further research for pathway genes elucidation is needed before the subsequent stage of heterologous pathway reconstruction. Besides, rational approaches provided understanding to know: how differential genetic expression and TFs regulate biosynthesis of taxol.

ABBREVIATIONS

10-DAB III	10-deacetylbaccatin III
ABA	Abscisic acid

AV	Atrioventricular
BAC III	Bbaccatin III
BAPT	Baccatin III 3-animo-3-phenylpropanoyl transferase
CCNSC	Cancer chemotherapy national service center
CMCs	Cambial meristematic cells
DBAT	10-deacetylbaccatin III 10-O-acetyltransferase
DBTNBT	3'-N-debenzoylTaxol N-benzoyltransferase
DDC	Dedifferentiated culture
DES	Diethyl sulfate
DMAPP	Dimethylallyl diphosphate
DMSO	Dimethyl sulfoxide
DT	10-deacetylTaxol
DXP	Deoxylulose 5-phosphate
ECG	Electrocardiogram
FDA	Food and drug administration
GDP	Guanosine diphosphate
GGPPS	Geranylgeranyl diphosphate synthase
GTP	Guanosine triphosphate
HPLC	High-performance liquid chromatography
HMG-CoA reductase	3-hydroxy-3-methylglutaryl-CoA reductase
IPPI	Isopentenyl diphosphate isomerase
IPP	Isopentenyl diphosphate
IUPAC	International union of pure and applied chemistry
JA	Jasmonic acid
kD	Killo dalton
MEP	2C-methyl-D-erythritol-4-phosphate pathway
MJ	Methyl jasmonate
MVA	Mevalonate pathway
NADPH	Nicotinamide adenine dinucleotide phosphate
NCED	9-cis-epoxycarotenoid dioxygenase
NCI	National cancer institute
ROS	Reactive oxygen species
T10βH	Taxane 10-β-hydroxylase
T13αH	Taxane 13-α- hydroxylase
T14βH	Taxane 14-β-hydroxylase

TBT	Taxane 2-α-O-benzoyltransferase
TDAT	Taxadiene-5-α-ol O-acetyltransferase
TXS	Taxadiene synthase
USDA	U.S. division of ggriculture
XDT	7-b-xylosyl-10-deacetylTaxol

CONSENT FOR PUBLICATION

Not applicable.

CONFLICT OF INTEREST

The authors confirm that this chapter contents have no conflict of interest.

ACKNOWLEDGEMENTS

All the authors have equally contributed to this work. This study was supported by grants from Forestry Science and Technology Innovation Project of Guangdong Province (2017KJCX044), the YangFang Project of Guangdong Province, China (Grant No. 2014YT02S044), Technology Planning Project of Guangdong Province, China (Grant No. 2014A070713005 and 2016A020208003), and Science and Technology Planning Project of Guangdong Province, China (2017B020205001).

REFERENCES

[1] Verpoorte, R. Secondary metabolism.*Metabolic engineering of plant secondary metabolism*; Springer, **2000**, pp. 1-29.
[http://dx.doi.org/10.1007/978-94-015-9423-3_1]

[2] Verpoorte, R.; Memelink, J. Engineering secondary metabolite production in plants. *Curr. Opin. Biotechnol.,* **2002**, *13*(2), 181-187.
[http://dx.doi.org/10.1016/S0958-1669(02)00308-7] [PMID: 11950573]

[3] Dewick, P.M. *Medicinal natural products: a biosynthetic approach*; John Wiley & Sons, **2002**.

[4] Colegate, S.M.; Molyneux, R.J. *Bioactive Natural Products: Detection, Isolation, and Structural Determination, 2nd Edi*; Crc Press, **2007**.
[http://dx.doi.org/10.1201/9781420006889]

[5] Visalakchi, S.; Muthumary, J. Taxol (anticancer drug) producing endophytic fungi: an overview. *Int. J. Pharma Bio Sci.,* **2010**.

[6] Kinghorn, A.D.; Chin, Y-W.; Swanson, S.M. Discovery of natural product anticancer agents from biodiverse organisms. *Curr. Opin. Drug Discov. Devel.,* **2009**, *12*(2), 189-196.
[PMID: 19333864]

[7] Cragg, G.M.; Newman, D.J. Plants as a source of anti-cancer agents. *J. Ethnopharmacol.,* **2005**, *100*(1-2), 72-79.
[http://dx.doi.org/10.1016/j.jep.2005.05.011] [PMID: 16009521]

[8] Cragg, G.M.; Newman, D.J.; Snader, K.M. Natural products in drug discovery and development. *J.*

Nat. Prod., **1997**, *60*(1), 52-60.
[http://dx.doi.org/10.1021/np9604893] [PMID: 9014353]

[9] Newman, D.J.; Cragg, G.M. Natural products as sources of new drugs over the last 25 years. *J. Nat. Prod.*, **2007**, *70*(3), 461-477.
[http://dx.doi.org/10.1021/np068054v] [PMID: 17309302]

[10] Perez, E.A. Paclitaxel in Breast Cancer. *Oncologist,* **1998**, *3*(6), 373-389.
[PMID: 10388129]

[11] Crown, J.; O'Leary, M.; Ooi, W-S. Docetaxel and paclitaxel in the treatment of breast cancer: a review of clinical experience. *Oncologist,* **2004**, *9* Suppl. 2, 24-32.
[http://dx.doi.org/10.1634/theoncologist.9-suppl_2-24] [PMID: 15161988]

[12] Ozols, R.F. Paclitaxel (Taxol)/carboplatin combination chemotherapy in the treatment of advanced ovarian cancer [J]. *Semin. Oncol.*, **2000**, *27*(3) Suppl. 7, 3-7.
[PMID: 10952119]

[13] Gréen, H. Strategies for individualization of Taxol (paclitaxel) treatment of ovarian cancer. *Department of clinical pharmacology,* **2002**.

[14] Bharadwaj, R.; Das, P.J.; Pal, P.; Mazumder, B. Topical delivery of paclitaxel for treatment of skin cancer. *Drug Dev. Ind. Pharm.*, **2016**, *42*(9), 1482-1494.
[http://dx.doi.org/10.3109/03639045.2016.1151028] [PMID: 26850463]

[15] Akerley, W., III Paclitaxel in advanced non-small cell lung cancer : an alternative high-dose weekly schedule. *Chest,* **2000**, *117*(4) Suppl. 1, 152S-155S.
[http://dx.doi.org/10.1378/chest.117.4_suppl_1.152S] [PMID: 10777471]

[16] Li, G.; Faibushevich, A.; Turunen, B.J.; Yoon, S.O.; Georg, G.; Michaelis, M.L.; Dobrowsky, R.T. Stabilization of the cyclin-dependent kinase 5 activator, p35, by paclitaxel decreases beta-amyloid toxicity in cortical neurons. *J. Neurochem.*, **2003**, *84*(2), 347-362.
[http://dx.doi.org/10.1046/j.1471-4159.2003.01526.x] [PMID: 12558997]

[17] Fu, Y.; Li, S.; Zu, Y.; Yang, G.; Yang, Z.; Luo, M.; Jiang, S.; Wink, M.; Efferth, T. Medicinal chemistry of paclitaxel and its analogues. *Curr. Med. Chem.*, **2009**, *16*(30), 3966-3985.
[http://dx.doi.org/10.2174/092986709789352277] [PMID: 19747129]

[18] Bajaj, N.R.; Garratt, K.N. Clinical studies with paclitaxel - eluting stent systems. *Curr. Pharm. Des.*, **2010**, *16*(36), 4025-4036.
[http://dx.doi.org/10.2174/138161210794454860] [PMID: 21208184]

[19] Woo, D.D.L.; Miao, S.Y.P.; Pelayo, J.C.; Woolf, A.S. Taxol inhibits progression of congenital polycystic kidney disease. *Nature,* **1994**, *368*(6473), 750-753.
[http://dx.doi.org/10.1038/368750a0] [PMID: 7908721]

[20] Unverdorben, M.; Vallbracht, C.; Cremers, B.; Heuer, H.; Hengstenberg, C.; Maikowski, C.; Werner, G.S.; Antoni, D.; Kleber, F.X.; Bocksch, W.; Leschke, M.; Ackermann, H.; Boxberger, M.; Speck, U.; Degenhardt, R.; Scheller, B. Paclitaxel-coated balloon catheter versus paclitaxel-coated stent for the treatment of coronary in-stent restenosis. *Circulation,* **2009**, *119*(23), 2986-2994.
[http://dx.doi.org/10.1161/CIRCULATIONAHA.108.839282] [PMID: 19487593]

[21] Xiao, J.; Liang, D.; Liu, Y.; Zhang, H.; Liu, Y.; Zhao, H.; Li, J.; Peng, L.; Zhou, Z.; Chen, Y.H. Taxol, a microtubule stabilizer, improves cardiac functional recovery during postischemic reperfusion in rat *in vitro*. *Cardiovasc. Ther.*, **2012**, *30*(1), 12-30.
[http://dx.doi.org/10.1111/j.1755-5922.2010.00163.x] [PMID: 20553295]

[22] Zhang, B.; Maiti, A.; Shively, S.; Lakhani, F.; McDonald-Jones, G.; Bruce, J.; Lee, E.B.; Xie, S.X.; Joyce, S.; Li, C.; Toleikis, P.M.; Lee, V.M.; Trojanowski, J.Q. Microtubule-binding drugs offset tau sequestration by stabilizing microtubules and reversing fast axonal transport deficits in a tauopathy model. *Proc. Natl. Acad. Sci. USA,* **2005**, *102*(1), 227-231.
[http://dx.doi.org/10.1073/pnas.0406361102] [PMID: 15615853]

[23] Goodman, J.; Walsh, V. *The Story of Taxol: Nature and Politics in the Pursuit of an Anti-Cancer Drug*; Cambridge University Press, **2001**.

[24] Wani, M.C.; Taylor, H.L.; Wall, M.E.; Coggon, P.; McPhail, A.T. Plant antitumor agents. VI. The isolation and structure of taxol, a novel antileukemic and antitumor agent from Taxus brevifolia. *J. Am. Chem. Soc.*, **1971**, *93*(9), 2325-2327.
[http://dx.doi.org/10.1021/ja00738a045] [PMID: 5553076]

[25] Suffness, M. Chapter 32. Taxol: From Discovery to Therapeutic Use. *Annu. Rep. Med. Chem.*, **1993**, *28*, 305-314.
[http://dx.doi.org/10.1016/S0065-7743(08)60902-1]

[26] Nikolic, V.D.; Savic, I.M.; Savic, I.M.; Nikolic, L.B.; Stankovic, M.Z.; Marinkovic, V.D. Paclitaxel as an anticancer agent: isolation, activity, synthesis and stability. *Cent. Eur. J. Med.*, **2011**, *6*(5), 527.

[27] Malik, S.; Cusidó, R.M.; Mirjalili, M.H.; Moyano, E.; Palazón, J.; Bonfill, M. Production of the anticancer drug taxol in Taxus baccata suspension cultures: A review. *Process Biochem.*, **2011**, *46*(1), 23-34.
[http://dx.doi.org/10.1016/j.procbio.2010.09.004]

[28] Leone, L.M.; Roberts, S.C. *Accessing anti-cancer natural products by plant cell culture*; Springer New York, **2013**, pp. 193-211.
[http://dx.doi.org/10.1007/978-1-4614-4654-5_8]

[29] Yared, J.A.; Tkaczuk, K.H. Update on taxane development: new analogs and new formulations. *Drug Des. Devel. Ther.*, **2012**, *6*, 371-384.
[PMID: 23251087]

[30] Żwawiak, J.; Zaprutko, L. A brief history of taxol. *Journal of Medical Science,* **2016**, *83*(1), 47-52.

[31] Cooper, G.M. *The Cell: A Molecular Approach. 2nd Edi*; ASM Press, **2000**.

[32] Desai, A.; Mitchison, T.J. Microtubule polymerization dynamics. *Annu. Rev. Cell Dev. Biol.*, **1997**, *13*, 83-117.
[http://dx.doi.org/10.1146/annurev.cellbio.13.1.83] [PMID: 9442869]

[33] Orr, G.A.; Verdier-Pinard, P.; McDaid, H.; Horwitz, S.B. Mechanisms of Taxol resistance related to microtubules. *Oncogene,* **2003**, *22*(47), 7280-7295.
[http://dx.doi.org/10.1038/sj.onc.1206934] [PMID: 14576838]

[34] Rao, S.; Krauss, N.E.; Heerding, J.M.; Swindell, C.S.; Ringel, I.; Orr, G.A.; Horwitz, S.B. 3′-(--azidobenzamido)taxol photolabels the N-terminal 31 amino acids of beta-tubulin. *J. Biol. Chem.*, **1994**, *269*(5), 3132-3134.
[PMID: 7906266]

[35] Bharadwaj, R.; Yu, H. The spindle checkpoint, aneuploidy, and cancer. *Oncogene,* **2004**, *23*(11), 2016-2027.
[http://dx.doi.org/10.1038/sj.onc.1207374] [PMID: 15021889]

[36] Brito, D.A.; Yang, Z.; Rieder, C.L. Microtubules do not promote mitotic slippage when the spindle assembly checkpoint cannot be satisfied. *J. Cell Biol.*, **2008**, *182*(4), 623-629.
[http://dx.doi.org/10.1083/jcb.200805072] [PMID: 18710927]

[37] Schiff, P.B.; Fant, J.; Horwitz, S.B. Promotion of microtubule assembly *in vitro* by taxol. *Nature,* **1979**, *277*(5698), 665-667.
[http://dx.doi.org/10.1038/277665a0] [PMID: 423966]

[38] Schiff, P.B.; Horwitz, S.B. Taxol stabilizes microtubules in mouse fibroblast cells. *Proc. Natl. Acad. Sci. USA,* **1980**, *77*(3), 1561-1565.
[http://dx.doi.org/10.1073/pnas.77.3.1561] [PMID: 6103535]

[39] Mullins, D.W.; Burger, C.J.; Elgert, K.D. Paclitaxel enhances macrophage IL-12 production in tumor-bearing hosts through nitric oxide. *J. Immunol.*, **1999**, *162*(11), 6811-6818.

[PMID: 10352302]

[40] Burkhart, C.A.; Berman, J.W.; Swindell, C.S.; Horwitz, S.B. Relationship between the structure of taxol and other taxanes on induction of tumor necrosis factor-α gene expression and cytotoxicity. *Cancer Res.,* **1994**, *54*(22), 5779-5782.
[PMID: 7954398]

[41] Pretto, F.; Elia, G.; Castioni, N.; Neri, D. Preclinical evaluation of IL2-based immunocytokines supports their use in combination with dacarbazine, paclitaxel and TNF-based immunotherapy. *Cancer Immunol. Immunother.,* **2014**, *63*(9), 901-910.
[http://dx.doi.org/10.1007/s00262-014-1562-7] [PMID: 24893857]

[42] Wang, T.H.; Wang, H.S.; Soong, Y.K. Paclitaxel-induced cell death: where the cell cycle and apoptosis come together. *Cancer,* **2000**, *88*(11), 2619-2628.
[http://dx.doi.org/10.1002/1097-0142(20000601)88:11<2619::AID-CNCR26>3.0.CO;2-J] [PMID: 10861441]

[43] Nguyen, D.M.; Chen, G.A.; Reddy, R.; Tsai, W.; Schrump, W.D.; Cole, G., Jr; Schrump, D.S. Potentiation of paclitaxel cytotoxicity in lung and esophageal cancer cells by pharmacologic inhibition of the phosphoinositide 3-kinase/protein kinase B (Akt)-mediated signaling pathway. *J. Thorac. Cardiovasc. Surg.,* **2004**, *127*(2), 365-375.
[http://dx.doi.org/10.1016/j.jtcvs.2003.09.033] [PMID: 14762343]

[44] Kampan, N. C.; Madondo, M. T.; McNally, O. M.; Quinn, M.; Plebanski, M. Paclitaxel and its evolving role in the management of ovarian cancer. *BioMed research international 2015,* **2015**.
[http://dx.doi.org/10.1155/2015/413076]

[45] Alexandre, J.; Hu, Y.; Lu, W.; Pelicano, H.; Huang, P. Novel action of paclitaxel against cancer cells: bystander effect mediated by reactive oxygen species. *Cancer Res.,* **2007**, *67*(8), 3512-3517.
[http://dx.doi.org/10.1158/0008-5472.CAN-06-3914] [PMID: 17440056]

[46] Hadzic, T.; Aykin-Burns, N.; Zhu, Y.; Coleman, M.C.; Leick, K.; Jacobson, G.M.; Spitz, D.R. Paclitaxel combined with inhibitors of glucose and hydroperoxide metabolism enhances breast cancer cell killing via H2O2-mediated oxidative stress. *Free Radic. Biol. Med.,* **2010**, *48*(8), 1024-1033.
[http://dx.doi.org/10.1016/j.freeradbiomed.2010.01.018] [PMID: 20083194]

[47] Gan, L.; Chen, S.; Wang, Y.; Watahiki, A.; Bohrer, L.; Sun, Z.; Wang, Y.; Huang, H. Inhibition of the androgen receptor as a novel mechanism of taxol chemotherapy in prostate cancer. *Cancer Res.,* **2009**, *69*(21), 8386-8394.
[http://dx.doi.org/10.1158/0008-5472.CAN-09-1504] [PMID: 19826044]

[48] Sevko, A.; Kremer, V.; Falk, C.; Umansky, L.; Shurin, M.R.; Shurin, G.V.; Umansky, V. Application of paclitaxel in low non-cytotoxic doses supports vaccination with melanoma antigens in normal mice. *J. Immunotoxicol.,* **2012**, *9*(3), 275-281.
[http://dx.doi.org/10.3109/1547691X.2012.655343] [PMID: 22449053]

[49] Sevko, A.; Michels, T.; Vrohlings, M.; Umansky, L.; Beckhove, P.; Kato, M.; Shurin, G.V.; Shurin, M.R.; Umansky, V. Anti-tumor Effect of Paclitaxel is Mediated by Inhibition of MDSCs and Chronic Inflammation in the Spontaneous Melanoma Model. *J. Immunol.,* **2013**, *190*(5), 2464-2471.
[http://dx.doi.org/10.4049/jimmunol.1202781] [PMID: 23359505]

[50] Markman, M.; Kennedy, A.; Webster, K.; Kulp, B.; Peterson, G.; Belinson, J. Paclitaxel-associated hypersensitivity reactions: experience of the gynecologic oncology program of the Cleveland Clinic Cancer Center. *J. Clin. Oncol.,* **2000**, *18*(1), 102-105.
[http://dx.doi.org/10.1200/JCO.2000.18.1.102] [PMID: 10623699]

[51] Weiss, R.B. Hypersensitivity reactions. *Semin. Oncol.,* **1992**, *19*(5), 458-477.
[PMID: 1384149]

[52] Sibaud, V.; Lebœuf, N.R.; Roche, H.; Belum, V.R.; Gladieff, L.; Deslandres, M.; Montastruc, M.; Eche, A.; Vigarios, E.; Dalenc, F.; Lacouture, M.E. Dermatological adverse events with taxane chemotherapy. *Eur. J. Dermatol.,* **2016**, *26*(5), 427-443.

[PMID: 27550571]

[53] Barbee, M.S.; Owonikoko, T.K.; Harvey, R.D. Taxanes: vesicants, irritants, or just irritating? *Ther. Adv. Med. Oncol.,* **2014**, *6*(1), 16-20. [http://dx.doi.org/10.1177/1758834013510546] [PMID: 24381657]

[54] Stanford, B.L.; Hardwicke, F. A review of clinical experience with paclitaxel extravasations. *Support. Care Cancer,* **2003**, *11*(5), 270-277. [PMID: 12690542]

[55] Pérez Fidalgo, J.A.; García Fabregat, L.; Cervantes, A.; Margulies, A.; Vidall, C.; Roila, F. ESMO Guidelines Working Group. Management of chemotherapy extravasation: ESMO--EONS clinical practice guidelines. *Eur. J. Oncol. Nurs.,* **2012**, *16*(5), 528-534. [http://dx.doi.org/10.1016/j.ejon.2012.09.004] [PMID: 23304728]

[56] Schulmeister, L. *In Extravasation management: Clinical update, Seminars in Oncology Nursing*; Elsevier, **2011**, pp. 82-90.

[57] Ascherman, J.A.; Knowles, S.L.; Attkiss, K. Docetaxel (taxotere) extravasation: a report of five cases with treatment recommendations. *Ann. Plast. Surg.,* **2000**, *45*(4), 438-441. [http://dx.doi.org/10.1097/00000637-200045040-00016] [PMID: 11037169]

[58] Bolognia, J.L.; Cooper, D.L.; Glusac, E.J. Toxic erythema of chemotherapy: a useful clinical term. *J. Am. Acad. Dermatol.,* **2008**, *59*(3), 524-529. [http://dx.doi.org/10.1016/j.jaad.2008.05.018] [PMID: 18694683]

[59] Spicknall, K.E.; Mutasim, D.F. Localized toxic erythema of chemotherapy during treatment with paclitaxel. *Int. J. Dermatol.,* **2014**, *53*(1), e3-e5. [http://dx.doi.org/10.1111/j.1365-4632.2012.05573.x] [PMID: 23451872]

[60] Park, S.B.; Lin, C.S.Y.; Krishnan, A.V.; Friedlander, M.L.; Lewis, C.R.; Kiernan, M.C. Early, progressive, and sustained dysfunction of sensory axons underlies paclitaxel-induced neuropathy. *Muscle Nerve,* **2011**, *43*(3), 367-374. [http://dx.doi.org/10.1002/mus.21874] [PMID: 21321953]

[61] Lee, J.J.; Swain, S.M. Peripheral neuropathy induced by microtubule-stabilizing agents. *J. Clin. Oncol.,* **2006**, *24*(10), 1633-1642. [http://dx.doi.org/10.1200/JCO.2005.04.0543] [PMID: 16575015]

[62] Argyriou, A.A.; Koltzenburg, M.; Polychronopoulos, P.; Papapetropoulos, S.; Kalofonos, H.P. Peripheral nerve damage associated with administration of taxanes in patients with cancer. *Crit. Rev. Oncol. Hematol.,* **2008**, *66*(3), 218-228. [http://dx.doi.org/10.1016/j.critrevonc.2008.01.008] [PMID: 18329278]

[63] Sahenk, Z.; Barohn, R.; New, P.; Mendell, J.R. Taxol neuropathy. Electrodiagnostic and sural nerve biopsy findings. *Arch. Neurol.,* **1994**, *51*(7), 726-729. [http://dx.doi.org/10.1001/archneur.1994.00540190110024] [PMID: 7912506]

[64] Melli, G.; Taiana, M.; Camozzi, F.; Triolo, D.; Podini, P.; Quattrini, A.; Taroni, F.; Lauria, G. Alpha-lipoic acid prevents mitochondrial damage and neurotoxicity in experimental chemotherapy neuropathy. *Exp. Neurol.,* **2008**, *214*(2), 276-284. [http://dx.doi.org/10.1016/j.expneurol.2008.08.013] [PMID: 18809400]

[65] Rovini, A.; Carré, M.; Bordet, T.; Pruss, R.M.; Braguer, D. Olesoxime prevents microtubule-targeting drug neurotoxicity: selective preservation of EB comets in differentiated neuronal cells. *Biochem. Pharmacol.,* **2010**, *80*(6), 884-894. [http://dx.doi.org/10.1016/j.bcp.2010.04.018] [PMID: 20417191]

[66] Verstappen, C.C.; Postma, T.J.; Geldof, A.A.; Heimans, J.J. Amifostine protects against chemotherapy-induced neurotoxicity: an *in vitro* investigation. *Anticancer Res.,* **2004**, *24*(4), 2337-2341. [PMID: 15330181]

[67] Kamineni, P.; Prakasa, K.; Hasan, S.P.; Akula, R.; Dawkins, F. Cardiotoxicities of paclitaxel in African Americans. *J. Natl. Med. Assoc.*, **2003**, *95*(10), 977-981.
[PMID: 14620711]

[68] Arbuck, S.G.; Strauss, H.; Rowinsky, E.; Christian, M.; Suffness, M.; Adams, J.; Oakes, M.; McGuire, W.; Reed, E.; Gibbs, H. A reassessment of cardiac toxicity associated with Taxol. *J. Natl. Cancer Inst. Monogr.*, **1993**, (15), 117-130.
[PMID: 7912518]

[69] Pestalozzi, B.C.; Sotos, G.A.; Choyke, P.L.; Fisherman, J.S.; Cowan, K.H.; O'Shaughnessy, J.A. Typhlitis resulting from treatment with taxol and doxorubicin in patients with metastatic breast cancer. *Cancer,* **1993**, *71*(5), 1797-1800.
[http://dx.doi.org/10.1002/1097-0142(19930301)71:5<1797::AID-CNCR2820710514>3.0.CO;2-B]
[PMID: 8095437]

[70] Risinger, A.L.; Riffle, S.M.; Lopus, M.; Jordan, M.A.; Wilson, L.; Mooberry, S.L. The taccalonolides and paclitaxel cause distinct effects on microtubule dynamics and aster formation. *Mol. Cancer,* **2014**, *13*(1), 41.
[http://dx.doi.org/10.1186/1476-4598-13-41] [PMID: 24576146]

[71] Tallon, B.; Blanchard, E.; Goldberg, L.J. Permanent chemotherapy-induced alopecia: case report and review of the literature. *J. Am. Acad. Dermatol.*, **2010**, *63*(2), 333-336.
[http://dx.doi.org/10.1016/j.jaad.2009.06.063] [PMID: 20471136]

[72] Paus, R.; Haslam, I.S.; Sharov, A.A.; Botchkarev, V.A. Pathobiology of chemotherapy-induced hair loss. *Lancet Oncol.*, **2013**, *14*(2), e50-e59.
[http://dx.doi.org/10.1016/S1470-2045(12)70553-3] [PMID: 23369683]

[73] Sparano, J.A.; Wang, M.; Martino, S.; Jones, V.; Perez, E.A.; Saphner, T.; Wolff, A.C.; Sledge, G.W., Jr; Wood, W.C.; Davidson, N.E. Weekly paclitaxel in the adjuvant treatment of breast cancer. *N. Engl. J. Med.*, **2008**, *358*(16), 1663-1671.
[http://dx.doi.org/10.1056/NEJMoa0707056] [PMID: 18420499]

[74] Trüeb, R.M. Chemotherapy-induced anagen effluvium: diffuse or patterned? *Dermatology (Basel),* **2007**, *215*(1), 1-2.
[http://dx.doi.org/10.1159/000102025] [PMID: 17587831]

[75] Hope, S.; Rugo, M.E.; Aimee, L.; Payne, S. Chemotherapy-induced alopecia. https://www.uptodate.com/contents/chemotherapy-induced-alopecia

[76] Chhetra Lalli, R.; Kaur, K.; Dadsena, S.; Chakraborti, A.; Srinivasan, R.; Ghosh, S. Maackia amurensis agglutinin enhances paclitaxel induced cytotoxicity in cultured non-small cell lung cancer cells. *Biochimie,* **2015**, *115*, 93-107.
[http://dx.doi.org/10.1016/j.biochi.2015.05.002] [PMID: 25978938]

[77] Cope, E.A. Taxaceae: The genera and cultivated species. *Bot. Rev.*, **1998**, *64*(4), 291-322.
[http://dx.doi.org/10.1007/BF02857621]

[78] Bedi, Y.; Ogra, R. KIRAN, K.; Kaul, B.; Kapil, R., Yew (Taxus spp.). A new look on utilization, cultivation and conservation. *Supplement to cultivation and utilization of medicinal plants,* **1996**, 443-456.

[79] Wheeler, N.C.; Jech, K.; Masters, S.; Brobst, S.W.; Alvarado, A.B.; Hoover, A.J.; Snader, K.M. Effects of genetic, epigenetic, and environmental factors on taxol content in Taxus brevifolia and related species. *J. Nat. Prod.*, **1992**, *55*(4), 432-440.
[http://dx.doi.org/10.1021/np50082a005] [PMID: 1355111]

[80] Németh-Kiss, V.; Forgács, E.; Cserháti, T.; Schmidt, G. Taxol content of various Taxus species in Hungary. *J. Pharm. Biomed. Anal.*, **1996**, *14*(8-10), 997-1001.
[http://dx.doi.org/10.1016/0731-7085(95)01682-1] [PMID: 8818006]

[81] Isah, T. Natural sources of taxol. *Br. J. Pharm. Res.*, **2015**, *6*(4), 214-227.

[http://dx.doi.org/10.9734/BJPR/2015/16293]

[82] Guéritte-Voegelein, F.; Guénard, D.; Potier, P. Taxol and derivatives: A biogenetic hypothesis. *J. Nat. Prod.,* **1987**, *50*(1), 9-18.
[http://dx.doi.org/10.1021/np50049a002] [PMID: 2885400]

[83] Stahlhut, R.; Park, G.; Petersen, R.; Ma, W.; Hylands, P. The occurrence of the anti-cancer diterpene taxol in Podocarpus gracilior Pilger (Podocarpaceae). *Biochem. Syst. Ecol.,* **1999**, *27*(6), 613-622.
[http://dx.doi.org/10.1016/S0305-1978(98)00118-5]

[84] Wang, Y-F.; Shi, Q-W.; Dong, M.; Kiyota, H.; Gu, Y-C.; Cong, B. Natural taxanes: developments since 1828. *Chem. Rev.,* **2011**, *111*(12), 7652-7709.
[http://dx.doi.org/10.1021/cr100147u] [PMID: 21970550]

[85] Chen, C.; Luo, S. New plant resources for 10 deacetylbacctin III. *Chinese Journal of Pharmaceuticals,* **1997**.

[86] Hoffman, A.; Khan, W.; Worapong, J.; Strobel, G.A.; Hriffin, D.; Arbogast, B.; Barofsky, D.; Boone, R.B.; Ning, L.; Zheng, P.; Daley, L.S. *Bioprospecting for taxol in angiosperm plant extracts using high performance liquid chromatographythermospray mass spectrometry to detect the anticancer agent and its related metabolites in filbert trees*; , **1998**, Vol. 13, pp. 22-31.

[87] Bestoso, F.; Ottaggio, L.; Armirotti, A.; Balbi, A.; Damonte, G.; Degan, P.; Mazzei, M.; Cavalli, F.; Ledda, B.; Miele, M. *In vitro* cell cultures obtained from different explants of Corylus avellana produce Taxol and taxanes. *BMC Biotechnol.,* **2006**, *6*(1), 45.
[http://dx.doi.org/10.1186/1472-6750-6-45] [PMID: 17150090]

[88] Kelsey, R.G.; Nan, C.V. Taxol and Cephalomannine Concentrations in the Foliage and Bark of Shade-Grown and Sun-Exposed Taxus brevifolia Trees. *J. Nat. Prod.,* **2004**, *55*(7), 912-917.
[http://dx.doi.org/10.1021/np50085a010]

[89] Ottaggio, L.; Bestoso, F.; Armirotti, A.; Balbi, A.; Damonte, G.; Mazzei, M.; Sancandi, M.; Miele, M. Taxanes from shells and leaves of Corylus avellana. *J. Nat. Prod.,* **2008**, *71*(1), 58-60.
[http://dx.doi.org/10.1021/np0704046] [PMID: 18163585]

[90] Phuc, D. T. H.; Popovich, D. G. *Screening for paclitaxel and other taxanes in kernel and shell of Corylus avellana (Hazelnut)*; , **2017**, 6, pp. (2)247-254.

[91] Miele, M.; Mumot, A.M.; Zappa, A.; Romano, P.; Ottaggio, L. Hazel and other sources of paclitaxel and related compounds. *Phytochem. Rev.,* **2012**, *11*(2-3), 211-225.
[http://dx.doi.org/10.1007/s11101-012-9234-8]

[92] Liu, X.K.; Liu, J.J. *New source for L-iditol and taxanes*; Nature Publishing Group, **2008**.

[93] Holton, R.A.; Kim, H.B.; Somoza, C.; Liang, F.; Biediger, R.J.; Boatman, P.D.; Shindo, M.; Smith, C.C.; Kim, S. First total synthesis of taxol. 2. Completion of the C and D rings. *J. Am. Chem. Soc.,* **1994**, *116*(4), 1599-1600.
[http://dx.doi.org/10.1021/ja00083a067]

[94] Nicolaou, K.C.; Yang, Z.; Liu, J.J.; Ueno, H.; Nantermet, P.G.; Guy, R.K.; Claiborne, C.F.; Renaud, J.; Couladouros, E.A.; Paulvannan, K. Total synthesis of taxol. *Nature,* **1994**, *367*(6464), 630-634.
[http://dx.doi.org/10.1038/367630a0] [PMID: 7906395]

[95] Ketchum, R.E.; Gibson, D.M.; Croteau, R.B.; Shuler, M.L. The kinetics of taxoid accumulation in cell suspension cultures of Taxus following elicitation with methyl jasmonate. *Biotechnol. Bioeng.,* **1999**, *62*(1), 97-105.
[http://dx.doi.org/10.1002/(SICI)1097-0290(19990105)62:1<97::AID-BIT11>3.0.CO;2-C] [PMID: 10099517]

[96] Masters, J.J.; Link, J.T.; Snyder, L.B.; Young, W.B.; Danishefsky, S.J. A Total Synthesis of Taxol. *Angew. Chem. Int. Ed.,* **1995**, *34*(16), 1723-1726.
[http://dx.doi.org/10.1002/anie.199517231]

[97] Danishefsky, S.J.; Masters, J.J.; Young, W.B.; Link, J.T.; Snyder, L.B.; Magee, T.V.; Jung, D.K.; Isaacs, R.C.A.; Bornmann, W.G.; Alaimo, C.A.; Coburn, C.A.; Di Grandi, M.J. Total Synthesis of Baccatin III and Taxol. *J. Am. Chem. Soc.,* **1996**, *118*(12), 2843-2859. [http://dx.doi.org/10.1021/ja952692a]

[98] Wender, P.A.; Badham, N.F.; Conway, S.P.; Floreancig, P.E.; Glass, T.E.; Houze, J.B.; Krauss, N.E.; Lee, D.; Marquess, D.G.; McGrane, P.L.; Meng, W.; Natchus, M.G.; Shuker, A.J.; Sutton, J.C.; Taylor, R.E. The pinene path to taxanes. 6. A concise stereocontrolled synthesis of taxol. *J. Am. Chem. Soc.,* **1997**, *119*(11), 2757-2758. [http://dx.doi.org/10.1021/ja963539z]

[99] Mukaiyama, T.; Shiina, I.; Iwadare, H.; Saitoh, M.; Nishimura, T.; Ohkawa, N.; Sakoh, H.; Nishimura, K.; Tani, Y.-i.; Hasegawa, M.; Yamada, K.; Saitoh, K. Asymmetric total synthesis of taxol\R chemistry *A European Journal,* **1999**, *5*(1), 121-161.

[100] Kusama, H.; Hara, R.; Kawahara, S.; Nishimori, T.; Kashima, H.; Nakamura, N.; Morihira, K.; Kuwajima, I. Enantioselective total synthesis of (−)-Taxol. *J. Am. Chem. Soc.,* **2000**, *122*(16), 3811-3820. [http://dx.doi.org/10.1021/ja9939439]

[101] Morihira, K.; Hara, R.; Kawahara, S.; Nishimori, T.; Nakamura, N.; Hiroyuki Kusama, A. Isao Kuwajima, Enantioselective total synthesis of taxol. *J. Org. Chem.,* **2005**, *69*(8), 2831-2843.

[102] Doi, T.; Fuse, S.; Miyamoto, S.; Nakai, K.; Sasuga, D.; Takahashi, T. A formal total synthesis of taxol aided by an automated synthesizer. *Chem. Asian J.,* **2006**, *1*(3), 370-383. [http://dx.doi.org/10.1002/asia.200600156] [PMID: 17441074]

[103] Doi, T.; Fuse, S.; Miyamoto, S.; Nakai, K.; Sasuga, D.; Takahashi, T. A formal total synthesis of taxol aided by an automated synthesizer. *Chem. Asian J.,* **2006**, *1*(3), 370-383. [http://dx.doi.org/10.1002/asia.200600156] [PMID: 17441074]

[104] Fukaya, K.; Tanaka, Y.; Sato, A.C.; Kodama, K.; Yamazaki, H.; Ishimoto, T.; Nozaki, Y.; Iwaki, Y.M.; Yuki, Y.; Umei, K.; Sugai, T.; Yamaguchi, Y.; Watanabe, A.; Oishi, T.; Sato, T.; Chida, N. Synthesis of paclitaxel. 1. synthesis of the ABC ring of paclitaxel by smI2-mediated cyclization. *Org. Lett.,* **2015**, *17*(11), 2570-2573. [http://dx.doi.org/10.1021/acs.orglett.5b01173] [PMID: 26010812]

[105] Fukaya, K.; Kodama, K.; Tanaka, Y.; Yamazaki, H.; Sugai, T.; Yamaguchi, Y.; Watanabe, A.; Oishi, T.; Sato, T.; Chida, N. Synthesis of paclitaxel. 2. construction of the ABCD ring and formal synthesis. *Org. Lett.,* **2015**, *17*(11), 2574-2577. [http://dx.doi.org/10.1021/acs.orglett.5b01174] [PMID: 26010999]

[106] Hirai, S.; Utsugi, M.; Iwamoto, M.; Nakada, M. Formal total synthesis of (-)-taxol through Pd-catalyzed eight-membered carbocyclic ring formation. *Chemistry,* **2015**, *21*(1), 355-359. [http://dx.doi.org/10.1002/chem.201404295] [PMID: 25346263]

[107] Mountford, P. G. *The Taxol®; Development of a green synthesis via plant cell fermentation*; Wiley□VCH Verlag GmbH & Co. KGaA, **2010**, pp. 145-160.

[108] Wuts, P.G. Semisynthesis of Taxol. *Curr. Opin. Drug Discov. Devel.,* **1998**, *1*(3), 329-337. [PMID: 19649807]

[109] Barua, N.C.; Boruwa, J.; Borah, J.C. Synthesis of the C-13 Side-Chain of Taxol. *Curr. Org. Synth.,* **2007**, *4*(2), 175-199. [http://dx.doi.org/10.2174/157017907780598899]

[110] Denis, J.N.; Greene, A.E.; Guenard, D.; Guerittevoegelein, F.; Mangatal, L.; Potier, P. Highly efficient, practical approach to natural taxol. *J. Am. Chem. Soc.,* **1988**, *110*(17), 5917-5919. [http://dx.doi.org/10.1021/ja00225a063]

[111] Holton, R.A. *Metal alkoxides*; Google Patents, **1993**.

[112] Kingston, D.G.I.; Chaudhary, A.G.; Gunatilaka, A.A.L.; Middleton, M.L. Synthesis of taxol from baccatin III via an oxazoline intermediate. *Tetrahedron Lett.,* **1994**, *35*(26), 4483-4484. [http://dx.doi.org/10.1016/S0040-4039(00)60706-2]

[113] Commerçon, A.; Bézard, D.; Bernard, F.; Bourzat, J.D. Improved protection and esterification of a precursor of the taxotere® and taxol side chains. *Tetrahedron Lett.,* **1992**, *33*(36), 5185-5188. [http://dx.doi.org/10.1016/S0040-4039(00)79128-3]

[114] Li, B.J.; Wang, H.; Gong, T.; Chen, J.J.; Chen, T.J.; Yang, J.L.; Zhu, P. Improving 10-deacetylbaccatin III-10-β-O-acetyltransferase catalytic fitness for Taxol production. *Nat. Commun.,* **2017**, *8*, 15544. [http://dx.doi.org/10.1038/ncomms15544] [PMID: 28516951]

[115] Chattopadhyay, S.K.; Sharma, R.P.; Kumar, S. *Process for the production of important taxol analogues 10-deacetyl taxol A, B, and C*; Google Patents, **2000**.

[116] Cheng, H.L.; Zhao, R.Y.; Chen, T.J.; Yu, W.B.; Wang, F.; Cheng, K.D.; Zhu, P. Cloning and characterization of the glycoside hydrolases that remove xylosyl groups from 7-β-xylosyl-10-deacetyltaxol and its analogues. *Mol. Cell. Proteomics,* **2013**, *12*(8), 2236-2248. [http://dx.doi.org/10.1074/mcp.M113.030619] [PMID: 23665501]

[117] Wang, K.; Wang, T.; Li, J.; Zou, J.; Chen, Y.; Dai, J. Microbial hydrolysis of 7-xylosyl--0-deacetyltaxol to 10-deacetyltaxol. *J. Mol. Catal., B Enzym.,* **2011**, *68*(3), 250-255. [http://dx.doi.org/10.1016/j.molcatb.2010.11.013]

[118] Liu, W.C.; Gong, T.; Zhu, P. Advances in exploring alternative Taxol sources. *RSC Advances,* **2016**, *6*(54), 48800-48809. [http://dx.doi.org/10.1039/C6RA06640B]

[119] Zhong, J.J. Plant cell culture for production of paclitaxel and other taxanes. *J. Biosci. Bioeng.,* **2002**, *94*(6), 591-599. [http://dx.doi.org/10.1016/S1389-1723(02)80200-6] [PMID: 16233355]

[120] Tabata, H. *Paclitaxel production by plant-cell-culture technology*; , **2004**, 87, pp. (87)1-23. [http://dx.doi.org/10.1007/b13538]

[121] Tabata, H. Production of paclitaxel and the related taxanes by cell suspension cultures of Taxus species. *Curr. Drug Targets,* **2006**, *7*(4), 453-461. [http://dx.doi.org/10.2174/138945006776359368] [PMID: 16611032]

[122] Khosroushahi, A.Y.; Valizadeh, M.; Ghasempour, A.; Khosrowshahli, M.; Naghdibadi, H.; Dadpour, M.R.; Omidi, Y. Improved Taxol production by combination of inducing factors in suspension cell culture of Taxus baccata. *Cell Biol. Int.,* **2006**, *30*(3), 262-269. [http://dx.doi.org/10.1016/j.cellbi.2005.11.004] [PMID: 16378737]

[123] Vongpaseuth, K.; Roberts, S.C. Advancements in the understanding of Paclitaxel metabolism in tissue culture. *Curr. Pharm. Biotechnol.,* **2007**, *8*(4), 219-236. [http://dx.doi.org/10.2174/138920107781387393] [PMID: 17691991]

[124] Frense, D. Taxanes: perspectives for biotechnological production. *Appl. Microbiol. Biotechnol.,* **2007**, *73*(6), 1233-1240. [http://dx.doi.org/10.1007/s00253-006-0711-0] [PMID: 17124581]

[125] Maheshwari, P.; Garg, S.; Kumar, A. Taxoids: Biosynthesis and *in vitro* production. *Biotechnol. Mol. Biol. Rev.,* **2008**, (4), 71-87.

[126] Expósito, O.; Bonfill, M.; Moyano, E.; Onrubia, M.; Mirjalili, M.H.; Cusidó, R.M.; Palazón, J. Biotechnological production of taxol and related taxoids: current state and prospects. *Anticancer. Agents Med. Chem.,* **2009**, *9*(1), 109-121. [http://dx.doi.org/10.2174/187152009787047761] [PMID: 19149486]

[127] Sabaterjara, A.B.; Tudela, L.R.; Lópezpérez, A.J.; Bucar, F.; Gibbons, S. *In vitro* culture of Taxus sp.:

strategies to increase cell growth and taxoid production. *Phytochem. Rev.*, **2010**, *9*(2), 343-356. [http://dx.doi.org/10.1007/s11101-010-9167-z]

[128] Onrubia, M.; Moyano, E.; Bonfill, M.; Cusidó, R.M.; Goossens, A.; Palazón, J. Coronatine, a more powerful elicitor for inducing taxane biosynthesis in Taxus media cell cultures than methyl jasmonate. *J. Plant Physiol.*, **2013**, *170*(2), 211-219. [http://dx.doi.org/10.1016/j.jplph.2012.09.004] [PMID: 23102875]

[129] Ramirez-Estrada, K.; Vidal-Limon, H.; Hidalgo, D.; Moyano, E.; Golenioswki, M.; Cusidó, R.M.; Palazon, J. Elicitation, an Effective Strategy for the Biotechnological Production of Bioactive High-Added Value Compounds in Plant Cell Factories. *Molecules*, **2016**, *21*(2), 182. [http://dx.doi.org/10.3390/molecules21020182] [PMID: 26848649]

[130] Christen, A.; Bland, J.; Gibson, D. In Cell cultures as a means to produce taxol. *Proc. Am. Assoc. Cancer Res.*, **1989**, 566.

[131] Kim, J-H.; Yun, J-H.; Hwang, Y-S.; Byun, S.Y.; Kim, D-I. Production of taxol and related taxanes in *Taxus brevifolia* cell cultures: effect of sugar. *Biotechnol. Lett.*, **1995**, *17*(1), 101-106. [http://dx.doi.org/10.1007/BF00134204]

[132] Cusidó, R.M.; Palazón, J.; Bonfill, M.; Navia-Osorio, A.; Morales, C.; Piñol, M.T. Improved paclitaxel and baccatin III production in suspension cultures of *Taxus media*. *Biotechnol. Prog.*, **2002**, *18*(3), 418-423. [http://dx.doi.org/10.1021/bp0101583] [PMID: 12052053]

[133] Bruňáková, K.; Babincova, Z.; Čellárová, E. Selection of callus cultures of Taxus baccata L. as a potential source of paclitaxel production. *Eng. Life Sci.*, **2004**, *4*(5), 465-469. [http://dx.doi.org/10.1002/elsc.200420050]

[134] Hussain, A.; Qarshi, I.A.; Nazir, H.; Ullah, I.; Rashid, M.; Shinwari, Z.K. *In vitro* callogenesis and organogenesis in *Taxus wallichiana* ZUCC, The Himalayan Yew. *Pak. J. Bot.*, **2013**, *45*(5), 1755-1759.

[135] Li, Y-L.; Huang, S-W.; Zhang, J-Y.; Bu, F-J.; Lin, T.; Zhang, Z-H.; Xiong, X-Y. A protocol of homozygous haploid callus induction from endosperm of Taxus chinensis Rehd. var. mairei. *Springerplus*, **2016**, *5*(1), 659. [http://dx.doi.org/10.1186/s40064-016-2320-4] [PMID: 27350901]

[136] Gibson, D.M.; Ketchum, R.E.; Vance, N.C.; Christen, A.A. Initiation and growth of cell lines of *Taxus brevifolia* (Pacific yew). *Plant Cell Rep.*, **1993**, *12*(9), 479-482. [http://dx.doi.org/10.1007/BF00236091] [PMID: 24196105]

[137] Bonfill, M.; Palazón, J.; Cusidó, R.M.; Joly, S.; Morales, C.; Piñol, M.T. Influence of elicitors on taxane production and 3-hydroxy-3-methylglutaryl coenzyme A reductase activity in *Taxus media* cells. *Plant Physiol. Biochem.*, **2003**, *41*(1), 91-96. [http://dx.doi.org/10.1016/S0981-9428(02)00013-X]

[138] Luo, J.; He, G-Y. Optimization of elicitors and precursors for paclitaxel production in cell suspension culture of *Taxus chinensis* in the presence of nutrient feeding. *Process Biochem.*, **2004**, *39*(9), 1073-1079. [http://dx.doi.org/10.1016/S0032-9592(03)00219-X]

[139] Kim, B.J.; Gibson, D.M.; Shuler, M.L. Effect of the plant peptide regulator, phytosulfokine-α, on the growth and Taxol production from *Taxus sp.* suspension cultures. *Biotechnol. Bioeng.*, **2006**, *95*(1), 8-14. [http://dx.doi.org/10.1002/bit.20934] [PMID: 16586507]

[140] Hirasuna, T.J.; Pestchanker, L.J.; Srinivasan, V.; Shuler, M.L. Taxol production in suspension cultures of *Taxus baccata*. *Plant Cell Tissue Organ Cult.*, **1996**, *44*(2), 95-102. [http://dx.doi.org/10.1007/BF00048185]

[141] Li, Y-C.; Tao, W-Y. Paclitaxel-producing fungal endophyte stimulates the accumulation of taxoids in

suspension cultures of *Taxus cuspidate. Sci. Hortic. (Amsterdam),* **2009**, *121*(1), 97-102. [http://dx.doi.org/10.1016/j.scienta.2009.01.016]

[142] Tapia, N.; Zamilpa, A.; Bonfill, M.; Ventura, E.; Cruz-Vega, D.; Del Villar, A.; Cruz-Sosa, F.; Osuna, L. Effect of the culture medium and biotic stimulation on taxane production in *Taxus globosa* Schltdl *in vitro* cultures. *Acta Physiol. Plant.,* **2013**, *35*(12), 3447-3455. [http://dx.doi.org/10.1007/s11738-013-1380-0]

[143] Furmanowa, M.; Olędzka, H.; Sykłowska-Baranek, K.; Józefowicz, J.; Gieracka, S. Increased taxane accumulation in callus cultures of *Taxus cuspidata* and *Taxus*× *media* by some elicitors and precursors. *Biotechnol. Lett.,* **2000**, *22*(18), 1449-1452. [http://dx.doi.org/10.1023/A:1005611114628]

[144] Kim, J.A.; Baek, K-H.; Son, Y.M.; Son, S.H.; Shin, H. Hairy root cultures of Taxus cuspidate for enhanced production of paclitaxel. *J. Korean Soc. Appl. Biol. Chem.,* **2009**, *52*(2), 144-150. [http://dx.doi.org/10.3839/jksabc.2009.027]

[145] Sykłowska-Baranek, K.; Pilarek, M.; Bonfill, M.; Kafel, K.; Pietrosiuk, A. Perfluorodecalin-supported system enhances taxane production in hairy root cultures of *Taxus x media* var. Hicksii carrying a taxadiene synthase transgene. *Plant Cell Tissue Organ Culture (PCTOC).,* **2015**, *120*(3), 1051-1059. [http://dx.doi.org/10.1007/s11240-014-0659-1]

[146] Lee, E-K.; Jin, Y-W.; Park, J.H.; Yoo, Y.M.; Hong, S.M.; Amir, R.; Yan, Z.; Kwon, E.; Elfick, A.; Tomlinson, S.; Halbritter, F.; Waibel, T.; Yun, B.W.; Loake, G.J. Cultured cambial meristematic cells as a source of plant natural products. *Nat. Biotechnol.,* **2010**, *28*(11), 1213-1217. [http://dx.doi.org/10.1038/nbt.1693] [PMID: 20972422]

[147] Fett-Neto, A. G.; DiCosmo, F.; Reynolds, W. F.; Sakata, K. Cell culture of Taxus as a source of the antineoplastic drug taxol and related taxanes. *Bio/technology (Nature Publishing Company),* **1992**, *10*(12), 1572-5. [http://dx.doi.org/10.1038/nbt1292-1572]

[148] Wickremesinhe, E.R.; Arteea, R.N. Taxus callus cultures: initiation, growth optimization, characterization and taxol production. *Plant Cell Tissue Organ Cult.,* **1993**, *35*(2), 181-193. [http://dx.doi.org/10.1007/BF00032968]

[149] Wang, S.; Wang, H.; Li, T.; Li, C.; Zhou, Y.; Zhong, X. The selection and stability analysis of stable and high Taxol-producing cell lines from Taxus cuspidata. *J. For. Res.,* **2017**, (1), 1-7. [http://dx.doi.org/10.1007/s11676-008-0001-z]

[150] Kajani, A.A.; Moghim, S.; Mofid, M.R. Optimization of the basal medium for improving production and secretion of taxanes from suspension cell culture of Taxus baccata L. *Daru,* **2012**, *20*(1), 54. [http://dx.doi.org/10.1186/2008-2231-20-54] [PMID: 23352123]

[151] Linden, J.; Haigh, J.; Mirjalili, N.; Phisaphalong, M. Gas concentration effects on secondary metabolite production by plant cell cultures.*Plant Cells*; Springer, **2001**, pp. 27-62. [http://dx.doi.org/10.1007/3-540-45302-4_2]

[152] Chen, Y.Q.; Zhu, W.H.; Wu, Y.Q.; Hu, Q. [Effects of culture conditions on callus growth and taxol formation of Taxus yunnanensis Cheng et L.K.Fu]. *Zhongguo Zhongyao Zazhi,* **2000**, *25*(5), 269-272. [PMID: 12512447]

[153] Zhao, J.; Davis, L.C.; Verpoorte, R. Elicitor signal transduction leading to production of plant secondary metabolites. *Biotechnol. Adv.,* **2005**, *23*(4), 283-333. [http://dx.doi.org/10.1016/j.biotechadv.2005.01.003] [PMID: 15848039]

[154] Bonfill, M.; Exposito, O.; Moyano, E.; Cusidó, R.; Palazón, J.; Pinol, M.T. Manipulation by culture mixing and elicitation of paclitaxel and baccatin III production in *Taxus baccata* suspension cultures. *In Vitro Cell. Dev. Biol. Plant,* **2006**, *42*(5), 422-426. [http://dx.doi.org/10.1079/IVP2006761]

[155] Yukimune, Y.; Tabata, H.; Higashi, Y.; Hara, Y. Methyl jasmonate-induced overproduction of

paclitaxel and baccatin III in Taxus cell suspension cultures. *Nat. Biotechnol.*, **1996**, *14*(9), 1129-1132. [http://dx.doi.org/10.1038/nbt0996-1129] [PMID: 9631065]

[156] Kim, S.; Choi, H.; Kim, J.; Lee, H.; Hong, S. Effect of osmotic pressure on paclitaxel production in suspension cell cultures of *Taxus chinensis*. *Enzyme Microb. Technol.*, **2001**, *28*(2-3), 202-209. [http://dx.doi.org/10.1016/S0141-0229(00)00292-1] [PMID: 11166813]

[157] Wang, Y.D.; Yuan, Y.J.; Lu, M.; Wu, J.C.; Jiang, J.L. Inhibitor studies of isopentenyl pyrophosphate biosynthesis in suspension cultures of the yew *Taxus chinensis var. mairei*. *Biotechnol. Appl. Biochem.*, **2003**, *37*(Pt 1), 39-43. [http://dx.doi.org/10.1042/BA20020061] [PMID: 12578550]

[158] Cusido, R.M.; Onrubia, M.; Sabater-Jara, A.B.; Moyano, E.; Bonfill, M.; Goossens, A.; Angeles Pedreño, M.; Palazon, J. A rational approach to improving the biotechnological production of taxanes in plant cell cultures of *Taxus spp*. *Biotechnol. Adv.*, **2014**, *32*(6), 1157-1167. [http://dx.doi.org/10.1016/j.biotechadv.2014.03.002] [PMID: 24681092]

[159] Bentebibel, S.; Moyano, E.; Palazón, J.; Cusidó, R.M.; Bonfill, M.; Eibl, R.; Piñol, M.T. Effects of immobilization by entrapment in alginate and scale-up on paclitaxel and baccatin III production in cell suspension cultures of *Taxus baccata*. *Biotechnol. Bioeng.*, **2005**, *89*(6), 647-655. [http://dx.doi.org/10.1002/bit.20321] [PMID: 15696535]

[160] Choi, H-K.; Kim, S-I.; Song, J-Y.; Son, J.S.; Hong, S.S.; Durzan, D.J.; Lee, H.J. Localization of paclitaxel in suspension culture of *Taxus chinensis*. *J. Microbiol. Biotechnol.*, **2001**, *11*(3), 458-462.

[161] Wilson, S.A.; Roberts, S.C. Recent advances towards development and commercialization of plant cell culture processes for the synthesis of biomolecules. *Plant Biotechnol. J.*, **2012**, *10*(3), 249-268. [http://dx.doi.org/10.1111/j.1467-7652.2011.00664.x] [PMID: 22059985]

[162] Roberts, S.C.; Naill, M.; Gibson, D.M.; Shuler, M.L. A simple method for enhancing paclitaxel release from *Taxus canadensis* cell suspension cultures utilizing cell wall digesting enzymes. *Plant Cell Rep.*, **2003**, *21*(12), 1217-1220. [http://dx.doi.org/10.1007/s00299-003-0575-z] [PMID: 12811504]

[163] Wang, C.; Wu, J.; Mei, X. Enhanced taxol production and release in *Taxus chinensis* cell suspension cultures with selected organic solvents and sucrose feeding. *Biotechnol. Prog.*, **2001**, *17*(1), 89-94. [http://dx.doi.org/10.1021/bp0001359] [PMID: 11170485]

[164] Cusido, R.; Palazon, J.; Navia-Osorio, A.; Mallol, A.; Bonfill, M.; Morales, C.; Teresa, M.; Ol, P. *Production of taxol and Baccatin III by a selected Taxus baccata callus line and its derived cell suspension culture*; , **1999**, 146, pp. 101-107.

[165] Palazón, J.; Cusidó, R.M.; Bonfill, M.; Morales, C.; Piñol, M.T. Inhibition of paclitaxel and baccatin III accumulation by mevinolin and fosmidomycin in suspension cultures of *Taxus baccata*. *J. Biotechnol.*, **2003**, *101*(2), 157-163. [http://dx.doi.org/10.1016/S0168-1656(02)00318-8] [PMID: 12568744]

[166] Strobel, G.A.; Stierle, A.A.; Stierle, D.B. *Taxol production by taxomyces andreanae*; US, **1994**.

[167] Strobel, G.; Yang, X.; Sears, J.; Kramer, R.; Sidhu, R.S.; Hess, W.M. Taxol from *Pestalotiopsis microspora*, an endophytic fungus of *Taxus wallachiana*. *Microbiology*, **1996**, *142*(Pt 2), 435-440. [http://dx.doi.org/10.1099/13500872-142-2-435] [PMID: 8932715]

[168] Li, J.Y.; Strobel, G.; Sidhu, R.; Hess, W.M.; Ford, E.J. Endophytic taxol-producing fungi from bald cypress, *Taxodium distichum*. *Microbiology*, **1996**, *142*(Pt 8), 2223-2226. [http://dx.doi.org/10.1099/13500872-142-8-2223] [PMID: 8760934]

[169] Li, J.Y.; Sidhu, R.S.; Ford, E.; Long, D.; Hess, W.; Strobel, G. The induction of taxol production in the endophytic fungus—*Periconia sp* from *Torreya grandifolia*. *J. Ind. Microbiol. Biotechnol.*, **1998**, *20*(5), 259-264. [http://dx.doi.org/10.1038/sj.jim.2900521]

[170] Gangadevi, V.; Muthumary, J. A novel endophytic Taxol-producing fungus *Chaetomella raphigera*

isolated from a medicinal plant, *Terminalia arjuna*. *Appl. Biochem. Biotechnol.*, **2009**, *158*(3), 675-684.
[http://dx.doi.org/10.1007/s12010-009-8532-0] [PMID: 19234679]

[171] Yan, B.; Bi, J.; Ji, Y.; Wang, W.; Zhao, Y.; Zhu, X. An endophytic taxol-producing fungus from cypress. *Acta Sci. Natur. Univ. Nankaiensis,* **2007**, *40*(6), 68-70.

[172] Sun, D.; Ran, X.; Wang, J. [Isolation and identification of a taxol-producing endophytic fungus from Podocarpus]. *Wei Sheng Wu Xue Bao,* **2008**, *48*(5), 589-595.
[PMID: 18652289]

[173] Bi, J.; Ji, Y.; Pan, J.; Yu, Y.; Chen, H.; Zhu, X. A new taxol-producing fungus (*Pestalotiopsis malicola*) and evidence for taxol as a transient product in the culture. *Afr. J. Biotechnol.,* **2011**, *10*(34), 6647-6654.

[174] Flores-Bustamante, Z.R.; Rivera-Orduña, F.N.; Martínez-Cárdenas, A.; Flores-Cotera, L.B. Microbial paclitaxel: advances and perspectives. *J. Antibiot. (Tokyo),* **2010**, *63*(8), 460-467.
[http://dx.doi.org/10.1038/ja.2010.83] [PMID: 20628412]

[175] Kusari, S.; Singh, S.; Jayabaskaran, C. Rethinking production of Taxol® (paclitaxel) using endophyte biotechnology. *Trends Biotechnol.,* **2014**, *32*(6), 304-311.
[http://dx.doi.org/10.1016/j.tibtech.2014.03.011] [PMID: 24810040]

[176] Suryanarayanan, T.; Thirunavukkarasu, N.; Govindarajulu, M.; Sasse, F.; Jansen, R.; Murali, T. Fungal endophytes and bioprospecting. *Fungal Biol. Rev.,* **2009**, *23*(1), 9-19.

[177] Zhao, K.; Ping, W-X.; Ma, X.; Liu, J.; Zhou, D.P. [Breeding of high-yield strain of taxol by mutagenesis of protoplast and primary discussion of genetic differences between mutants and their parent strain]. *Wei Sheng Wu Xue Bao,* **2005**, *45*(3), 355-358.
[PMID: 15989225]

[178] Zhao, K.; Zhou, D.P.; Ping, W.X.; Liu, J.; Ma, X.; Jin, T. [Study on breeding up high-yield strain of taxol by protoplast mutagenesis]. *Chin. J. Biotechnol.,* **2005**, *21*(5), 848-851.

[179] Xu, F.; Tao, W.; Cheng, L.; Guo, L. Strain improvement and optimization of the media of taxol-producing fungus *Fusarium maire*. *Biochem. Eng. J.,* **2006**, *31*(1), 67-73.
[http://dx.doi.org/10.1016/j.bej.2006.05.024]

[180] Zhao, K.; Li, Z.; Ge, N.; Li, X.; Wang, X.; Zhou, D. Investigation of fermentation conditions and optimization of medium for taxol production from taxol-producing fungi. *J. Med. Plants Res.,* **2011**, *5*(29), 6528-6535.

[181] Li, J-Y.; Sidhu, R.S.; Bollon, A.; Strobel, G.A. Stimulation of taxol production in liquid cultures of *Pestalotiopsis microspora*. *Mycol. Res.,* **1998**, *102*(4), 461-464.
[http://dx.doi.org/10.1017/S0953756297005078]

[182] Yang, Y.; Zhao, H.; Barrero, R.A.; Zhang, B.; Sun, G.; Wilson, I.W.; Xie, F.; Walker, K.D.; Parks, J.W.; Bruce, R.; Guo, G.; Chen, L.; Zhang, Y.; Huang, X.; Tang, Q.; Liu, H.; Bellgard, M.I.; Qiu, D.; Lai, J.; Hoffman, A. Genome sequencing and analysis of the paclitaxel-producing endophytic fungus *Penicillium aurantiogriseum* NRRL 62431. *BMC Genomics,* **2014**, *15*(1), 69.
[http://dx.doi.org/10.1186/1471-2164-15-69] [PMID: 24460898]

[183] Li, Y-C.; Tao, W-Y.; Cheng, L. Paclitaxel production using co-culture of Taxus suspension cells and paclitaxel-producing endophytic fungi in a co-bioreactor. *Appl. Microbiol. Biotechnol.,* **2009**, *83*(2), 233-239.
[http://dx.doi.org/10.1007/s00253-009-1856-4] [PMID: 19172266]

[184] Zhao, K.; Sun, L.; Ma, X.; Li, X.; Wang, X.; Ping, W.; Zhou, D. Improved taxol production in *Nodulisporium sylviforme* derived from inactivated protoplast fusion. *Afr. J. Biotechnol.,* **2011**, *10*(20), 4175-4182.

[185] Zhao, K.; Ping, W.; Zhang, L.; Liu, J.; Lin, Y.; Jin, T.; Zhou, D. Screening and breeding of high taxol

producing fungi by genome shuffling. *Sci. China C Life Sci.,* **2008**, *51*(3), 222-231. [http://dx.doi.org/10.1007/s11427-008-0037-5] [PMID: 18246310]

[186] Zhou, X.; Zhu, H.; Liu, L.; Lin, J.; Tang, K. A review: recent advances and future prospects of taxol-producing endophytic fungi. *Appl. Microbiol. Biotechnol.,* **2010**, *86*(6), 1707-1717. [http://dx.doi.org/10.1007/s00253-010-2546-y] [PMID: 20358192]

[187] Kathiravan, G.; Sri Raman, V. *In vitro* TAXOL production, by *Pestalotiopsis breviseta*--a first report. *Fitoterapia,* **2010**, *81*(6), 557-564. [http://dx.doi.org/10.1016/j.fitote.2010.01.021] [PMID: 20149851]

[188] Kumaran, R.S.; Muthumary, J.; Hur, B-K. Taxol from Phyllosticta citricarpa, a leaf spot fungus of the angiosperm *Citrus medica. J. Biosci. Bioeng.,* **2008**, *106*(1), 103-106. [http://dx.doi.org/10.1263/jbb.106.103] [PMID: 18691540]

[189] Kumaran, R.S.; Kim, H.J.; Hur, B-K. Taxol-producing [corrected] fungal endophyte, Pestalotiopsis species isolated from Taxus cuspidata. *J. Biosci. Bioeng.,* **2010**, *110*(5), 541-546. [http://dx.doi.org/10.1016/j.jbiosc.2010.06.007] [PMID: 20634132]

[190] Sreekanth, D.; Syed, A.; Sarkar, S.; Sarkar, D.; Santhakumari, B.; Ahmad, A.; Khan, I. Production, purification and characterization of taxol and 10DAB III from a new endophytic fungus Gliocladium sp. isolated from the Indian yew tree, Taxus baccata. *J. Microbiol. Biotechnol.,* **2009**, *19*(11), 1342-1347. [PMID: 19996685]

[191] Wang, Y.; Tang, K. A new endophytic taxol-and baccatin III-producing fungus isolated from *Taxus chinensis var. mairei. Afr. J. Biotechnol.,* **2011**, *10*(72), 16379-16386.

[192] Somjaipeng, S.; Medina, A.; Kwaśna, H.; Ordaz Ortiz, J.; Magan, N. Isolation, identification, and ecology of growth and taxol production by an endophytic strain of *Paraconiothyrium variabile* from English yew trees (*Taxus baccata*). *Fungal Biol.,* **2015**, *119*(11), 1022-1031. [http://dx.doi.org/10.1016/j.funbio.2015.07.007] [PMID: 26466877]

[193] Zaiyou, J.; Li, M.; Guifang, X.; Xiuren, Z. Isolation of an endophytic fungus producing baccatin III from *Taxus wallichiana var. mairei. J. Ind. Microbiol. Biotechnol.,* **2013**, *40*(11), 1297-1302. [http://dx.doi.org/10.1007/s10295-013-1320-4] [PMID: 23958913]

[194] Garyali, S.; Kumar, A.; Reddy, M.S. Enhancement of taxol production from endophytic fungus *Fusarium redolens. Biotechnol. Bioprocess Eng.; BBE,* **2014**, *19*(5), 908-915. [http://dx.doi.org/10.1007/s12257-014-0160-z]

[195] Srinivasan, K.; Muthumary, J. Taxol production from Pestalotiopsis sp an endophytic fungus isolated from *Catharanthus roseus. Journal of Ecobiotechnology,* **2009**, *1*(1)

[196] Gohar, U.F.; Mukhtar, H. HAQ, I. U., Isolation and screening of endophytic fungi for the reduction of taxol. *Pak. J. Bot.,* **2015**, *47*, 355-358.

[197] Xiong, Z.Q.; Yang, Y.Y.; Zhao, N.; Wang, Y. Diversity of endophytic fungi and screening of fungal paclitaxel producer from Anglojap yew, *Taxus x media. BMC Microbiol.,* **2013**, *13*(1), 71. [http://dx.doi.org/10.1186/1471-2180-13-71] [PMID: 23537181]

[198] Zhao, K.; Ping, W.; Li, Q.; Hao, S.; Zhao, L.; Gao, T.; Zhou, D. Aspergillus niger var. taxi, a new species variant of taxol-producing fungus isolated from *Taxus cuspidata* in China. *J. Appl. Microbiol.,* **2009**, *107*(4), 1202-1207. [http://dx.doi.org/10.1111/j.1365-2672.2009.04305.x] [PMID: 19486395]

[199] Senthilkumar, N.; Murugesan, S.; Mohan, V.; Muthumary, J. Taxol producing fungal endophyte, *Colletotrichum gleospoiroides* (Penz.) from *Tectona grandis* L. *Curr. Biot.,* **2013**, *7*, 3-15.

[200] Doss, V.; Govindharajanb, K.; Ravichandran, D. Screening of Taxol, an Anticancer Drug produced from *Pestaloptiopsis stellata* isolated from *Ficus infectoria. Life Sci. J.,* **2016**, *13*(10)

[201] Soliman, S.S.; Tsao, R.; Raizada, M.N. Chemical inhibitors suggest endophytic fungal paclitaxel is

derived from both mevalonate and non-mevalonate-like pathways. *J. Nat. Prod.,* **2011**, *74*(12), 2497-2504.
[http://dx.doi.org/10.1021/np200303v] [PMID: 22103292]

[202] Elavarasi, A.; Rathna, G.S.; Kalaiselvam, M. Taxol producing mangrove endophytic fungi *Fusarium oxysporum* from *Rhizophora annamalayana. Asian Pac. J. Trop. Biomed.,* **2012**, *2*(2), S1081-S1085.
[http://dx.doi.org/10.1016/S2221-1691(12)60365-7]

[203] Chakravarthi, B.V.; Das, P.; Surendranath, K.; Karande, A.A.; Jayabaskaran, C. Production of paclitaxel by *Fusarium solani isolated* from *Taxus celebica. J. Biosci.,* **2008**, *33*(2), 259-267.
[http://dx.doi.org/10.1007/s12038-008-0043-6] [PMID: 18535360]

[204] Liu, K.; Ding, X.; Deng, B.; Chen, W. Isolation and characterization of endophytic taxol-producing fungi from *Taxus chinensis. J. Ind. Microbiol. Biotechnol.,* **2009**, *36*(9), 1171-1177.
[http://dx.doi.org/10.1007/s10295-009-0598-8] [PMID: 19484278]

[205] Zhang, P.; Zhou, P-P.; Yu, L-J. An endophytic taxol-producing fungus from *Taxus media, Cladosporium cladosporioides* MD2. *Curr. Microbiol.,* **2009**, *59*(3), 227-232.
[http://dx.doi.org/10.1007/s00284-008-9270-1] [PMID: 19484305]

[206] Kumaran, R.S.; Choi, Y.K.; Lee, S.; Jeon, H.J.; Jung, H.; Kim, H.J. Isolation of taxol, an anticancer drug produced by the endophytic fungus, *Phoma betae. Afr. J. Biotechnol.,* **2012**, *11*(4), 950-960.

[207] Gangadevi, V.; Muthumary, J. Isolation of Colletotrichum gloeosporioides, a novel endophytic taxol-producing fungus from the leaves of a medicinal plant, *Justicia gendarussa. Mycologia Balcanica,* **2008**, *5*, 1-4.

[208] Kumaran, S. R; Muthumary, J.; Hur, B., Production of Taxol fromPhyllosticta spinarum, an endophytic fungus of *Cupressus sp. Eng. Life Sci.,* **2008**, *8*(4), 438-446.
[http://dx.doi.org/10.1002/elsc.200800019]

[209] Kumaran, R.S.; Muthumary, J.; Kim, E-K.; Hur, B-K. Production of taxol from Phyllosticta dioscoreae, a leaf spot fungus isolated from *Hibiscus rosa-sinensis. Biotechnol. Bioprocess Eng.; BBE,* **2009**, *14*(1), 76.
[http://dx.doi.org/10.1007/s12257-008-0041-4]

[210] Pandi, M.; Kumaran, R.S.; Choi, Y-K.; Kim, H.J.; Muthumary, J. Isolation and detection of taxol, an anticancer drug produced *from Lasiodiplodia theobromae*, an endophytic fungus of the medicinal plant *Morinda citrifolia. Afr. J. Biotechnol.,* **2011**, *10*(8), 1428-1435.

[211] Zaiyou, J.; Li, M.; Xiqiao, H. An endophytic fungus efficiently producing paclitaxel isolated from *Taxus wallichiana var. mairei. Medicine (Baltimore),* **2017**, *96*(27)e7406
[http://dx.doi.org/10.1097/MD.0000000000007406] [PMID: 28682896]

[212] Kani, B.C.; Kumar, S.S.; Pandi, M. Screening and Characterization of Fungal Taxol from Leaf Spot Fungi. *American Journal of Bioscience and Bioengineering,* **2017**, *5*(6), 113.
[http://dx.doi.org/10.11648/j.bio.20170506.11]

[213] Das, A.; Rahman, M.I.; Ferdous, A.S.; Amin, A.; Rahman, M.M.; Nahar, N.; Uddin, M.A.; Islam, M.R.; Khan, H. An endophytic Basidiomycete, Grammothele lineata, isolated from *Corchorus olitorius*, produces paclitaxel that shows cytotoxicity. *PLoS One,* **2017**, *12*(6)e0178612
[http://dx.doi.org/10.1371/journal.pone.0178612] [PMID: 28636663]

[214] Mirjalili, M.H.; Farzaneh, M.; Bonfill, M.; Rezadoost, H.; Ghassempour, A. Isolation and characterization of *Stemphylium sedicola* SBU-16 as a new endophytic taxol-producing fungus from *Taxus baccata* grown in Iran. *FEMS Microbiol. Lett.,* **2012**, *328*(2), 122-129.
[http://dx.doi.org/10.1111/j.1574-6968.2011.02488.x] [PMID: 22211912]

[215] Kuzuyama, T. Mevalonate and nonmevalonate pathways for the biosynthesis of isoprene units. *Biosci. Biotechnol. Biochem.,* **2002**, *66*(8), 1619-1627.
[http://dx.doi.org/10.1271/bbb.66.1619] [PMID: 12353619]

[216] Gräwert, T.; Groll, M.; Rohdich, F.; Bacher, A.; Eisenreich, W. Biochemistry of the non-mevalonate

isoprenoid pathway. *Cell. Mol. Life Sci.,* **2011**, *68*(23), 3797-3814. [http://dx.doi.org/10.1007/s00018-011-0753-z] [PMID: 21744068]

[217] Banerjee, A.; Sharkey, T.D. Methylerythritol 4-phosphate (MEP) pathway metabolic regulation. *Nat. Prod. Rep.,* **2014**, *31*(8), 1043-1055. [http://dx.doi.org/10.1039/C3NP70124G] [PMID: 24921065]

[218] Eisenreich, W.; Menhard, B.; Hylands, P.J.; Zenk, M.H.; Bacher, A. Studies on the biosynthesis of taxol: the taxane carbon skeleton is not of mevalonoid origin. *Proc. Natl. Acad. Sci. USA,* **1996**, *93*(13), 6431-6436. [http://dx.doi.org/10.1073/pnas.93.13.6431] [PMID: 8692832]

[219] Lansing, A.; Haertel, M.; Gordon, M.; Floss, H. Biosynthetic studies on taxol. *Planta Medica,* **1991**, *57*(S 2), A83-A83. [http://dx.doi.org/10.1055/s-2006-960355]

[220] Zamir, L.O.; Nedea, M.E.; Garneau, F.X. Biosynthetic building blocks of *Taxus canadensis* taxanes. *Tetrahedron Lett.,* **1992**, *33*(36), 5235-5236. [http://dx.doi.org/10.1016/S0040-4039(00)79141-6]

[221] Palazón, J.; Cusidó, R.M.; Bonfill, M.; Mallol, A.; Moyano, E.; Morales, C.; Piñol, M.T. Elicitation of different *Panax ginseng* transformed root phenotypes for an improved ginsenoside production. *Plant Physiol. Biochem.,* **2003**, *41*(11-12), 1019-1025. [http://dx.doi.org/10.1016/j.plaphy.2003.09.002]

[222] Croteau, R.; Ketchum, R.E.; Long, R.M.; Kaspera, R.; Wildung, M.R. Taxol biosynthesis and molecular genetics. *Phytochemistry Reviews Proceedings of the Phytochemical Society of Europe,* **2006**, *5*(1), p. 75. [http://dx.doi.org/10.1007/s11101-005-3748-2]

[223] Howat, S.; Park, B.; Oh, I.S.; Jin, Y-W.; Lee, E-K.; Loake, G.J. Paclitaxel: biosynthesis, production and future prospects. *N. Biotechnol.,* **2014**, *31*(3), 242-245. [http://dx.doi.org/10.1016/j.nbt.2014.02.010] [PMID: 24614567]

[224] Nims, E.; Dubois, C.P.; Roberts, S.C.; Walker, E.L. Expression profiling of genes involved in paclitaxel biosynthesis for targeted metabolic engineering. *Metab. Eng.,* **2006**, *8*(5), 385-394. [http://dx.doi.org/10.1016/j.ymben.2006.04.001] [PMID: 16793302]

[225] Tyo, K.E.; Alper, H.S.; Stephanopoulos, G.N. Expanding the metabolic engineering toolbox: more options to engineer cells. *Trends Biotechnol.,* **2007**, *25*(3), 132-137. [http://dx.doi.org/10.1016/j.tibtech.2007.01.003] [PMID: 17254656]

[226] Ajikumar, P.K.; Tyo, K.; Carlsen, S.; Mucha, O.; Phon, T.H.; Stephanopoulos, G. Terpenoids: opportunities for biosynthesis of natural product drugs using engineered microorganisms. *Mol. Pharm.,* **2008**, *5*(2), 167-190. [http://dx.doi.org/10.1021/mp700151b] [PMID: 18355030]

[227] Dejong, J.M.; Liu, Y.; Bollon, A.P.; Long, R.M.; Jennewein, S.; Williams, D.; Croteau, R.B. Genetic engineering of taxol biosynthetic genes in Saccharomyces cerevisiae. *Biotechnol. Bioeng.,* **2006**, *93*(2), 212-224. [http://dx.doi.org/10.1002/bit.20694] [PMID: 16161138]

[228] Wang, W.; Meng, C.; Zhu, P.; Cheng, K. Preliminary study on metabolic engineering of yeast for producing taxadiene. *Journal of Chinese biotechnology,* **2005**, *25*(8), 103.

[229] Jennewein, S.; Park, H.; DeJong, J.M.; Long, R.M.; Bollon, A.P.; Croteau, R.B. Coexpression in yeast of Taxus cytochrome P450 reductase with cytochrome P450 oxygenases involved in Taxol biosynthesis. *Biotechnol. Bioeng.,* **2005**, *89*(5), 588-598. [http://dx.doi.org/10.1002/bit.20390] [PMID: 15672381]

[230] Engels, B.; Dahm, P.; Jennewein, S. Metabolic engineering of taxadiene biosynthesis in yeast as a first step towards Taxol (Paclitaxel) production. *Metab. Eng.,* **2008**, *10*(3-4), 201-206.

[http://dx.doi.org/10.1016/j.ymben.2008.03.001] [PMID: 18485776]

[231] Ding, M.Z.; Yan, H.F.; Li, L.F.; Zhai, F.; Shang, L.Q.; Yin, Z.; Yuan, Y.J. Biosynthesis of Taxadiene in *Saccharomyces cerevisiae* : selection of geranylgeranyl diphosphate synthase directed by a computer-aided docking strategy. *PLoS One,* **2014**, *9*(10)e109348 [http://dx.doi.org/10.1371/journal.pone.0109348] [PMID: 25295588]

[232] Huang, Q.; Roessner, C.A.; Croteau, R.; Scott, A.I. Engineering *Escherichia coli* for the synthesis of taxadiene, a key intermediate in the biosynthesis of taxol. *Bioorg. Med. Chem.,* **2001**, *9*(9), 2237-2242. [http://dx.doi.org/10.1016/S0968-0896(01)00072-4] [PMID: 11553461]

[233] Ajikumar, P.K.; Xiao, W-H.; Tyo, K.E.; Wang, Y.; Simeon, F.; Leonard, E.; Mucha, O.; Phon, T.H.; Pfeifer, B.; Stephanopoulos, G. Isoprenoid pathway optimization for Taxol precursor overproduction in *Escherichia coli. Science,* **2010**, *330*(6000), 70-74. [http://dx.doi.org/10.1126/science.1191652] [PMID: 20929806]

[234] Meng, H.; Wang, Y.; Hua, Q.; Zhang, S.; Wang, X. In silico analysis and experimental improvement of taxadiene heterologous biosynthesis in *Escherichia coli. Biotechnol. Bioprocess Eng.; BBE,* **2011**, *16*(2), 205-215. [http://dx.doi.org/10.1007/s12257-010-0329-z]

[235] Boghigian, B.A.; Salas, D.; Ajikumar, P.K.; Stephanopoulos, G.; Pfeifer, B.A. Analysis of heterologous taxadiene production in K- and B-derived *Escherichia coli. Appl. Microbiol. Biotechnol.,* **2012**, *93*(4), 1651-1661. [http://dx.doi.org/10.1007/s00253-011-3528-4] [PMID: 21850432]

[236] Biggs, B.W.; Lim, C.G.; Sagliani, K.; Shankar, S.; Stephanopoulos, G.; De Mey, M.; Ajikumar, P.K. Overcoming heterologous protein interdependency to optimize P450-mediated Taxol precursor synthesis in *Escherichia coli. Proc. Natl. Acad. Sci. USA,* **2016**, *113*(12), 3209-3214. [http://dx.doi.org/10.1073/pnas.1515826113] [PMID: 26951651]

[237] Biggs, B.W.; Rouck, J.E.; Kambalyal, A.; Arnold, W.; Lim, C.G.; De Mey, M.; O'Neil-Johnson, M.; Starks, C.M.; Das, A.; Ajikumar, P.K. Orthogonal assays clarify the oxidative biochemistry of Taxol P450 CYP725A4. *ACS Chem. Biol.,* **2016**, *11*(5), 1445-1451. [http://dx.doi.org/10.1021/acschembio.5b00968] [PMID: 26930136]

[238] Edgar, S.; Li, F-S.; Qiao, K.; Weng, J-K.; Stephanopoulos, G. Engineering of taxadiene synthase for improved selectivity and yield of a key taxol biosynthetic intermediate. *ACS Synth. Biol.,* **2017**, *6*(2), 201-205. [http://dx.doi.org/10.1021/acssynbio.6b00206] [PMID: 27794603]

[239] Bian, G.; Yuan, Y.; Tao, H.; Shi, X.; Zhong, X.; Han, Y.; Fu, S.; Fang, C.; Deng, Z.; Liu, T. Production of taxadiene by engineering of mevalonate pathway in *Escherichia coli* and endophytic fungus *Alternaria alternata* TPF6. *Biotechnol. J.,* **2017**, *12*(4) [http://dx.doi.org/10.1002/biot.201600697] [PMID: 28217906]

[240] Han, K-H.; Fleming, P.; Walker, K.; Loper, M.; Chilton, W.S.; Mocek, U.; Gordon, M.P.; Floss, H.G. Genetic transformation of mature Taxus: an approach to genetically control the *in vitro* production of the anticancer drug, taxol. *Plant Sci.,* **1994**, *95*(2), 187-196. [http://dx.doi.org/10.1016/0168-9452(94)90092-2]

[241] Luan, E.C.; Allen, S.E.; Bolyard, M.G. Transient gus expression in zygotic embryos of Taxus brevifolia. In: *Vitro-Plant*; , **1996**; 32, p. (2)81-85.

[242] Ho, C-K.; Chang, S-H.; Lung, J.; Tsai, C-J.; Chen, K-P. The strategies to increase taxol production by using *Taxus mairei* cells transformed with TS and DBAT genes. *Int J Appl Sci Eng,* **2005**, *3*(3), 179-185.

[243] Ketchum, R.E.; Wherland, L.; Croteau, R.B. Stable transformation and long-term maintenance of transgenic Taxus cell suspension cultures. *Plant Cell Rep.,* **2007**, *26*(7), 1025-1033. [http://dx.doi.org/10.1007/s00299-007-0323-x] [PMID: 17333018]

[244] Syklowska-Baranek, K.; Pietrosiuk, A.; Kokoszka, A.; Furmanowa, M. Enhancement of taxane production in hairy root culture of *Taxus x media var. Hicksii. J. Plant Physiol.,* **2009**, *166*(17), 1950-1954.
[http://dx.doi.org/10.1016/j.jplph.2009.05.001] [PMID: 19573947]

[245] Exposito, O.; Syklowska-Baranek, K.; Moyano, E.; Onrubia, M.; Bonfill, M.; Palazon, J.; Cusido, R.M. Metabolic responses of *Taxus media* transformed cell cultures to the addition of methyl jasmonate. *Biotechnol. Prog.,* **2010**, *26*(4), 1145-1153.
[http://dx.doi.org/10.1002/btpr.424] [PMID: 20730769]

[246] Li, S-t.; Fu, C.h.; Zhang, M.; Zhang, Y.; Xie, S.; Yu, L.j. Enhancing taxol biosynthesis by overexpressing a 9-cis-epoxycarotenoid dioxygenase gene in transgenic cell lines of *Taxus chinensis. Plant Mol. Biol. Report.,* **2012**, *30*(5), 1125-1130.
[http://dx.doi.org/10.1007/s11105-012-0436-4]

[247] Sykłowska-Baranek, K.; Grech-Baran, M.; Naliwajski, M.; Bonfill, M.; Pietrosiuk, A. Paclitaxel production and PAL activity in hairy root cultures of *Taxus xmedia var. Hicksii* carrying a taxadiene synthase transgene elicited with nitric oxide and methyl jasmonate. *Acta Physiol. Plant.,* **2015**, *37*(10), 218.
[http://dx.doi.org/10.1007/s11738-015-1949-x]

[248] Besumbes, O.; Sauret-Güeto, S.; Phillips, M.A.; Imperial, S.; Rodríguez-Concepción, M.; Boronat, A. Metabolic engineering of isoprenoid biosynthesis in Arabidopsis for the production of taxadiene, the first committed precursor of Taxol. *Biotechnol. Bioeng.,* **2004**, *88*(2), 168-175.
[http://dx.doi.org/10.1002/bit.20237] [PMID: 15449291]

[249] Rontein, D.; Onillon, S.; Herbette, G.; Lesot, A.; Werck-Reichhart, D.; Sallaud, C.; Tissier, A. CYP725A4 from yew catalyzes complex structural rearrangement of taxa-4(5),11(12)-diene into the cyclic ether 5(12)-oxa-3(11)-cyclotaxane. *J. Biol. Chem.,* **2008**, *283*(10), 6067-6075.
[http://dx.doi.org/10.1074/jbc.M708950200] [PMID: 18167342]

[250] Kovacs, K.; Zhang, L.; Linforth, R.S.; Whittaker, B.; Hayes, C.J.; Fray, R.G. Redirection of carotenoid metabolism for the efficient production of taxadiene [taxa-4(5),11(12)-diene] in transgenic tomato fruit. *Transgenic Res.,* **2007**, *16*(1), 121-126.
[http://dx.doi.org/10.1007/s11248-006-9039-x] [PMID: 17106766]

[251] Anterola, A.; Shanle, E.; Perroud, P-F.; Quatrano, R. Production of taxa-4(5),11(12)-diene by transgenic Physcomitrella patens. *Transgenic Res.,* **2009**, *18*(4), 655-660.
[http://dx.doi.org/10.1007/s11248-009-9252-5] [PMID: 19241134]

[252] Cha, M.; Shim, S-H.; Kim, S-H.; Kim, O-T.; Lee, S-W.; Kwon, S-Y.; Baek, K-H. Production of taxadiene from cultured ginseng roots transformed with taxadiene synthase gene. *BMB Rep.,* **2012**, *45*(10), 589-594.
[http://dx.doi.org/10.5483/BMBRep.2012.45.10.085] [PMID: 23101514]

[253] Hasan, M.M.; Kim, H.S.; Jeon, J-H.; Kim, S.H.; Moon, B.; Song, J.Y.; Shim, S.H.; Baek, K.H. Metabolic engineering of *Nicotiana benthamiana* for the increased production of taxadiene. *Plant Cell Rep.,* **2014**, *33*(6), 895-904.
[http://dx.doi.org/10.1007/s00299-014-1568-9] [PMID: 24463610]

[254] Li, M.; Jiang, F.; Yu, X.; Miao, Z. Engineering isoprenoid biosynthesis in Artemisia Annua L. for the production of taxadiene: a key intermediate of taxol. *BioMed research international 2015,* **2015**.

[255] Zhang, J.; Chiodini, R.; Badr, A.; Zhang, G. The impact of next-generation sequencing on genomics. *J. Genet. Genomics,* **2011**, *38*(3), 95-109.
[http://dx.doi.org/10.1016/j.jgg.2011.02.003] [PMID: 21477781]

[256] Unamba, C.I.; Nag, A.; Sharma, R.K. Next generation sequencing technologies: the doorway to the unexplored genomics of non-model plants. *Front. Plant Sci.,* **2015**, *6*, 1074.
[http://dx.doi.org/10.3389/fpls.2015.01074] [PMID: 26734016]

[257] Jennewein, S.; Wildung, M.R.; Chau, M.; Walker, K.; Croteau, R. Random sequencing of an induced Taxus cell cDNA library for identification of clones involved in Taxol biosynthesis. *Proc. Natl. Acad. Sci. USA,* **2004**, *101*(24), 9149-9154.
[http://dx.doi.org/10.1073/pnas.0403009101] [PMID: 15178753]

[258] Hao, D.; Yang, L.; Xiao, P. The first insight into the Taxus genome via fosmid library construction and end sequencing. *Mol. Genet. Genomics,* **2011**, *285*(3), 197-205.
[http://dx.doi.org/10.1007/s00438-010-0598-4] [PMID: 21207064]

[259] Hao, C.; Ge, G.; Xiao, P.; Zhang, Y.; Yang, L. The first insight into the tissue specific taxus transcriptome via Illumina second generation sequencing. *PLoS One,* **2011**, *6*(6)e21220
[http://dx.doi.org/10.1371/journal.pone.0021220] [PMID: 21731678]

[260] Wu, Q.; Sun, C.; Luo, H.; Li, Y.; Niu, Y.; Sun, Y.; Lu, A.; Chen, S. Transcriptome analysis of *Taxus cuspidata* needles based on 454 pyrosequencing. *Planta Med.,* **2011**, *77*(4), 394-400.
[http://dx.doi.org/10.1055/s-0030-1250331] [PMID: 20862637]

[261] Li, S.T.; Zhang, P.; Zhang, M.; Fu, C.H.; Zhao, C.F.; Dong, Y.S.; Guo, A.Y.; Yu, L.J. Transcriptional profile of *Taxus chinensis* cells in response to methyl jasmonate. *BMC Genomics,* **2012**, *13*(1), 295.
[http://dx.doi.org/10.1186/1471-2164-13-295] [PMID: 22748077]

[262] Lenka, S.K.; Boutaoui, N.; Paulose, B.; Vongpaseuth, K.; Normanly, J.; Roberts, S.C.; Walker, E.L. Identification and expression analysis of methyl jasmonate responsive ESTs in paclitaxel producing *Taxus cuspidata* suspension culture cells. *BMC Genomics,* **2012**, *13*(1), 148.
[http://dx.doi.org/10.1186/1471-2164-13-148] [PMID: 22530557]

[263] Sun, G.; Yang, Y.; Xie, F.; Wen, J-F.; Wu, J.; Wilson, I.W.; Tang, Q.; Liu, H.; Qiu, D. Deep sequencing reveals transcriptome re-programming of *Taxus* × *media* cells to the elicitation with methyl jasmonate. *PLoS One,* **2013**, *8*(4)e62865
[http://dx.doi.org/10.1371/journal.pone.0062865] [PMID: 23646152]

[264] He, C.T.; Li, Z.L.; Zhou, Q.; Shen, C.; Huang, Y-Y.; Mubeen, S.; Yang, J-Z.; Yuan, J.G.; Yang, Z.Y. Transcriptome profiling reveals specific patterns of paclitaxel synthesis in a new *Taxus yunnanensis* cultivar. *Plant Physiol. Biochem.,* **2018**, *122*, 10-18.
[http://dx.doi.org/10.1016/j.plaphy.2017.10.028] [PMID: 29169081]

[265] Mubeen, S.; Li, Z.L.; Huang, Q.M.; He, C.T.; Yang, Z.Y. Comparative Transcriptome Analysis Revealed the Tissue-Specific Accumulations of Taxanes among Three Experimental Lines of *Taxus yunnanensis. J. Agric. Food Chem.,* **2018**, *66*(40), 10410-10420.
[http://dx.doi.org/10.1021/acs.jafc.8b03502] [PMID: 30208705]

[266] Qiu, D.; Pan, X.; Wilson, I.W.; Li, F.; Liu, M.; Teng, W.; Zhang, B. High throughput sequencing technology reveals that the taxoid elicitor methyl jasmonate regulates microRNA expression in Chinese yew (*Taxus chinensis*). *Gene,* **2009**, *436*(1-2), 37-44.
[http://dx.doi.org/10.1016/j.gene.2009.01.006] [PMID: 19393185]

[267] Li, S.; Zhang, P.; Zhang, M.; Fu, C.; Yu, L. Functional analysis of a WRKY transcription factor involved in transcriptional activation of the DBAT gene in *Taxus chinensis. Plant Biol (Stuttg),* **2013**, *15*(1), 19-26.
[http://dx.doi.org/10.1111/j.1438-8677.2012.00611.x] [PMID: 22686366]

[268] Lenka, S.K.; Nims, N.E.; Vongpaseuth, K.; Boshar, R.A.; Roberts, S.C.; Walker, E.L. Jasmonate-responsive expression of paclitaxel biosynthesis genes in *Taxus cuspidata* cultured cells is negatively regulated by the bHLH transcription factors TcJAMYC1, TcJAMYC2, and TcJAMYC4. *Front. Plant Sci.,* **2015**, *6*, 115.
[http://dx.doi.org/10.3389/fpls.2015.00115] [PMID: 25767476]

[269] Zhang, M.; Li, S.; Nie, L.; Chen, Q.; Xu, X.; Yu, L.; Fu, C. Two jasmonate-responsive factors, TcERF12 and TcERF15, respectively act as repressor and activator of tasy gene of taxol biosynthesis in *Taxus chinensis. Plant Mol. Biol.,* **2015**, *89*(4-5), 463-473.
[http://dx.doi.org/10.1007/s11103-015-0382-2] [PMID: 26445975]

CHAPTER 5

Cytotoxicity Through Molecular Targets Involved in Apoptosis. Where Should We Further Search for Mushrooms Functionalities in Future Cancer Treatment?

Dejan Stojković[1], Jelena Živković[2], Danijela Stanisavljević[3], Marija Smiljković[1], Jelena Popović[3], Milena Stevanović[3, 4, 5], Jasmina Glamočlija[1] and **Marina Soković[1, *]**

[1] *Department of Plant Physiology, Institute for Biological Research "Siniša Stanković", University of Belgrade, Bulevar Despota Stefana 142, 11000, Belgrade, Serbia*

[2] *Institute for Medicinal Plant Research "Dr. Josif Pančić", Tadeuša Košćuška 1, 11000, Belgrade, Serbia*

[3] *Institute of Molecular Genetics and Genetic Engineering, University of Belgrade, Vojvode Stepe 444a, PO Box 23, 11010, Belgrade, Serbia*

[4] *Faculty of Biology, University of Belgrade, Studentski trg 16, PO box 43, 11000, Belgrade, Serbia*

[5] *Serbian Academy of Sciences and Arts, Knez Mihailova 35, 11001, Belgrade, Serbia*

Abstract: Apoptosis is considered as a classical way of programmed cell death and important control mechanism of cell homeostasis. Cancer cells acquire different instruments to circumvent programmed cell death. This promotes uncontrolled growth and frequently confers chemoresistance to tumor cells. Activation of apoptotic signaling pathway has been a target of anti-cancer drugs in an induction of cytotoxicity. The mechanism of apoptosis is complex and includes many pathways. This chapter will focus on the current knowledge of apoptosis-triggering approaches in cancer therapy, as well as on mushroom extracts and isolated compounds acting as initiators of apoptosis through regulation of genes expression involved in cancer cell death. Furthermore, we pointed out directions for novel search for mushroom functionalities in this experimental field and discuss the possible further steps for exploration on the *in vitro* and *in vivo* levels.

Keywords: Cytotoxicity, Apoptosis, Molecular targets, Mushrooms, Cancer cells.

[*] **Corresponding author Marina Soković:** Institute for Biological Research "Siniša Stanković", University of Belgrade, Bulevar Despota Stefana 142, 11000 Belgrade, Serbia, Tel : +381112078419 ; E-mail: mris@ibiss.bg.ac.rs

INTRODUCTION

Cancer represents a group of more than 100 various diseases which are characterized by uncontrolled cellular growth, local tissue invasion and distant metastases. It presents second leading cause of death worldwide next to cardiovascular diseases [1]. According to American Cancer Society, mortality caused by cancer would increase up to 13 million in 2030, together with 22 million new cancer cases which makes cancer one of the most destructive diseases worldwide [2]. Regardless of considerable achievements in the development of anticancer therapeutics, the incidence of cancer is still increasing globally [3]. Presently, existing cytotoxic therapies such as chemotherapy, γ-irradiation and immunotherapy are to a large degree dependant on activation or reactivation of the apoptosis mechanism. Accordingly, failure of cell to undergo apoptosis leads to resistance to anticancer drugs [4].

Cancer is a multifaceted process, the formation of which is followed by three stages of cell transformation: initiation, promotion, and progression. Each of them is associated with oxidative stress. During the initiation phase, free radicals are the major cause of structural changes in DNA and consequent gene mutations. In the promotional phase, they block cellular communication, resulting in an increase in proliferation and/or a decrease in apoptosis in the initiated cell population. Finally, oxidative stress also has effects on the progression of cancer, causing additional DNA changes in an already transformed cell population. Reactive oxygen species (ROS) can also increase the rate of cell migration, affecting both invasiveness and tumor metastases [5].

On the other hand, increased production of ROS- leads to - aging and death of tumor cells, thus induction of ROS can also be considered as anti-cancer approach. How ROS will affect the cell depends on the type of cells and tissue, the concentration of ROS, and the activity of the antioxidant enzymes [5].

The aim of each therapeutic approach is to target tumor cells with minimal adverse effect to normal cell function. The problem lies in the fact that normal cells also have the possibility to employ the apoptotic program and they often do so more easily compared to their tumorigenic correlatives. The therapeutic plan could rely on modulation of expression and/or function of apoptotic-related molecules that are particularly fundamental for control of tumor cell function or molecules that are controlled in a diverse way in tumor cells and in normal cells [6].

There are various mechanisms of cell death: apoptosis, necrosis, autophagy, senescence and mitotic catastrophe [7]. In contrast to necrotic cells, which are damaged by external factors and lysed after diffusion of inflammatory molecules, apoptotic cells initiate pathways leading to their suicide and consequent macrophage phagocytosis [8].

Apoptosis is considered as the normal physiological way of noninflammatory programmed cell death [9]. The apoptotic threshold of the cell is determined with the net balance of all pro-and anti-apoptotic "control mechanisms". Programmed cell death exists when the pro-apoptotic signals overstep anti-apoptotic buffering capacity of the cell [10].

Until now, research indicates that there are two main types of apoptotic pathways: the extrinsic or death receptor pathway and the intrinsic or mitochondrial pathway. However, although their mechanisms differ these two pathways are connected and molecules from one pathway can impact the other [11]. Caspases are central components in the apoptosis mechanism since they are both responsible for the initiation and execution of apoptosis [12]. The caspases can be roughly subdivided into two groups: 1) those connected to caspase 1 (*e.g.* caspase-1, -4, -5, -13, and -14) that are mainly included in cytokine production during inflammation and 2) those that have an essential role in apoptosis (*e.g.* caspase-2, -3. -6, -7, -8, -9 and -10). In the second group caspase-2, -8, -9 and -10 are mainly in charged for the initiation of the apoptotic pathway, while caspase-3, -6 and -7 are responsible for the final cleavage of cell components during apoptosis [12].

INTRINSIC PATHWAY

Intrinsic apoptosis pathway is also called mitochondrial because it depends on factors that are released from mitochondria. This pathway regulates cell death in response to various stimuli such as cellular stresses and developmental signals [13]. Today it is clearly determined that as a result of a stress signal (such as DNA damage), cytoplasmatic p53 rapidly translocates to mitochondria, where it interacts with multi-domain members of the anti and proapoptotic Bcl-2 family members to either inhibit or activate them. This direct action of p53 results in mitochondrial outer membrane permeability, releasing the enzymatic apoptotic machinery of caspases and leading to chromatin degradation [14].

Proteins from Bcl-2 family can have pro- or anti- apoptotic activities, and when different stimuli converge on mitochondria these proteins can lead to mitochondrial outer membrane permeabilisation [15]. Members of Bcl-2 family, Bax and Bak, homooligomerize and form mitochondrial permeability transition pore through which different proteins are released in cytosol [16]. Bak is constitutively located in outer mitochondria membrane, while Bax is predominant in cytosol. In response to apoptotic stimuli they both change conformation and Bax than locates at mitochondrial outer membrane where it forms pore with Bak

[16]. When permeability is increased proteins are released in cytosol and among them cytochrome C is the most studied. Cytochrome c in cytosole binds APAF 1 (Apoptotic protease activating factor 1) and induces conformational changes that expose a nucleotide-binding site in the nucleotide binding and oligomerization (NACHT) domain of APAF1. Once nucleotide binding site is exposed, deoxy-ATP binds it and induces second conformational change that exposes CARD (caspase activation and recruitment domain) and oligomerization domains [17]. APAF 1 than oligomerizes with cytochrome c and regrutes and activates caspase-9, and all three of them form apoptosome [18]. Caspase-9 activates caspase-3, effector caspase necessary for efficient cell killing [19]. Besides caspase-3, also caspase-6 and caspase-7 are executioner caspases that induce changes in morphological and other properties of cell characteristic for apoptosis by cleaving various substrates. Executioner caspases exist as inactive dimers that are activated upon proteolytic cleavage of both monomers at loops containing specific cleavage sites [20]. Caspase-3 cleaves the inhibitor of the caspase-activated deoxyribonuclease, which is responsible for nuclear apoptosis. Downstream caspases cleave protein kinases, cytosceletal proteins, DNA repair proteins and inhibitory subunits of endonucleases family. Cytosceleton, cell cycle and signaling pathways are also affected by caspase activation and all of these changes in summary are changes that are observed as typical for apoptosis [21]. Apoptotic cell death can be also caspase independent. It can be mediated by the release of pro-apoptotic proteins (endonuclease G, apoptosis inducing factor, HtrA2/OMI) from the mitochondria. Endonuclease G is released from mitochondria in cytosole and then locates in nucleus where it cleaves nuclear DNA. Apoptosis inducing factor is NADH oxidase located in mitochondria and when mitochondrial membrane permeabilization is increased it locates in cytosole and nucleus where it induces cellular damage [22].

There is increasing search for efficient anticancer agents for treating neoplastic disease and there are studies investigating targeting of apoptosis pathway as anticancer therapy. In high percent of all cancers there is evidence for overexpression of antiapoptotic Bcl-2 or Bcl-xL which makes tumor cell resistant to most cytotoxic anticancer drugs [23, 24]. Bcl2 and Bcl-xl are antiapoptotic members of Bcl protein family which act by blocking the mitochondrial release of cytochrome C [12]. Usage of antisense oligonucleotides [24] or development of small molecules that would interfere with Bcl-2/Bcl-xL function, are currently investigated [25].

EXTRINSIC PATHWAY

Extracellular signals are responsible for apoptosis initiation via extrinsic pathway [26]. Death receptors serve as signal transporters from extracellular death ligands to the cellular apoptotic machinery initiating the caspase cascade [27]. As transmembrane receptors, death receptors belong to the superfamily of tumor-necrosis factor receptors (TNFR) and they activate apoptosis upon ligand binding [28]. In that way they activate caspases as the main executioners of apoptosis [29]. These ligand-bound death receptors connected with extrinsic apoptotic pathway include Fas (CD95 or APO1), TNFR1, DR3, DR4 (TRAIL-R1), DR5 (TRAIL- R2) and DR6 [30]. Among death ligands, TRAIL nowadays present the most encouraging candidates for clinical trials since they primarily trigger apoptosis in malignant or transformed cells, whereas normal cells are relatively resistant. Also, contrary to FasL or TNF, increased signaling through DR4 and DR5 is not connected with undesirable toxicity levels *in vivo* [27].

Tumour cells have developed various mechanisms in order to modify the extrinsic or intrinsic pathway mechanism. The capacity of neoplastic cells to conquer abundant pro-apoptotic signals is a valuable target for cancer chemotherapeutics [31].

TARGETING APOPTOSIS IN CANCER TREATMENT

Targeting Bcl-2 and Bax

The family of B-cell lymphoma-2 (Bcl-2) proteins has a central role in the control of cell life and death and the interest for Bcl-2 as a cancer drug target raised when the researchers pointed out to link among blocking apoptosis and chemoresistance [32]. Promising treatment strategies involve application of therapeutic agents in order to inhibit the Bcl-2 proteins or to suppress the associated upregulated anti-apoptotic proteins or genes [12]. Bcl-2 protein family includes three subgroups of proteins that either promote cell survival (*e.g.*, Bcl-2 and Bcl-xL), initiate cell killing (*e.g.*, Bcl-2-interacting mediator of cell death (Bim), p53 upregulated mediator of apoptosis (Puma) or Bcl-2-interacting domain (Bid)) or activate the effector pathways of programmed cell death (Bax, Bak) [33]. It is believed that a balance between antiapoptotic and proapoptotic Bcl-2 family members control the apoptotic response by regulating mitochondrial membrane integrity [34].

Predominance of anti-apoptotic members of the Bcl-2 family of proteins is a phenomenon that usually and naturally appears in cancer cells. For almost 50% of the cancers, over-expression of anti-apoptotic Bcl-2 or Bcl-xL is specific. Also, failure of Bax expression is found in some colorectal cancers and hematopoietic malignancies, whereas the expression of a highly apoptogenic variant of Bax (Baxw) is in correlation with an increased survival of patients with glioblastoma multiforme, an aggressive form of brain tumors [35].

Targeting Death Receptors

As members of the tumor necrosis factor (TNF) receptor superfamily, death receptors are defined by cysteine-rich extracellular domain. They also involve a homologous cytoplasmatic sequence known as death domain which represents recognition point for the apoptotic machinery. TNF family of cytokines comprises of three ligands for death receptors: Fas ligand (FasL), TNF and TNF related apoptosis inducing ligand (TRAIL) [36]. Both, chemotherapy and radiotherapy use the intrinsic pathway for apoptosis induction. Defects in the intrinsic pathway are usual cause of resistance toward these therapies. Their combination with TRAIL receptor targeting agents might prevent this resistance [37]. TNF-α-related apoptosis-inducing ligand (TRAIL/Apo2L), alone or in combination with the existing therapies, is the most perspective candidate since it is able to promote apoptosis in numerous types of malignant cells while saving most normal tissues. On the contrary to some other representatives of the TNF superfamily (such as TNFα), which can produce severe toxic side effects, TRAIL is efficient in selectively killing a wide range of tumour cells from lung, breast, kidney, colon, prostate, thyroid and skin cancers, without causing significant organ toxicity and inflammation *in vivo* [38].

Also, binding of TRAIL to death receptors DR5 (TRAIL-R2) and DR4 (TRAIL-R1) acts as a trigger for apoptosis. On the contrary to tumour cells, normal cells express mainly decoy receptors DcR1 (TRAIL-R3) and DcR2 (TRAIL-R4) which do not transfer cell death signals [39].

Caspase Activators

The extrinsic pathway cause to the activation of pro-Caspases-8 and/or -10 into active Caspases-8 and/or -10 at the Death Inducing Signaling Complex (DISC). On the other hand, internal and external stresses in intrinsic pathway promote release of cytochrome-c from the mitochondria, which, together with Apaf-1, activates pro-Caspase-9 into Caspase-9. These three caspases acting as a group (pro-Caspases-10, 8 and 9) are known as the initiator caspases since they can initiate the activation of the effector pro-Caspases 3 and 7 into active Caspases-3 and -7 (hereafter Caspases-3 and -7) causing the apoptotic cascade [40].

As central regulators of apoptosis, controlled activation of caspases represents attractive target for cancer therapy.

Modulation of the p53 Tumor Suppressor

p53 protein is involved in the regulation of cell life and death processes, such as apoptosis, cell cycle arrest, senescence and DNA repair [41]. P53 involvement in

DNA damage-related programs is regarded as the major, if not a sole mechanism by which p53 exerts its tumour suppressor function [42]. Due to its important role in conserving stability by preventing genome mutation, p53 has also been described as the "guardian of the genome" [43]. The major consequence of p53 deregulation is tumour initiation and progression. So far, many different mechanisms that lead to its deregulation were described [44, 45].

The essential role of p53 as a tumor suppressor has become evident when sequencing of thousands of cancer genomes revealed that mutations in *TP53* gene are the most common lesions in different cancer types [46]. The most common mutations are the missense mutations within the DNA binding domain, comprising 75% of all p53 mutations, which impair direct interactions with DNA, while other types of mutations affect the proper p53 protein folding [47].

Complex network that regulates p53 level and activity is comprised of number of proteins [48]. Mdm2 and MdmX proto-oncogenes are important regulators of p53 function. In a negative feedback loop, they inhibit p53 transcriptional activity by binding to its N terminal trans-activation domain. Mdm2 promotes p53 rapid degradation by binding to a small domain [49 - 51], while Mdmx is unable to degrade p53 as it does not possess E3 ligase activity [52]. Inhibition of Mdm2 and MdmX expressions can result in the induction of p53 activity and apoptosis. Realizing the important role of p53 in major cellular processes, the race has started for finding a way to reactivate p53 protein, as a promising strategy to treat a cancer. The major aim in this struggle is the incessant reconstitution of p53 function, which can result in regression of various types of tumours, as already described for lymphomas, soft tissue sarcomas and hepatocellular carcinomas [53 - 55].

In this struggle, many different approaches were applied, and achievements will be summarized in this section, especially those addressed to targeting mutant p53 and reactivation of *wt*p53 by targeting Mdm2 and MdmX inhibitors. The special emphasis will be addressed to natural compounds from fungi and their potential to restore function of this important protein.

Targeting Mutant p53 to Restore its Wild-Type Function

It is well known that many different cancer types expressed mutant p53 protein that contributes to more aggressive malignant phenotype [56]. In case of repairing mutant p53, several approaches have been applied, including mutant p53 refolding to the wild-type conformation, induction of mutant p53 proteasomal degradation or focusing on protein–protein interactions [44, 56, 57].

Reactivation of Wild-type p53 by Targeting Mdm2 and MdmX Inhibitors

The level of p53 activity must be very tightly controlled to sustain healthy cell phenotype and to achieve tumour cell elimination without causing toxicity to normal proliferative tissues, which underline tight control of p53 and all other components of this signaling pathway. The function of p53 in tumours without p53 mutations is frequently impaired due to enhanced activity of two inhibitors, Mdm2 and its homologue MdmX. The high level of these inhibitors is achieved through gene amplification, increased transcription, enhanced mRNA stability and altered post-translational modifications [58]. The protein-protein interactions have become the most interesting aspect of p53 signaling for drug targeting and many efforts have been made to find a proper way to block a p53-Mdm2 and p53-MdmX interactions.

Natural Bioactive Compounds from Fungi That Modulate p53 Activity

Looking toward new strategies for targeting p53, there is a continued interest in the search for natural bioactive compounds, like extracts of mushrooms. Polysaccharide fraction PAP-3 from fruiting bodies of Abalone mushroom was highly active in inhibiting proliferation of MCF7 cells leading to elevated levels of p53 protein [59]. Another known polysaccharide with antiproliferative effect on MCF7 cells is SCH isolated from medicinal mushroom *Schizophyllum commune*. This polysaccharide leads to p53 accumulation in a dose dependent manner [60]. Also, dichloromethane fraction (DCMF) from mushroom *Auricularia auricula-judae* ethanol extract and an immunomodulatory protein isolated from *Flammulina velutipes* resulted in cell cycle arrest through increased p53 expression [61, 62].

Some extracts from medicinal mushroom *Ganoderma lucidum* showed anticancer activity on colon and ovarian cancer cells, leading to induction of apoptosis and p53 expression through activation of caspase-3 [63, 64]. Hispolon, bioactive compound of *Phellinus linteus* was shown to have a potential use in cancer treatment since it down-regulated the expression of the Mdm2 [65]. Recently, it was shown that some steroids from mushrooms have potential anti-tumour effect through inhibiting Mdm2 [66]. The ethanol extract of *Innotus obliquus* (Chaga mushroom) induced G1 cell cycle arrest in HT-29 human colon cancer cells, decreased protein expression of CDK2, CDK4, and cyclin D1, and increased expression of p21, p27, and p53 [67].

Taken together, bioactive compounds isolated from mushrooms have promising therapeutic potential trough various, but still not fully understood mechanisms that lead to proper function of highly important tumour suppressor protein p53.

Mushrooms as Part of Regular Diet - Potential Role in Cancer Prevention

Recently, numerous food products have been named "superfoods", in order to emphasize their beneficial effect to overall health together with high nutritional value [68]. Among more than 2000 mushroom species found all over the world, around 25 of them are used in human diet. There is a blurry line between edible and medicinal mushroom since many of them are usually both [69]. They have been abundantly used in Oriental medicine, but during the last decade's numerous studies are conducted in order to shed light onto specific biological properties and to identify mushroom ingredients responsible for their activities. According to Patel i Goyal [70], mushrooms are considered as "biotherapeutics" of new generation as well as "nutraceutical food" [69]. Medicinal mushrooms could be used in common diet as encapsulated powder, extracts, but also as tea [71].

Healthy nutrition is important precondition for cancer prevention. As reviewed by Donaldson [72], healthy diet together with adequate lifestyle might reduce cancer incidence for almost 40%. Some studies have suggested that more than 90% of colon cancers are linked to inadequate diet [73], while various diseases including lung cancer could be prevented by natural products [74].

Diet reach in mushrooms is associated with decreased cancer risk in few studies. Four mushrooms (*Corrinellus shiitake*, *Flammulina velutipes*, *Hypsizigus marmoreus*, *Pholiota nameko*) have been explored as anticancer agents in hospital based case-control study. Increased intake of these mushrooms was associated with reduced risk of stomach cancer [75]. Case–control study, conducted in southeast China, found significant correlation between mushroom consumption and lower risk for breast cancer development [76], together with study conducted among Korean women [77]. A hospital-based case-control study in China, found a link between decreased risk of epithelial ovarian cancer and mushroom consumption, especially white button mushroom (*Agaricus bisporus*).

Diverse antioxidants have impact on chemoprevention of various cancers. They can reduce incidence of prostate cancer [78], breast cancer [79] as well as gastric cancer [80]. Since mushrooms are valuable source of antioxidants [81], diet reach in these "nutraceuticals" could serve, at least in part, as cancer prophylaxis. One more reason to include them in regular diet is selenium - an essential micronutrient found in mushrooms. Absence of selenium in human nutrition is associated with different conditions including some cancers [82]. Besides serving in cancer prevention, diet rich in mushroom can also help in reduction of chemotherapy and radiation side effects. They can reduce nausea, anemia and bone marrow suppression [70]. Antitumor properties of medicinal mushrooms have been used to develop the new formulations for cancer treatment - biological response modifiers (BRMs). These supplements are applied along with conventional treatment [83]. Chemopreventive properties of mushrooms are mostly linked to fungal polysaccharides [71].

Most of the literature data on anticancer properties of mushrooms is based on *in vitro* experiments. For the ones that are most studied, like *Ganoderma lucidum*, there are some data from *in vivo* studies and clinical trials. Polysacharides from *Ganoderma lucidum* were used for the development of product named Ganopoly®. This formulation was tested on advanced-stage cancer patients where 12 week treatment (1800 mg, 3 times daily) lead to significant improvement of patient's immune status [84]. In the recent years, *Ganoderma* species are considered safe for use as an alternative in the treatment of leukemia, different carcinomas, but also in some other diseases including diabetes. It is estimated that millions of people are using products based on this fungus every day, both as prevention or as a cure for some of the diseases. These products are based either on fruiting bodes, mycelium or spores [85]. *Ganoderma lucidum* is maybe the most famous mushroom for its anticancer effects partly due to positive effect on immune system, cancer cell cytotoxicity and reduction of angiogenesis [69]. Clinical trial was conducted also in order to explore potential beneficial effect of Sun mushroom (*Agaricus sylvaticus*) on colorectal cancer patients. It was proven that tablets containing this mushroom (30 mg/kg/day) had excellent effect in reducing fasting glycemia levels, trait that could potentially lead to interfered carcinogenesis process [86].

Mushrooms as Apoptosis Inducers in Cancer Cells

In the next pages we will focus on mushroom species investigated in the past few years (2014-2018) for their cytotoxic potential with presented molecular targets. The most important observation about mushrooms citotoxicities are summarized in the Table **1**.

Inonotus obliquus (Ach. ex Pers.) Pilát (1942)

Inonotus obliquus (Fig. **1**), Chaga mushroom, can be found in Russia, China, Japan, Eastern and Northern Europe, and Alaska as a parasite on birch (*Betula platyphylla* var. *japonica*) where it looks like burnt charcoal. Mushroom *I. obliquus* is well known for wide range of biological and pharmacological activities including antibacterial, anti-inflammatory, antiallergic and other, justifying the fact that it has been used as medicinal mushroom for the treatment of different conditions in many countries. In Russian ethnomedicine it is used to treat different cancers, including breast, gastrointestinal and lung cancers [87].

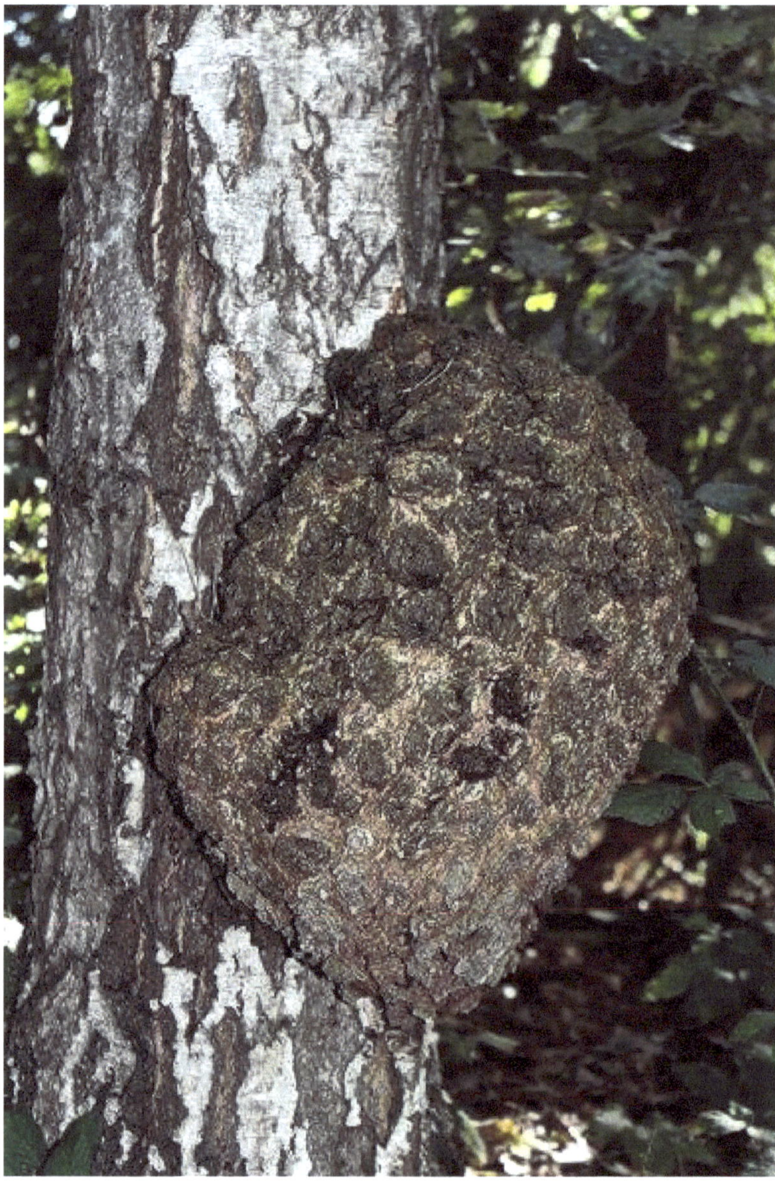

Fig (1). *Inonotus obliquus.*

Methanolic extract of *Inonotus obliquus* is able to induce apoptosis by caspase-3 activation in lung cancer cells leading to reduced viability of the cells (IC_{50} 2.03 mg/mL). Some of the triterpenoids presented in the extract might be the cause of anticancer properties, since they showed IC_{50} 75.1 - 227.4 µM [87]. Human lung carcinoma cells can also be inhibited by inotodiol extracted from *Inonotus obliquus*, since 20 mg/L are inducing morphological changes typical for apoptotic cells, as well as by altering expression of apoptosis related genes (upregulating p53 gene expression and downregulating Bcl-2 gene) [88]. Two lignin metabolites were isolated from *I. obliquus* hot water extract. These metabolites were active in inhibiting A549 lung cancer line (IC_{50} 160.5 μg/mL and 222.9 μg/mL). Both compounds were reducing nuclear translocation component p65, leading to inhibition of nuclear transcription factor, NF-kB [89].

Inonotus taiwanensis Sheng H. Wu, Y.T. Lin & C.L. Chern (2018)

Inonotus taiwanensis is recently described fungus from Taiwan and could be found on trunk of *Trema tomentosa* [90]. Polysaccharidic extract induces apoptotic cell death in human acute monocytic leukemia THP-1 and U937 cell lines *in vitro* (IC_{50} 137 μg/mL and 255 μg/mL). This extract induces cell cycle arrest, endonuclease G-mediated apoptosis and autophagy inhibition [91].

Phellinus igniarius (L.) Quél. (1886)

Phellinus igniarius is a perennial mushroom found on different woods, mostly in Asian countries. It has been used as medicinal mushroom in East Asian countries for curing bloody gonorrhea, festering wounds, diarrhea and menoxenia [92].

Phellinus igniarius ethanolic extract exhibited antitumor activities against different cell lines (HepG-2, AGS, SGC-7901, Hela and A-549) (IC_{50} 110.7 - 531.7 μg/mL), with the most promising activity towards gastric cancer cells (IC_{50} 110.7 μg/mL). Extract induced apoptosis leading to typical cell morphology changes (chromatin condensation, nuclear fragmentation), as well as downregulation of cyclin D1 expression and eventually led to cell death by activation of caspase-9, -3 and PARP cleavage. Extract also upregulated expression of Bax and downregulated expression of Bcl-2, and since it showed anticancer potential both *in vitro* and *in vivo* it represents a promising candidate for further investigation [92].

Ganoderma resinaceum Boud. (1889)

Ganoderma resinaceum is a mushroom belongs to Ganodermataceae family, known for its numerous health promoting activities. *G. resinaceum* extract has been proven to possess antimicrobial and antioxidant activities [93].

G. resinaceum ethyl acetate extract showed antitumor activity towards human ovarian cancer cell line and less prominent activity towards human breast cancer cell line in tested concentrations of 0.01 mg/mL and 0.1 mg/mL. A phytosterol, α-spinasterol is isolated from *Ganoderma resinaceum* and it has been proven to possess anticancer properties. This phytosterol is able to highly reduce growth of

MCF-7 cells (human breast cancer cell line, IC_{50} 1 μM) and to lesser extent SKOV-3 cells (human ovarian cancer cell line, IC_{50} 10 μM). Antitumor activities of α-spinasterol could be due upregulated expression of p53 and Bax and downregulated expression of cyclin dependent kinase cdk4/6 [94].

Ganoderma applanatum (Pers.) Pat. (1887)

Ganoderma applanatum (Fig. **2**) is a medicinal fungi growing on trees, as saprobe or parasite. It has different biological properties including antimicrobial, anti-fibrotic and anti-tumor [95].

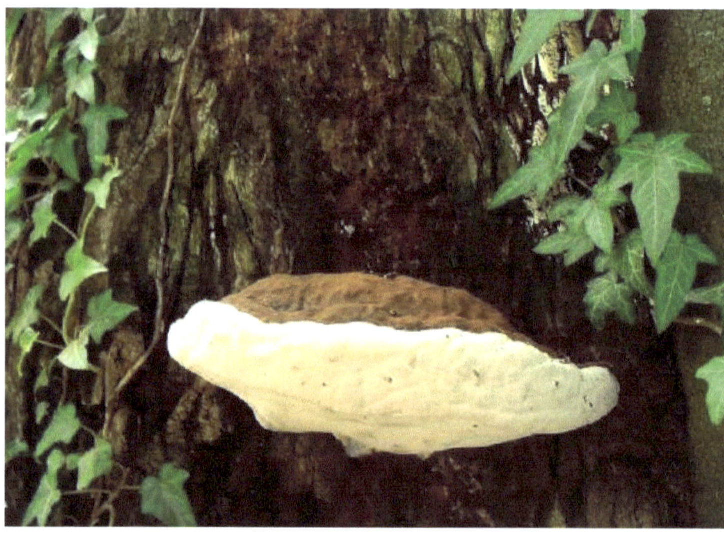

Fig. (2). *Ganoderma applanatum.*

Methanolic extract was efficient in inhibiting Caco-2 cell line (colon cancer) showing IC_{50} of 160 μg/mL. Possible mode of anti-tumor activity includes an increase in Bax expression, decrease in Bcl-2 expression, as well as up-regulation of caspase, Casp-3. Anti-tumor properties of this mushroom was confirmed *in vivo*, since application of extract at concentration 200 μg/mL during five days, was able to decrease mass of developed Ehrlich tumor [95].

Cantharellus cibarius Fr. (1821)

Cantharelus cibarius (Fig. **3**), gold chanterelles, is one of the most popular edible mushroom due to its properties like high nutritional value, high protein content and pleasant odour and taste [96].

C. cibarius aqueous methanol extract in concentrations of 1 - 20 mg/mL, led to

0.00 - 78.02% of cell death, showing IC_{50} < 1 mg/mL in human lung adenocarcinoma cell line A549. Piceatannol, stilbene, is thought to be at least in part responsible for this activity, since it is able to significantly reduce viability of A549 cell line when applied in concentration of 0.0075 mg/mL [97].

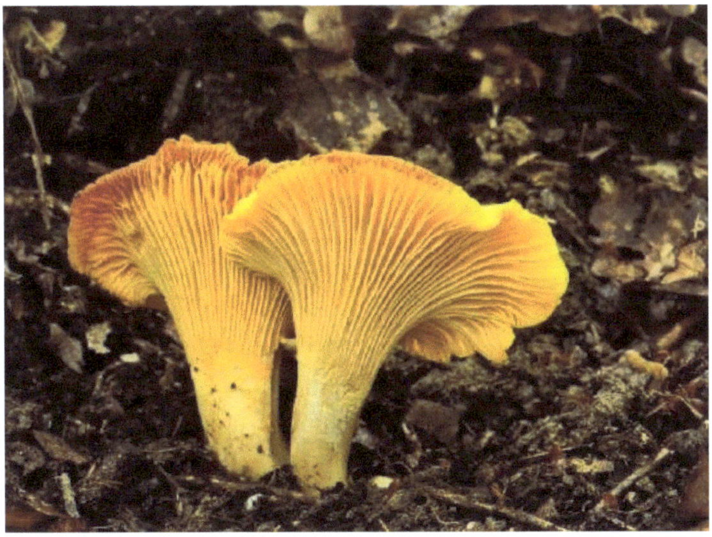

Fig. (3). *Cantharelus cibarius.*

Pleurotus sajor-caju **(Fr.) Singer (1951)**

Pleurotus sajor-caju is edible mushroom often used as food supplement. Most promising was n-hexane mushroom extract exhibiting IC_{50} 0.05 mg/mL towards colorectal cancer cells. Its mode of anti-tumor action includes ROS generation, breakdown of mitochondrial membrane potential, as well as increased expression of p53, Bax and Caspase-3 together with decrease of Bcl-2. Compound that is possibly related to these antitumor properties is ergosta-5,7,22-trien-3β-ol since it is shown *in silico* that it could inhibit Bcl-2 [98].

Lignosus rhinocerus **(Cooke) Ryvarden (1972)**

Lignosus rhinocerus, tiger milk mushroom, has medicinal value and it is efficient in the treatment of wounds, fever, asthma and other conditions. Sclerotia extract has been proven to have activities such as anti-inflammatory, antimicrobial, and antihypertensive [99].

Protein fraction obtained from mushroom's sclerotia cold water extract has IC_{50} 3.00 μg/mL towards human breast adenocarcinoma cell line (MCF7). This cytotoxic effect is due to activation of both extrinsic and intrinsic apoptosis pathways. Apoptosis is mediated by upregulation of caspase-8 and -9 activities and a downregulation of Bcl-2 [100]. Sesquiterpenes were isolated form *L. rhinocerotis* and of them (+)-torreyol could be considered as cytotoxic agent since it shows IC_{50} of 3.5 μg/mL towards MCF7 cells (breast cancer cell line) [100].

Morchella esculenta (L.) Pers. (1801)

Morchella esculenta (L.) Pers. (Fig. **4**), morel mushroom or sponge morel, is edible mushroom distributed throughout the world and widely used in gourmet cuisine for its pleasant flavor and beneficial nutritional properties. It is also used in traditional medicine to treat excessive sputum, gastrointestinal disorder and shortness of breath, and is known for range of biological activities including antioxidant, antimicrobial and others [101].

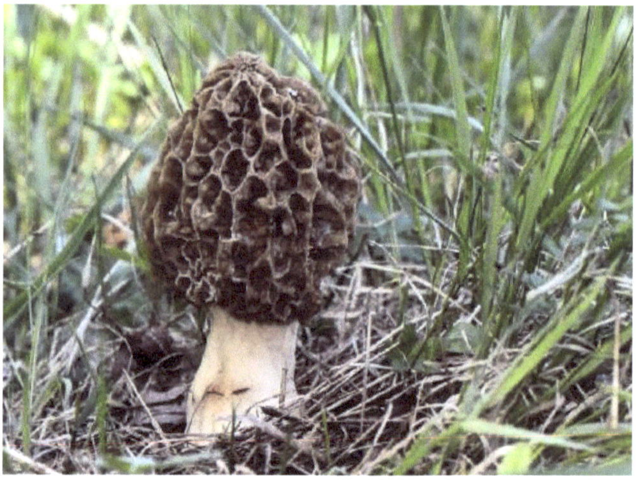

Fig. (4). *Morchella esculenta.*

M. esculenta methanolic extract inhibited human lung cancer cells with IC_{50} 0.49 - 1.35 mg/mL, causing apoptosis with characteristic changes in morphology of the cells, including cell rounding, shrinkage, membrane blabbing and detachment of cells. It was shown that fatty acids and sterols (IC_{50} 156.9 - 278 M) are moderately responsible for cytotoxic activities of mushroom extract towards lung cancer cells [101].

Lentinus squarrosulus Mont. (1842)

L. squarrosulus is edible paleotropic mushroom species growing on tree trunks, old stumps, tree roots. Its range of biological activities includes antioxidant, antiproliferative, and immunomodulatory [102].

Lentinus squarrosulus aqueous extract was used for the isolation of peptide fractions which exhibited IC_{50} 2.8-26.84 μg/mL in different lung cancer cell lines. Mushroom peptide extract (20 mg/mL) induced apoptosis via both intrinsic and extrinsic apoptosis pathways, downregulating Bcl-2 and upregulating BAX, as well as decreasing levels of death receptor inhibitor c-FLIP [103].

Ramaria botrytis (Pers.) Ricken (1918)

Ramaria botrytis (Fig. **5**), edible mushroom found in eastern Asia, Europe and North America is used in culinary practice due to its pleasant taste. Mushroom possesses antimicrobial and antioxidant activities. The mushroom was used for the isolation of novel ubiquitin-like antitumour protein (RBUP). This protein showed antitumor activity towards A549 cells (human non-small-cell lung cancer), mediated through apoptosis (IC_{50} 15.93 μM) possibly through its hemagglutinating and DNase activities [104].

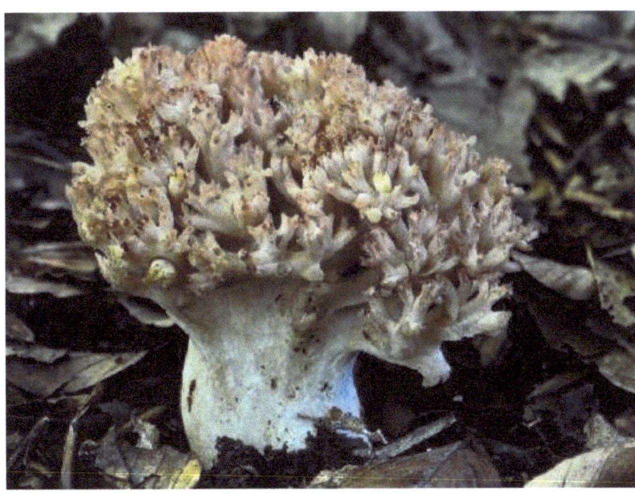

Fig. (5). *Ramaria botrytis.*

Coprinus comatus (O.F.Müll.) Pers. (1797)

C. comatus (Fig. **6**), chicken drumstick mushroom or shaggy-mane, is an edible mushroom with biological properties such as antioxidant and antimicrobial [105]. Protein Y3 is glycan binding protein isolated from *C. comatus*. This protein is exhibiting antitumor activities due to its potential to inhibit human T-cell leukemia Jurkat cells by inducing caspase-dependent apoptosis. Treatment at 0.1 μM Y3 protein for 4h induced 45% Jurkat cells to enter early stage apoptosis, while 23% of cells were in late-phase apoptosis. This action is achieved through caspase mediated apoptosis by induced activation of caspases 3, 8, and 9 [106].

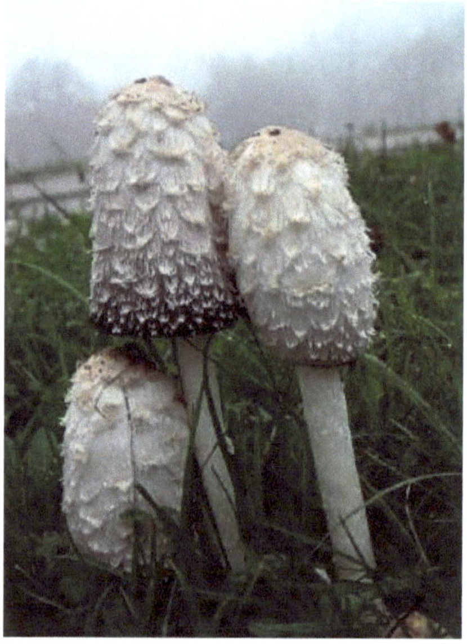

Fig. (6). *Coprinus comatus.*

Grifola frondosa (Dicks.) Gray (1821)

G. frondosa (Fig. **7**) is edible mushroom used also as a food supplement. It has medicinal properties mainly due to improvement of organism immune defense [107]. D-fraction polysaccharide was obtained from *Grifola frondosa*, maitake mushroom, and had IC_{50} 0.80 mg/mL towards human hepatocarcinoma SMMC-7721 cell line. This fraction is active in combination with vitamin C, where together they induce the release of cytochrome c, upregulation of BAX, downregulation of Bcl-2 and activation of poly-(ADP-ribose)-polymerase (PARP) [108].

Cyclocybe aegerita (V. Brig.) Vizzini 2014

Agrocybe aegerita (syn. *Cyclocybe aegerita*) (Fig. **8**), black poplar mushroom, is an edible mushroom found in North America, Europe and Asia where it colonizes woods and bark, most commonly stumps of poplar trees. It possesses antioxidant and antimicrobial activities [109].

Ageritin is ribotoxin isolated from *A. aegerita*. It has shown cytotoxic activities towards three different CNS cancer cell lines (SK-N-BE(2)-C, U-251 and C6) (ID_{50} 4.58 μg/mL - 9.46 μg/mL). Ageritin acts through extrinsic apoptotic pathway, since it activates caspase-8 [110].

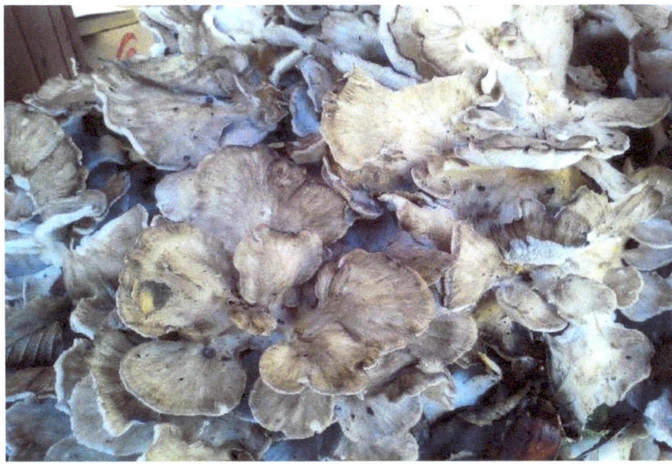

Fig. (7). *Grifola frondosa.*

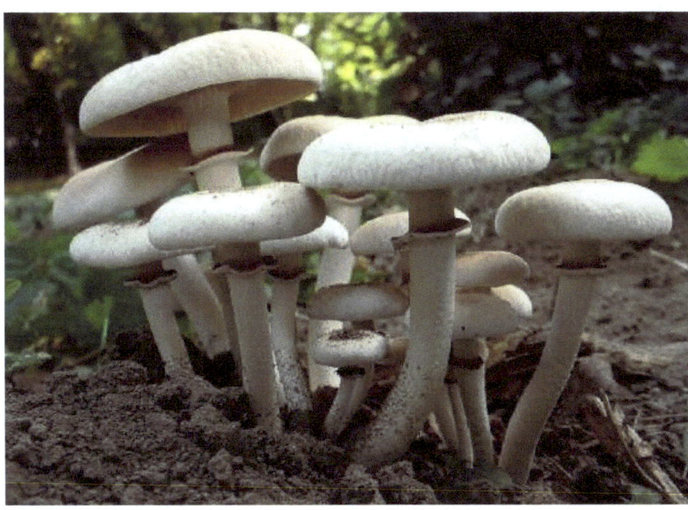

Fig. (8). *Agrocybe aegerita.*

Antrodia salmonea Chang & Chou (2004)

Antrodia salmonea is an edible and medicinal mushroom in Taiwan. Its aqueous extract inhibits cell viability and growth of human triple-negative breast cancer (MDA-MB-231) cells (IC_{50} 142 – 348 μg/mL). Inhibition of apoptosis is mediated through both extrinsic and intrinsic death pathways and signs like increased DNA fragmentation and increased Bax-Bcl-2 ratio [111]. *A. salmonea* is also inducing G2 cell-cycle arrest (through reducing the concentrations of cyclin B1, cyclin A, cyclin E, and CDC2 proteins) and decreases expression of COX-2 while it induces PARP cleavage. Antitumour effect of this mushroom is also confirmed *in vivo*, since it was able to lower incidence of tumors and to decrease their growth [112].

Antrodia cinnamomea Chang & Chou (1995)

Antrodia cinnamomea (syn. *Antrodia camphorata*) is medicinal mushroom used in Taiwan to treat stomach pain, food poisoning, liver cancer and other diseases. Compound pinicolol B, lanosta-7,9(11),24-trien-3β,15α,21-triol, was isolated from this mushroom and it showed antitumour activity towards nasopharyngeal carcinoma cell lines TW02 and TW04 (IC_{50} 63.3 - 115.0 μM) [113]. Ethanolic extract of fruiting body showed IC_{50} values of 50 μg/mL towards B16-F0 cells (skin melanoma) and is also able to reduce migration of these cells in time dependent manner. Treatment with this extract leads to nuclear condensation [114].

Agaricus lanipes (F.H. Møller & Jul. Schäffer) Singer (1949)

Agaricus lanipes is edible mushroom found on neutral and calcareous ground together with pine trees. Methanolic extract of *A. lanipes* exhibited antitumour properties towards A549 lung cancer cells (IC_{50} 250 μg/mL). This extract did not cause any change in expression of p53, caspase-9 and p21, so its mode of proapoptotic action is still to be investigated [115].

Polyporus squamosus (Huds.) Quélet (1886)

Polyporus squamosus (Fig. **9**) is an edible mushroom found in Europe, Asia, North America and Australia and is often used as a spice. It has range of biological activities including antioxidant, immunomodulatory, and antimicrobial [116].

Lectin PSL1a (0.5 and 5 μg/mL) isolated from *P. squamosus* shows cytotoxic activities towards mammalian cancer cells (HeLa, HEp-2, SKBR-3 and PC3 cells). Its apoptosis inducing properties might be related to the ability of this lectin to disrupt focal adhesion of cells and to interfere with integrin signaling [117].

Pulveroboletus ravenelii (Berk. & M.A. Curtis) Murrill (1909)

P. ravanelii is an edible mushroom found in Korea, Japan and China and it is used in traditional Chinese medicine. Methanolic extract of this mushroom is able to induce apoptosis in different cancer cell lines (lung adenocarcinoma cell lines (A549, NCI-H1264, NCI-H1299 and Calu-6), pancreatic ductal adenocarcinoma cell lines (PANC-1 and MIA PaCa-2) and hepatocellular carcinoma cell line (Hep G2) with IC_{50} 219.8 to 490.5 mg/mL. Vulpine acid is considered to be involved in this proapoptotic activity (IC_{50} 21.65 - 146.17 μM) [118].

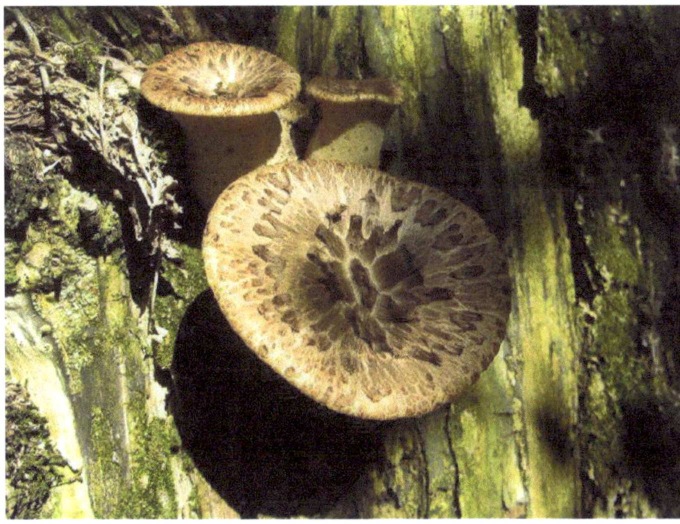

Fig. (9). *Polyporus squamosus.*

Trametes versicolor **(syn.** ***Coriolus versicolor)*** **(L.) Lloyd (1920)**

T. versicolor (Fig. **10**) is a mushroom with range of biological properties including hepatoprotective, anti-inflammatory, antioxidant and many more [119]. Tramesan (TR) is a polysaccharide fraction isolated from the liquid culture of *T. versicolor*. Tramesan is able to decrease cell count of human myeloid (OCI-AML3) and lymphoid (Jurkat) leukemia cells when applied in concentration 1 mg/mL, but it did not significantly increase the number of cells undergoing apoptosis. When applied on AML cells in concentration of 0.5 – 2 mg/mL it was able to increase apoptosis [120].

Ganoderma lucidum **(Curtis) P. Karst. (1881)**

G. lucidum (Fig. **11**) is used in traditional Chinese medicine for many years as well as in other Asian countries for curing the conditions like bronchitis, asthma, hypertension and many others. Its range of biological activities includes antimicrobial and antioxidant [121].

Ergosterol peroxide and ganodermanondiol were isolated from the mushroom fruiting bodies; both of them were active against HL-60 lymphoma cells (LC_{50} 3.5 and 2.9 μg/mL, respectively) and against MCF7 breast cancer epithelial cells (LC_{50} 20 μg/ml) [122]. Ribonuclease was isolated from this mushroom and it exhibited apoptosis inducing effects towards HT29 and HCT116 colorectal cancer cells (IC_{50} 2.8 and 0.1 μM, respectively). Apoptosis inducing properties of ribonuclease include both caspase -9 regulated pathways (HCT116 cells) and pathways independent of caspase -9 (HT29 cells) [123]. Mycelium of *G. lucidum* is producing 1,3-β-D-glucan (G) and its sulfated derivative (GS). GS showed more promising antitumour properties since it caused 40% proliferating inhibition of U937 cells (human Caucasian histiocytic lymphoma cell line) when applied in concentration of 60 μg/mL, while G caused only 10% decrease [124]. Different triterpenoids (ganolucidic acid E, lucidumol A, ganodermanontriol, 7-ox--ganoderic acid Z, 15-hydroxy-ganoderic acid S, and ganoderic acid DM) isolated from *G. lucidum* are active against human carcinoma cells (Caco-2, HepG2, and HeLa) exhibiting LC_{50} 20.87 - 84.36 μM. Despite its sensitivity to triterpenoids treatment, it is still not clear if these compounds are inducing apoptosis in HepG2 cells since no accumulation of sub-G1 cells was recorded. Sub-G1 accumulation was featured only in Caco-2 and HeLa cells [125].

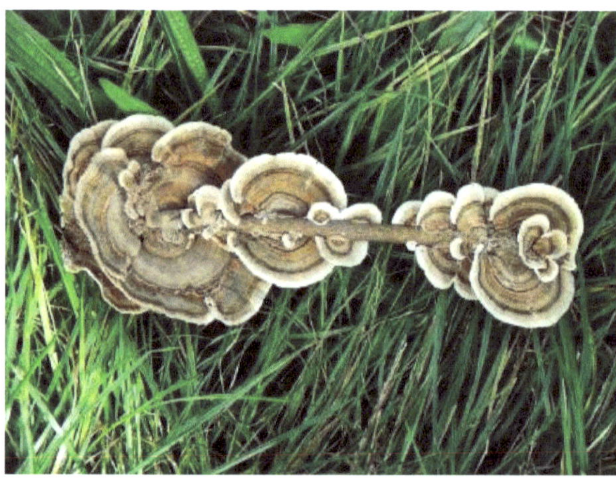

Fig. (10). *Trametes versicolor.*

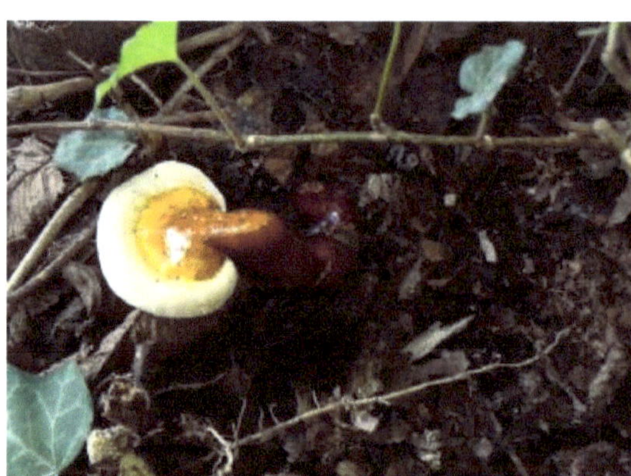

Fig. (11). *Ganoderma lucidum.*

Agaricus blazei Murill. (1945)

Agaricus blazei is mushroom highly appreciated as delicacy, but also as a medicine and food supplement. It boosts immune system and protects against infections and malignancies. It is also promising antimicrobial agent [126].

Formulation called Andosan™ was prepared and contained 82% of *A. blazei* extract, the rest were extracts of mushrooms *Hericeum erinaceus* and *Grifola frondosa.* Andosan (0.5–5.0%) showed *in vitro* cytotoxic effect towards Caco-2 cell line (human colon cancer cell line). Andosan was also efficient *in vivo*, it reduced incidence of adenocarcinomas in intestines, as well as tumour number and size in mice fed with tap water with 10% Andosan [127]. Agarol is ergosterol derivate obtained from *A. blazei*. It induced cytotoxicity with IC_{50} values of 0.26 µg/mL (A549, human lung cancer), 0.34 µg/mL (MKN45, gastric cancer cell line), 1.72 µg/mL (HSC-3, oral squamous cell carcinoma) and 1.94 µg/mL (HSC-4, Tongue squamous cell carcinoma). Treatment with agarol leads to caspase-independent apoptosis pathways in A549 cells; it decreases levels of Bcl-2 and increases levels of Bax together with cleavage of PARP in A549 cells. Apoptosis induced by agarol is mediated also with increase of ROS levels and activation of p53 [128].

Fulviformes fastuosus

F. fastuosus is a terrestrial mushroom widely distributed in Sri Lanka. Compound isolated from this mushroom, ergone (ergosta-4,6,8 (14),22-tetraen-3-one), exhibited cytotoxic properties towards RD cells (human rhabdomyosarcoma cell lines) with IC_{50} 1.49 mM, and against against HepG-2 cells (human liver cancer cell line) with IC_{50} 68.32mM. Cells treated with high concentration of ergone exhibited morphological features typical for apoptosis (cellular shrinkage, oval or irregular shape, fragmented nuclei, apoptotic bodies formation and condensation of cytoplasm) [129].

Ganoderma colossum (Fr.) C.F. Baker (1918)

G. collosum is a rare member of *Ganoderma* mushrooms and can be found in tropical and subtropical forests. It has been used in Asia for its medicinal benefits. Cytotoxic compounds Colo H and colossolactone G were isolated from this mushroom. Colo H had stronger cytotoxic properties (IC_{50} 32.8 - 68.5 µM), while Colossolactone G had lower cytotoxic potential (IC_{50} 64.7 - 102.6 µM) towards various cancer cell lines (lung cancer, breast cancer, colon cancer and hepatoma cells). Difference in activities between two compounds is the consequence of hydrophyl group at C-23 of Colo H molecule. Colo-H acts by downregulationg expression of genes involved in cell cycle progression, organelle organization and regulation of cellular component organization; while upregulating genes involved in oxidation reduction. Colo H is able to significantly increase levels of intracellular ROS; it leads to DNA damage and it also increases levels of p53 [130].

Calvatia gigantea (Batsch) Lloyd (1904)

C. gigantea (Fig. **12**), puffball, is an edible mushroom with anesthetic effect. Methanolic extract of *C. gigantea* was efficient in inhibiting A549, lung cancer cell line (IC_{50} 500 μg/mL). Mode of apoptosis and cell cycle arrest included downregulation of CCND1, CCND2, CDK4, Akt and Bcl-2 together with upregulation of Bax, p53, caspase-3 and caspase-9 expression [131].

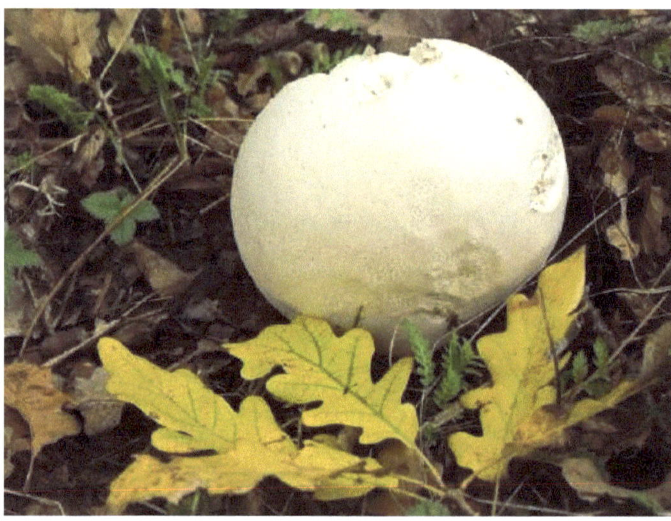

Fig. (12). *Calvatia gigantean.*

Termitomyces clypeatus R.Heim (1951)

T. clypeatus is an edible mushroom commonly found in India, especially during the rainy season. It is used in ethnomedicine for the treatment of pox. Serine proteases were isolated from this mushroom and exhibited cytotoxic activity towards human liver cancer cells, HepG2 (IC_{50} 75 nM). Induction of apoptosis events is caused by upregulation of p53 and Bax proteins following by activation of caspase-3 [132].

Armillaria mellea (Vahl) P.Kumm. (1871)

Armillaria mellea (Fig. **13**), honey mushroom, is an edible medicinal mushroom commonly found throughout the Northern hemisphere. It has ethnopharmacological significance in Chinese medicine in the treatments of headache and hypertension. Methanolic extract of *A. mellea* did not show cytotoxic effects towards MCF7, NCI-H460, HCT-15 and HepG2 cell lines [133]. Armillarikin was isolated from this mushroom and was active against hepatocellular carcinoma Huh7, HA22T, and HepG2 cells in concentrations up to 50 μM. Cytotoxic activities of armillaria were mediated by activation of procaspase-3, -8, -9 and upregulation of histones involved in apoptosis and cell cycle arrest, accumulation of ROS and collapse of mitochondrial function [134].

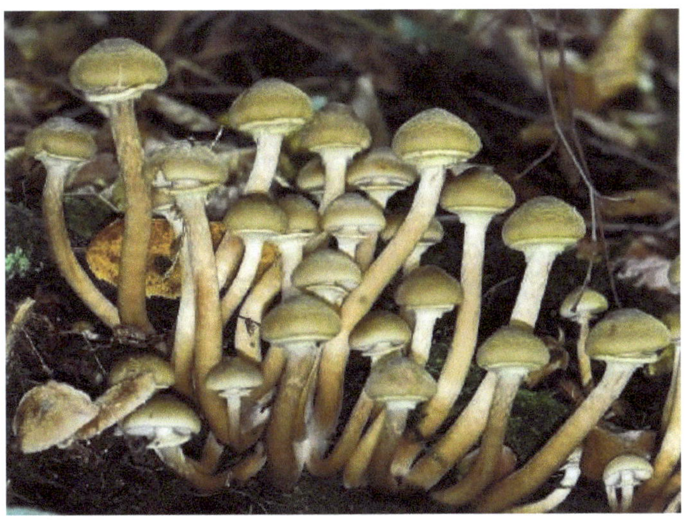

Fig. (13). *Armillaria mellea.*

Pyropolyporus fomentarius (L.) Teng (1963)

P. fomentarius - syn. *Fomes fomentarius* (Fig. **14**) is been used for centuries in traditional medicines, for example in the form of hemostatic. It is used in preparation of health promoting tonic drink in Japan and in traditional Chinese medicine for conditions like gastroenteric disorders and hepatocirrhosis [135]. Ethanolic extract of *P. fomentarius* exhibited cytotoxic activity towards L1210 murine leukemia cells (IC_{50} 69.35 μg/mL). Extract is interfering with mitochondrial potential, cleaving caspase-3, caspase-9, decreasing levels of Bcl-2 and increasing ratio of Bax/Bcl2, all leading to mitochondrial related apoptosis events [136]. Petroleum ether fraction of *P. fomentarius* exhibited cytotoxic activities towards S180 cells, sarcoma cancer cell line (IC_{50} 528.12 and 318.43 μg/mL, for 24h and 48h, respectively). Mode of action includes loss of mitochondrial potential and ROS accumulation in the treated cells. *P. fomentarius* was efficient *in vivo*; it caused reduction of sarcoma weight when applied in concentrations of 120 or 240 mg/kg [137]. Chloroform fraction of this mushroom

(20 μg/mL) is able to inhibit proliferation of K563 cells, causing overload of intracellular calcium, increase of intracellular ROS and mitochondria damage [135].

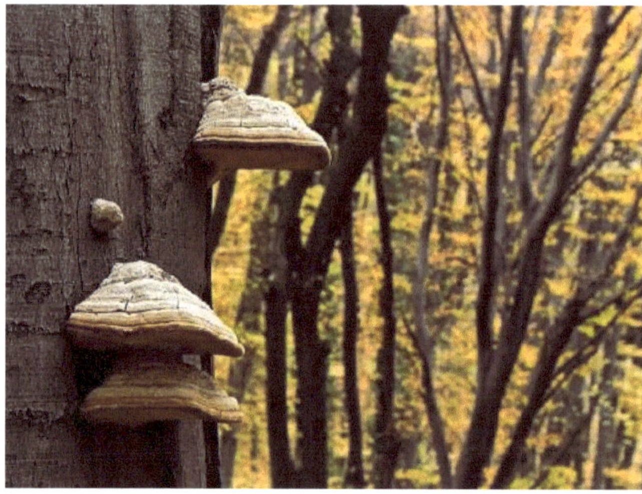

Fig. (14). *Pyropolyporus fomentarius.*

Leccinum vulpinum Watling (1961)

L. vulpinum is a promising source of essential nutrients and compounds with various biological activities, including antioxidant properties [138]. Extract of *L. vulpinun* was tested on MCF-7, NCI-H460, HCT-15 and AGS cell lines and the lowest GI_{50} concentrations were obtained in HCT-15 (human colon carcinoma) and MCF-7 (breast cancer) cell lines (53 μg/mL and 99 μg/mL, respectively). This extract is inducing apoptosis through mitochondrial pathway. It induces an increase in p53 tumour suppressor protein and p21 protein, as well as decrease in Bcl-2 and Bcl-xL. Extract caused a decrease in procaspase-9 levels and significantly decreased total PARP levels and induced DNA damage [139].

Tricholoma matsutake (S. Ito & S. Imai) Singer (1943)

T. matsutake is ectomycorrhizal mushroom with range of biological activities such as antimicrobial and immunostimulatory. Water extract of this mushroom is active against cells of liver cancer by inducing apoptosis through caspase dependent mitochondrial pathway (48 h IC_{50} in HepG2 and SMMC-7721 cells 5.3 mg/mL and 3.4 mg/mL, respectively). It is increasing levels of ROS when applied in concentration of 2.5 and 5 mg/mL, after 6h treatment. Extract is also reducing cell viability and interfering with potential of mitochondrial membrane. Mode of apoptosis action includes increased levels of cleaved PARP, Bad and Bax with decreased levels of Bcl-2. Extract is increasing activities of caspase-3, caspase-8, and caspase-9 in tumour cells. It is also efficient *in vivo*, 14 days treatment of mice (1g/kg) with this mushroom leads to reduced tumour growth [140].

Hericium erinaceum (Bull.) Persoon (1797)

H. erinaceum (Fig. **15**), lion`s mane mushroom is an edible mushroom used also for its medicinal properties in East Asia. Compounds obtained from this mushroom, hericerin A and hericerin, were active against HL-60 human acute promyelocytic leukaemia cells (IC_{50} 3.06 and 5.47 μM, respectively). They increased the proportion of cells in the sub-G1 fraction (M1) of cell cycle. The compounds were also down-regulating p-AKT and c-myc levels together with increasing expression of Bax, decreasing expression of Bcl-2, increasing expression of caspase-3 followed by cleavage of PARP [141].

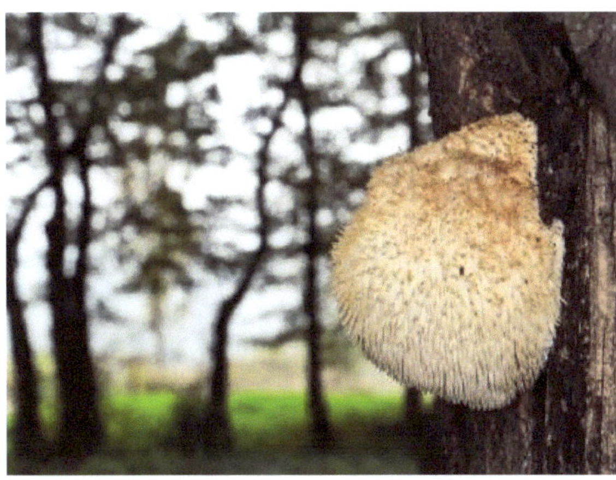

Fig. (15). *Hericium erinaceum.*

Amauroderma rude (Berk.) Torrend (1920)

Amauroderma rude is common in tropical areas and is newly described, so not many information regarding its activities are available [142]. Both ethanol extract and chloroform fraction of this mushroom were active against breast cancer cell line, with chloroform fraction showing better activity (tested concentration were up to 300 μg/mL). Ergosterol was isolated and is thought to be responsible for its cytotoxic activities since it increased cell death of cancer cells when applied in concentration 50–100 μM. It increases the expression of Foxo3 (activator of pro-apoptotic genes) both mRNA and protein and increases expression of Fas and Fas L (involved in the cell extrinsic apoptotic pathway). *in vivo* experiments showed that mice treated with ergosterol (50 mg/kg/mouse) have better chance of surviving cancer [143].

Cordyceps militaris (L.) Fr. (1818)

C. militaris (Fig. **16**) is a parasitic mushroom that grows on insects. It has been used for anti-aging, hypertension, hyperglycemia and other conditions [144]. Adenosine analog, cordycepin, was isolated from *C. militaris* and was active against leukemia cell lines NB-4 and U937 (IC_{50} 18.4 µg/mL (73.2 µM) and 22.7 µg/mL (90.4 µM), respectively). Cordycepin mode of action included increased expression of p53 leading to efflux of cytochrome c in cytosol which then activates caspase-9, all together leading to intrinsic pathway of apoptosis. Treatment of cells with cordycepin is also leading to decreased expression of cyclin A2, cyclin E, and CDK2, DNA damage and degradation of Cdc25A [145]. Cultivated fruiting bodies of this mushroom are exhibiting higher cytotoxic potential on cancer cell line (Huh7, HCT116, HL-60 and PC-3) compared to cultured mycelia of *C. militaris* (concentrations tested 7.8–125 µg/mL). Extract of fruiting bodies significantly increases levels of DNA fragmentation in treated cells; it causes activation of caspase-3 leading to PARP cleavage. Cordycepin is thought to be responsible for these apoptotic events, since in concentration of 25 µg/mL it is able to induce DNA fragmentation, it also activates caspase-3 cleaves PARP [144].

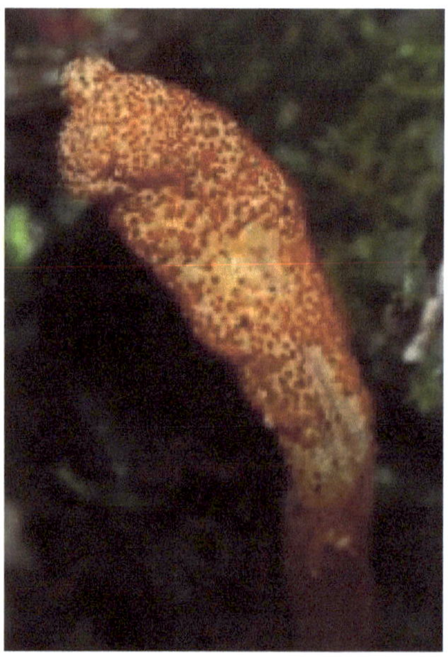

Fig. (16). *Cordyceps militaris.*

Cordyceps bassiana Z.Z. Li, C.R. Li, B. Huang & M.Z. Fan (2001)

C. bassiana (Fig. **17**) is a pathogen of insects, used for its beneficial medicinal properties in treatment of conditions such as epilepsy and stroke [146]. Buthanol fraction of this mushroom was active in inhibiting proliferation of A549 cells in tested concentrations 100 and 200 μg/mL. Out of this fraction, 5 compounds were isolated. Compound named KTH-13 (4-isopropyl-2,6-bis(1-phenylethyl)phenol) showed potent antiproliferative potential against C6 glioma cells (IC_{50} 64.9 μM) by inducing apoptosis. Its activity might be through mitochondrial pathway. Cells treated with this compound had higher concentration of cleaved caspase-3, -7, -9, but not caspase -8. It also increased Bax/Bcl2 ratio [147].

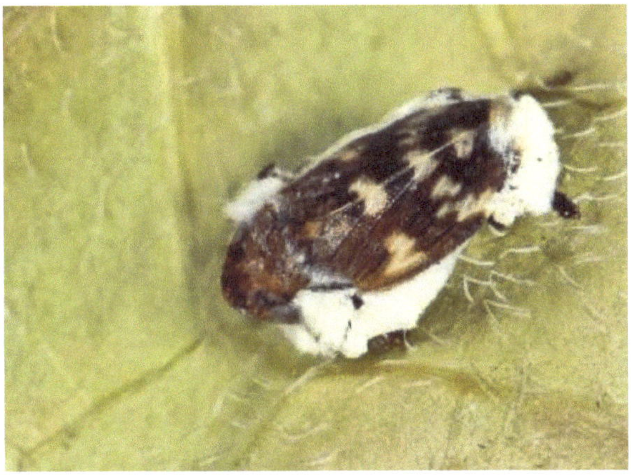

Fig. (17). *Cordyceps bassiana.*

Pleurotus eryngii var. *ferulae* (Lanzi) Sacc. 1887

P. eryngii var. *ferulae* shortly – *P. ferulae* is an edible mushroom growing on living rhizome trunks. It has been used for treating cancer in traditional medicine, but it also possesses activities such as antimicrobial, antioxidant and others. Ethanolic extract of *P. ferulae* caused morphological changes typical for apoptosis with IC_{50} 1.4 mg/mL on melanoma cell line B16F10. Extract was able to increase activity of caspase-3; it damaged mitochondria and inhibited migration of cancer cells. Even *in vivo* treatments found this extract to be promising anticancer candidate, since mice treated with extract (1000 mg/kg per day) had tumours but with reduced growth, size and weight. Levels of gene expression were altered after treatment with *P. ferulae* extract, levels of Akt, PI3K, Bcl-2, Bcl-xl were reduced, and levels of Bax and Bid were increased, as well as Bad, caspase-8 and caspase-9 [148].

Lentinus crinitus (L.) Fr. (1825)

L. crinitus is an edible mushroom and source of panepoxydone, compound with cytotoxic activity in various cell lines (IC_{50} 4, 5, 6 and 15 μM towards MDA-MB-

453, MCF-7, MDA-MB-468 and MDA-MB-231 cell lines, respectively). It also inhibits migration and invasion of tumour cells. Treatment with panepoxydone leads to decreased levels of Bcl-2, survivin, cyclin D, caspase-3, FOXM1 and decreased phosphorylation of inhibitor of NF-kB, while levels of Bax, cleaved PARP are increased. Increase of Bax/Bcl2 ratio is the highest in MDAMB-453 cells [149].

Sarcodon aspratus (Berk.) S. Ito (1955)

Sarcodon aspratus is an edible mushroom distributed in China, Korea and Japan. In Korea it is a traditional dish and a digestive [150]. Ergosterol peroxide isolated from *S. aspratus* had shown cytotoxic effect towards DU 145, PC 3, M2182 prostate cancer cells (applied concentrations up to 200 μM/mL). It acts through extrinsic apoptosis pathway by activation of PARP cleavage, Bax and caspase 8/3, and inhibition of procaspase 8, Bcl-2, Bcl-XL expression [151].

Meripilus giganteus (Pers.) Karst. (1882)

Meripilus giganteus Karst. (Fig. **18**) is a wild growing basidiomycete with an edible fruiting body, belonging to the family Meripilaceae. It is a parasitic species on trees, being also characterized as saprobic. It is frequently found on *Quercus* and *Fagus* species, but it can also be found on some hardwoods and coniferous species [152].

Treatment of cervical carcinoma cell line (HeLa) with *M. giganteus* methanol extract led to reduction in cell's viability in MTT assay (IC_{50} 0.41 mg/mL after 48 h), induced process of apoptosis and inhibited cell's migration *in vitro* [152]. Cells treated with *M. giganteus* extract exhibited typical features of apoptosis such as nuclear condensation, fragmentation and formation of apoptotic bodies. Treatment of HeLa cells with the extract caused an increase in p53 and Bax protein levels and apoptosis-specific cleavage of PARP-1 [153].

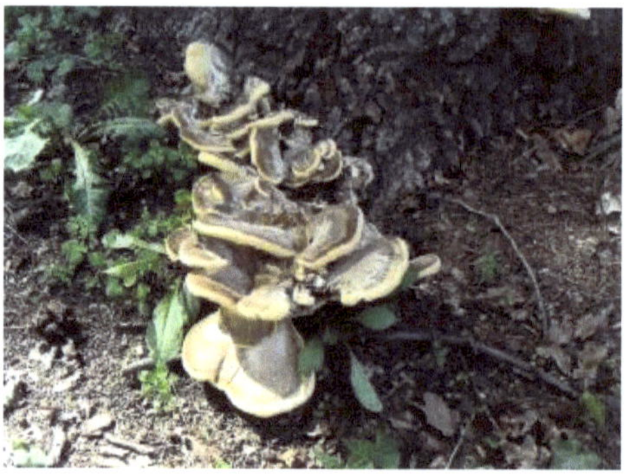

Fig. (18). *Meripilus giganteus.*

Table 1. Mushroom extracts and compounds with most prominent cytotoxic potential.

Fungi	Inhibitory Concentration	Compound Responsible for Cytotoxicity	Inhibitory Concentration of Compound	References
Inonotus obliquus	IC_{50} 2.03 mg/mL	triterpenoids, inotodiol, lignin metabolites	IC_{50} 75.1 - 227.4 μM, 20 mg/L, IC_{50} 160.5 μg/mL and 222.9 μg/mL	[87 - 89]
Inonotus taiwanensis	IC_{50} 137 μg/mL, 255 μg/mL			[91]
Phellinus igniarius	110.7 - 531.7 μg/mL			[92]
Ganoderma resinaceum	0.01 mg/mL and 0.1 mg/mL	α-spinasterol	IC_{50} 1 - 10 μM	[94]
Ganoderma applanatum	IC_{50} 160 μg/mL			[95]
Cantharellus cibarius	IC_{50} < 1 mg/mL	Piceatannol	0.0075 mg/mL	[97]
Pleurotus sajor-caju	IC_{50} 0.05 mg/mL	ergosta-5,7,22-trien-3β-ol		[98]
Lignosus rhinocerus		Protein fraction	IC_{50} 3.00 μg/mL	[100]
Morchella esculenta	IC_{50} 0.49 - 1.35 mg/mL	1O-octadecanoyl-sn-glycerol, (3β,5α,8α,22E,24S)-5,- -epidioxyergosta-6,9(11),22-trien-3-ol, (3β,5α,22E)-Ergost- -7,22,24(28)-trien-3-ol	IC_{50} 156.9 to 278 M	[101]
Lentinus squarrosulus		Peptides	IC_{50} 2.8-26.84 μg/mL	[103]
Ramaria botrytis		ubiquitin-like antitumour protein (RBUP)	IC_{50} 15.93 μM	[104]
Coprinus comatus		Glycan binding protein Y3	0.1 μM	[106]
Lignosus rhinocerotis		(+)-torreyol	3.5 μg/mL	[100]
Grifola frondosa		D-fraction polysaccharide	IC_{50} 0.80 mg/mL	[108]
Agrogybe aegerita		Ageritin	ID_{50} 4.58 μg/mL - 9.46 μg/mL	[110]
Antrodia salmonea	IC_{50} 142 – 348 μg/mL			[111]
Antrodia cinnamomea	IC_{50} 50 μg/mL	pinicolol B	IC_{50} 63.3 - 115.0 μM	[113, 114]
Agaricus lanipes	IC_{50} 250 μg/mL			[115]

(Table 1) cont.....

Fungi	Inhibitory Concentration	Compound Responsible for Cytotoxicity	Inhibitory Concentration of Compound	References
Polyporus squamosus		Lectin PSL1a	0.5 and 5 μg/mL	[117]
Pulveroboletus ravenelii	IC_{50} 219.8 - 490.5 mg/mL	Vulpinic acid	IC50 21.65 - 146.17 μM	[118]
Trametes versicolor		Tramesan	0.5 - 2mg/mL	[120]
Ganoderma lucidum		Ergosterol peroxide, ganodermanondiol, ribunucelase, sulfated (1,3)-β-D-Glucan, triterpenoids	LC_{50} 3.5 - 20 μg/mL, IC_{50} 2.8 and 0.1 μM, 60 μg/mL, LC_{50} 20.87 - 84.36 μM	[122 - 125]
Fulviformes fastuosus		Ergone	1.49 mM - 68.32 mM	[129]
Ganoderma colossum		Colo H and colossolactone G	IC_{50} 32.8 - 68.5 μM, IC_{50} 64.7 - 102.6 μM	[130]
Calvatia gigantea	IC_{50} 500 μg/mL			[131]
Termitomyces clypeatus				[132]
Armillaria mellea	No extract activity	Armillarikin	50 μM	[133, 134]
Pyropolyporus fomentarius	IC_{50} 69.35 μg/mL, IC_{50} 528.12 and 318.43 μg/mL, 20 μg/mL			[135 - 137]
Leccinum vulpinum	GI_{50} 53 μg/mL and 99 μg/mL			[139]
Agaricus blazei	10% Andosan formulation	Agarol	0.26 μg/mL - 1.94 μg/mL	[127, 128]
Tricholoma matsutake	IC_{50} 5.3 mg/mL and 3.4 mg/mL			[140]
Hericium erinaceum		hericerin A and hericerin	IC_{50} 3.06 and 5.47 μM	[141]

(Table 1) cont.....

Fungi	Inhibitory Concentration	Compound Responsible for Cytotoxicity	Inhibitory Concentration of Compound	References
Amauroderma rude	tested concentrations up to 300 μg/mL	Ergosterol	50–100 μM	[143]
Cordyceps militaris	7.8–125 μg/mL	Cordycepin	IC_{50} 18.4 μg/mL (73.2 μM) and 22.7 μg/mL (90.4 μM)	[144, 145]
Cordyceps bassiana	100 and 200 μg/mL	4-isopropyl-2,6-bis(1-phenylethyl)phenol	IC_{50} 64.9 μM	[147]
Pleurotus ferulae	IC_{50} 1.4 mg/mL			[148]
Lentinus crinitus		Panepoxydone	IC_{50} 4 - 15 μM	[149]
Sarcodon aspratus	applied concentrations up to 200 μM/mL	Ergosterol peroxide		[151]

WHERE SHOULD WE FURTHER SEARCH FOR MUSHROOMS FUNCTIONALITIES?

As reviewed in the previous paragraphs of this chapter, mushroom species present valuable source of antitumor agents and expressed cytotoxic activities *in vitro* and *in vivo*. Literature indicates that mushroom species are able to induce apoptosis in cancer cell lines, by regulating expression of important markers of apoptosis, as reviewed in this chapter. Mushrooms such as *Innonotus obliquus*, *Ganoderma resinaceum*, *Pleurotus sajor-caju*, *Ganoderma collosum*, Calvatia gigantean, *Termitomyces clypeatus*, *Leccinum vulpinum*, *Cordyceps militaris*, *Meripilus giganteus* induce apoptosis by regulating expression of p53; species like *Phellinus igniarius*, *Ganoderma applanatum*, *Lignosus rhinocerus*, *Lentinus squarrosulus*, *Grifola frondosa*, *Antrodia salmonea*, *Agaricus blazei*, *Fomes fomentarius*, *Hericium erinaceum*, *Cordyceps bassiana*, *Pleurotus ferulae*, *Lentinus crinitus* directly regulate Bax/Bcl2 expression: *Coprinus comatus*, *Ganoderma lucidum* and *Armillaria mellea* regulate expression of Cas-9 and directly influence on apoptotic activation in cancer cell lines (Fig. **19**).

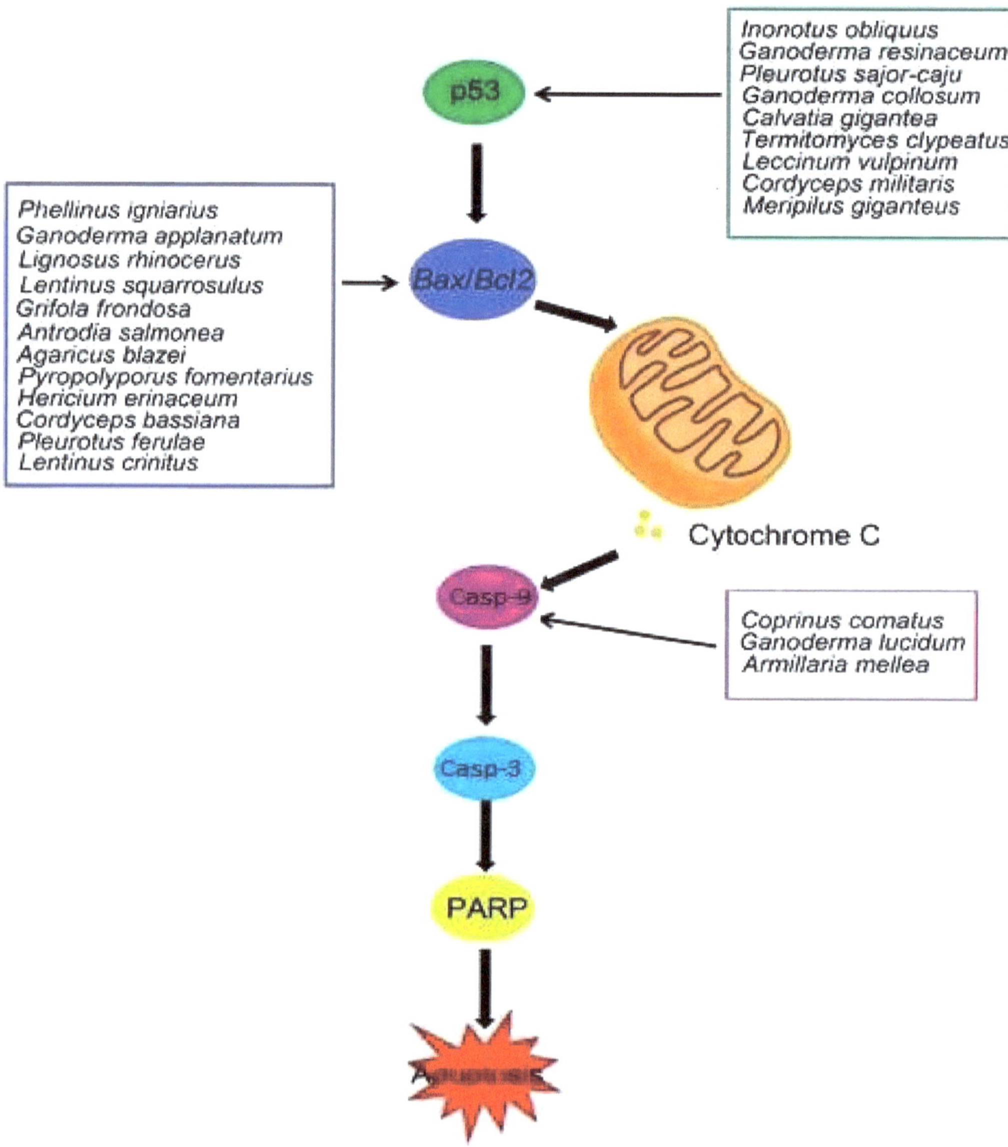

Fig. (19). Mushrooms induce apoptosis by regulating expression of apoptotic signaling molecules.

Bioactive compounds of flavonoid nature present in mushrooms could also stimulate the expression of p53 and can mediate p53 signaling pathway [154]. It is evident that literature data on this interesting subject is scarce having in mind that Kingdom of Fungi counts for more than 5 mil. species. Further, modes of cytotoxic action should be elucidated and effects of mushroom extracts and compounds on markers of apoptosis as potential targets should be studied in more details. There are numerous studies described by our group [155 - 160] indicating that consumable mushrooms are not cytotoxic to nontumor cell lines. It should be further examined if mushroom species that are nontoxic to non-tumor cells have cytotoxic potential to cancer cell lines and further elucidate, based on current studies, if potential mechanism is involved in apoptosis induction. It was shown that different proteins like protein kinases, acethyltransferases, methyl-transferases, ubiquitin-like modifying enzymes and some members of SOX family can trigger posttranslational modification of p53 and activate this tumour suppressor [161]. In the light of that fact it should be further investigated whether mushroom extracts can influence on this enzyme that could activate p53 by posttranslational modification. We should further search for the compounds responsible for cytotoxic potential, based on cytotoxic activity guided isolation. This area of investigation is hot topic and might bring solutions to still not solved problems related to cancer treatment in the near future. Mushroom functionalities related to cancer treatment are still not explored in their full light and that should be the object of our future scientific quest.

CONSENT FOR PUBLICATION

Not applicable.

CONFLICT OF INTEREST

The authors confirm that this chapter contents have no conflict of interest.

ACKNOWLEDGEMENTS

We are very thankful to Dr. Dragisa Savic from the National Park Fruska Gora for providing the majority of the photographs used in this chapter (*A. mellea, A. aegerita, C. gigantea, C. cibarius, C. comatus, C. bassiana, F. fomentarius*, *G. applanatum, H. erinaceus, M. esculenta, R. botrytis*). This work was supported by the Ministry of Education, Science and Technological Development, Republic of Serbia (Grants No 173032 and 173051).

REFERENCES

[1] Madhusudan, S.; Middleton, M.R. The emerging role of DNA repair proteins as predictive, prognostic and therapeutic targets in cancer. *Cancer Treat. Rev.*, **2005**, *31*(8), 603-617. [http://dx.doi.org/10.1016/j.ctrv.2005.09.006] [PMID: 16298073]

[2] Pujol, M.; Gavilondo, J.; Ayala, M.; Rodríguez, M.; González, E.M.; Pérez, L. Fighting cancer with plant-expressed pharmaceuticals. *Trends Biotechnol.*, **2007**, *25*(10), 455-459. [http://dx.doi.org/10.1016/j.tibtech.2007.09.001] [PMID: 17869360]

[3] Tanaka, T. Role of apoptosis in the chemoprevention of cancer. *J. Exp. Clin. Medicine (Taiwan)*, **2013**, *5*(3), 89-91.

[http://dx.doi.org/10.1016/j.jecm.2013.04.001]

[4] Sui, X.; Chen, R.; Wang, Z.; Huang, Z.; Kong, N.; Zhang, M.; Han, W.; Lou, F.; Yang, J.; Zhang, Q.; Wang, X.; He, C.; Pan, H. Autophagy and chemotherapy resistance: a promising therapeutic target for cancer treatment. *Cell Death Dis.*, **2013**, *4*e838
[http://dx.doi.org/10.1038/cddis.2013.350] [PMID: 24113172]

[5] Todorović, A. *Ekspresija antioksidativnih enzima i transkripcionog faktora Nrf2 kod pacijentkinja sa benigno, premaligno i maligno transformisanim endometrijumom. Doktorska disertacija. Univerzitet u Beogradu; Biološki fakultet*; , **2013**.

[6] Kasibhatla, S.; Tseng, B. Why target apoptosis in cancer treatment? *Mol. Cancer Ther.*, **2003**, *2*(6), 573-580.
[PMID: 12813137]

[7] Ricci, M.S.; Zong, W.X. Chemotherapeutic approaches for targeting cell death pathways. *Oncologist*, **2006**, *11*(4), 342-357.
[http://dx.doi.org/10.1634/theoncologist.11-4-342] [PMID: 16614230]

[8] Di Pietro, C.; Piro, S.; Tabbì, G.; Ragusa, M.; Di Pietro, V.; Zimmitti, V.; Cuda, F.; Anello, M.; Consoli, U.; Salinaro, E.T.; Caruso, M.; Vancheri, C.; Crimi, N.; Sabini, M.G.; Cirrone, G.A.; Raffaele, L.; Privitera, G.; Pulvirenti, A.; Giugno, R.; Ferro, A.; Cuttone, G.; Lo Nigro, S.; Purrello, R.; Purrello, F.; Purrello, M. Cellular and molecular effects of protons: apoptosis induction and potential implications for cancer therapy. *Apoptosis*, **2006**, *11*(1), 57-66.
[http://dx.doi.org/10.1007/s10495-005-3346-1] [PMID: 16374542]

[9] Schultz, D.R.; Harrington, W.J., Jr Apoptosis: programmed cell death at a molecular level. *Semin. Arthritis Rheum.*, **2003**, *32*(6), 345-369.
[http://dx.doi.org/10.1053/sarh.2003.50005] [PMID: 12833244]

[10] Rückert, F.; Samm, N.; Lehner, A.K.; Saeger, H.D.; Grützmann, R.; Pilarsky, C. Simultaneous gene silencing of Bcl-2, XIAP and Survivin re-sensitizes pancreatic cancer cells towards apoptosis. *BMC Cancer*, **2010**, *10*, 379.
[http://dx.doi.org/10.1186/1471-2407-10-379] [PMID: 20646298]

[11] Elmore, S. Apoptosis: a review of programmed cell death. *Toxicol. Pathol.*, **2007**, *35*(4), 495-516.
[http://dx.doi.org/10.1080/01926230701320337] [PMID: 17562483]

[12] Wong, R.S.Y. Apoptosis in cancer: from pathogenesis to treatment. *J. Exp. Clin. Cancer Res.*, **2011**, *30*(11), 87.
[http://dx.doi.org/10.1186/1756-9966-30-87] [PMID: 21943236]

[13] Brenner, D.; Mak, T.W. Mitochondrial cell death effectors. *Curr. Opin. Cell Biol.*, **2009**, *21*(6), 871-877.
[http://dx.doi.org/10.1016/j.ceb.2009.09.004] [PMID: 19822411]

[14] Vaseva, A.V.; Moll, U.M. The mitochondrial p53 pathway. *Biochim. Biophys. Acta*, **2009**, *1787*(5), 414-420.
[http://dx.doi.org/10.1016/j.bbabio.2008.10.005] [PMID: 19007744]

[15] Eichhorn, S.W.; Guo, H.; McGeary, S.E.; Rodriguez-Mias, R.A.; Shin, C.; Baek, D.; Hsu, S.H.; Ghoshal, K.; Villén, J.; Bartel, D.P. mRNA destabilization is the dominant effect of mammalian microRNAs by the time substantial repression ensues. *Mol. Cell*, **2014**, *56*(1), 104-115.
[http://dx.doi.org/10.1016/j.molcel.2014.08.028] [PMID: 25263593]

[16] Brunelle, J.K.; Letai, A. Control of mitochondrial apoptosis by the Bcl-2 family. *J. Cell Sci.*, **2009**, *122*(Pt 4), 437-441.
[http://dx.doi.org/10.1242/jcs.031682] [PMID: 19193868]

[17] Acehan, D.; Jiang, X.; Morgan, D.G.; Heuser, J.E.; Wang, X.; Akey, C.W. Three-dimensional structure of the apoptosome: implications for assembly, procaspase-9 binding, and activation. *Mol. Cell*, **2002**, *9*(2), 423-432.

[http://dx.doi.org/10.1016/S1097-2765(02)00442-2] [PMID: 11864614]

[18] Bratton, S.B.; Salvesen, G.S. Regulation of the Apaf-1-caspase-9 apoptosome. *J. Cell Sci.*, **2010**, *123*(Pt 19), 3209-3214.
[http://dx.doi.org/10.1242/jcs.073643] [PMID: 20844150]

[19] Brentnall, M.; Rodriguez-Menocal, L.; De Guevara, R.L.; Cepero, E.; Boise, L.H. Caspase-9, caspase-3 and caspase-7 have distinct roles during intrinsic apoptosis. *BMC Cell Biol.*, **2013**, *14*, 32.
[http://dx.doi.org/10.1186/1471-2121-14-32] [PMID: 23834359]

[20] McStay, G.P.; Green, D.R. Measuring apoptosis: caspase inhibitors and activity assays. *Cold Spring Harb. Protoc.*, **2014**, *2014*(8), 799-806.
[http://dx.doi.org/10.1101/pdb.top070359] [PMID: 25086023]

[21] Ghobrial, I.M.; Witzig, T.E.; Adjei, A.A. Targeting apoptosis pathways in cancer therapy. *CA Cancer J. Clin.*, **2005**, *55*(3), 178-194.
[http://dx.doi.org/10.3322/canjclin.55.3.178] [PMID: 15890640]

[22] Galluzzi, L.; Aaronson, S.A.; Abrams, J.; Alnemri, E.S.; Andrews, D.W.; Baehrecke, E.H.; Bazan, N.G.; Blagosklonny, M.V.; Blomgren, K.; Borner, C.; Bredesen, D.E.; Brenner, C.; Castedo, M.; Cidlowski, J.A.; Ciechanover, A.; Cohen, G.M.; De Laurenzi, V.; De Maria, R.; Deshmukh, M.; Dynlacht, B.D.; El-Deiry, W.S.; Flavell, R.A.; Fulda, S.; Garrido, C.; Golstein, P.; Gougeon, M.L.; Green, D.R.; Gronemeyer, H.; Hajnóczky, G.; Hardwick, J.M.; Hengartner, M.O.; Ichijo, H.; Jäättelä, M.; Kepp, O.; Kimchi, A.; Klionsky, D.J.; Knight, R.A.; Kornbluth, S.; Kumar, S.; Levine, B.; Lipton, S.A.; Lugli, E.; Madeo, F.; Malomi, W.; Marine, J.C.; Martin, S.J.; Medema, J.P.; Mehlen, P.; Melino, G.; Moll, U.M.; Morselli, E.; Nagata, S.; Nicholson, D.W.; Nicotera, P.; Nuñez, G.; Oren, M.; Penninger, J.; Pervaiz, S.; Peter, M.E.; Piacentini, M.; Prehn, J.H.; Puthalakath, H.; Rabinovich, G.A.; Rizzuto, R.; Rodrigues, C.M.; Rubinsztein, D.C.; Rudel, T.; Scorrano, L.; Simon, H.U.; Steller, H.; Tschopp, J.; Tsujimoto, Y.; Vandenabeele, P.; Vitale, I.; Vousden, K.H.; Youle, R.J.; Yuan, J.; Zhivotovsky, B.; Kroemer, G. Guidelines for the use and interpretation of assays for monitoring cell death in higher eukaryotes. *Cell Death Differ.*, **2009**, *16*(8), 1093-1107.
[http://dx.doi.org/10.1038/cdd.2009.44] [PMID: 19373242]

[23] Amundson, S.A.; Myers, T.G.; Scudiero, D.; Kitada, S.; Reed, J.C.; Fornace, A.J., Jr An informatics approach identifying markers of chemosensitivity in human cancer cell lines. *Cancer Res.*, **2000**, *60*(21), 6101-6110.
[PMID: 11085534]

[24] Donovan, M.; Cotter, T.G. Control of mitochondrial integrity by Bcl-2 family members and caspase-independent cell death. *Biochim. Biophys. Acta*, **2004**, *1644*(2-3), 133-147.
[http://dx.doi.org/10.1016/j.bbamcr.2003.08.011] [PMID: 14996498]

[25] Anderson, M.A.; Huang, D.; Roberts, A. Targeting BCL2 for the treatment of lymphoid malignancies. *Semin. Hematol.*, **2014**, *51*(3), 219-227.
[http://dx.doi.org/10.1053/j.seminhematol.2014.05.008] [PMID: 25048785]

[26] Pfeffer, C.M.; Singh, A.T.K. Apoptosis: A target for anticancer therapy. *Int. J. Mol. Sci.*, **2018**, *19*(2), 1-10.
[PMID: 29393886]

[27] Sayers, T.J. Targeting the extrinsic apoptosis signaling pathway for cancer therapy. *Cancer Immunol. Immunother.*, **2011**, *60*(8), 1173-1180.
[http://dx.doi.org/10.1007/s00262-011-1008-4] [PMID: 21626033]

[28] Jia, L.T.; Chen, S.Y.; Yang, A.G. Cancer gene therapy targeting cellular apoptosis machinery. *Cancer Treat. Rev.*, **2012**, *38*(7), 868-876.
[http://dx.doi.org/10.1016/j.ctrv.2012.06.008] [PMID: 22800735]

[29] Sartorius, U.; Schmitz, I.; Krammer, P.H. Molecular mechanisms of death-receptor-mediated apoptosis. *ChemBioChem*, **2001**, *2*(1), 20-29.
[http://dx.doi.org/10.1002/1439-7633(20010105)2:1<20::AID-CBIC20>3.0.CO;2-X] [PMID:

11828422]

[30] Elrod, H.A.; Sun, S.Y. Modulation of death receptors by cancer therapeutic agents. *Cancer Biol. Ther.*, **2008**, *7*(2), 163-173.
[http://dx.doi.org/10.4161/cbt.7.2.5335] [PMID: 18059181]

[31] Hensley, P.; Mishra, M.; Kyprianou, N. Targeting caspases in cancer therapeutics. *Biol. Chem.*, **2013**, *394*(7), 831-843.
[http://dx.doi.org/10.1515/hsz-2013-0128] [PMID: 23509217]

[32] Croce, C.M.; Reed, J.C. Finally, An Apoptosis-Targeting Therapeutic for Cancer. *Cancer Res.*, **2016**, *76*(20), 5914-5920.
[http://dx.doi.org/10.1158/0008-5472.CAN-16-1248] [PMID: 27694602]

[33] Kelly, P.N.; Strasser, A. The role of Bcl-2 and its pro-survival relatives in tumourigenesis and cancer therapy. *Cell Death Differ.*, **2011**, *18*(9), 1414-1424.
[http://dx.doi.org/10.1038/cdd.2011.17] [PMID: 21415859]

[34] Brown, S.P.; Taygerly, J.P. Small-Molecule Antagonists of Bcl-2 Family Proteins. *Annu. Rep. Med. Chem.*, **2012**, *47*, 253-266.
[http://dx.doi.org/10.1016/B978-0-12-396492-2.00017-5]

[35] Ola, M.S.; Nawaz, M.; Ahsan, H. Role of Bcl-2 family proteins and caspases in the regulation of apoptosis. *Mol. Cell. Biochem.*, **2011**, *351*(1-2), 41-58.
[http://dx.doi.org/10.1007/s11010-010-0709-x] [PMID: 21210296]

[36] Mocellin, S. Targeting death receptors to fight cancer: from biological rational to clinical implementation. *Curr. Med. Chem.*, **2010**, *17*(25), 2713-2728.
[http://dx.doi.org/10.2174/092986710791859342] [PMID: 20586721]

[37] Oldenhuis, C.N.; Stegehuis, J.H.; Walenkamp, A.M.; de Jong, S.; de Vries, e.g. Targeting TRAIL death receptors. *Curr. Opin. Pharmacol.*, **2008**, *8*(4), 433-439.
[http://dx.doi.org/10.1016/j.coph.2008.06.011] [PMID: 18625341]

[38] Di Pietro, R. Signaling Pathways Leading to TRAIL Resistance.*Advances in Cancer Therapy*; Gali-Muhtasib, H., Ed.; IntechOpen, **2011**, pp. 201-226.

[39] Shoeb, M.; Ramana, K.V.; Srivastava, S.K. Aldose reductase inhibition enhances TRAIL-induced human colon cancer cell apoptosis through AKT/FOXO3a-dependent upregulation of death receptors. *Free Radic. Biol. Med.*, **2013**, *63*, 280-290.
[http://dx.doi.org/10.1016/j.freeradbiomed.2013.05.039] [PMID: 23732517]

[40] Mandal, R.; Raab, M.; Matthess, Y.; Becker, S.; Knecht, R.; Strebhardt, K. pERK 1/2 inhibit Caspase-8 induced apoptosis in cancer cells by phosphorylating it in a cell cycle specific manner. *Mol. Oncol.*, **2014**, *8*(2), 232-249.
[http://dx.doi.org/10.1016/j.molonc.2013.11.003] [PMID: 24342355]

[41] Speidel, D. The role of DNA damage responses in p53 biology. *Arch. Toxicol.*, **2015**, *89*(4), 501-517.
[http://dx.doi.org/10.1007/s00204-015-1459-z] [PMID: 25618545]

[42] Vogelstein, B.; Lane, D.; Levine, A.J. Surfing the p53 network. *Nature*, **2000**, *408*(6810), 307-310.
[http://dx.doi.org/10.1038/35042675] [PMID: 11099028]

[43] Lane, D.P. Cancer. p53, guardian of the genome. *Nature*, **1992**, *358*(6381), 15-16.
[http://dx.doi.org/10.1038/358015a0] [PMID: 1614522]

[44] Khoo, K.H.; Verma, C.S.; Lane, D.P. Drugging the p53 pathway: understanding the route to clinical efficacy. *Nat. Rev. Drug Discov.*, **2014**, *13*(3), 217-236.
[http://dx.doi.org/10.1038/nrd4236] [PMID: 24577402]

[45] Muller, P.A.; Vousden, K.H. Mutant p53 in cancer: new functions and therapeutic opportunities. *Cancer Cell*, **2014**, *25*(3), 304-317.
[http://dx.doi.org/10.1016/j.ccr.2014.01.021] [PMID: 24651012]

[46] Kandoth, C.; McLellan, M.D.; Vandin, F.; Ye, K.; Niu, B.; Lu, C.; Xie, M.; Zhang, Q.; McMichael, J.F.; Wyczalkowski, M.A.; Leiserson, M.D.M.; Miller, C.A.; Welch, J.S.; Walter, M.J.; Wendl, M.C.; Ley, T.J.; Wilson, R.K.; Raphael, B.J.; Ding, L. Mutational landscape and significance across 12 major cancer types. *Nature,* **2013**, *502*(7471), 333-339. [http://dx.doi.org/10.1038/nature12634] [PMID: 24132290]

[47] Leroy, B.; Fournier, J.L.; Ishioka, C.; Monti, P.; Inga, A.; Fronza, G.; Soussi, T. The TP53 website: an integrative resource centre for the TP53 mutation database and TP53 mutant analysis. *Nucleic Acids Res.,* **2013**, *41*(Database issue), D962-D969. [http://dx.doi.org/10.1093/nar/gks1033] [PMID: 23161690]

[48] Bai, L.; Zhu, W-G. p53: Structure, Function and Therapeutic Applications. *J Cancer Mol.,* **2006**, *2*(4), 141-153.

[49] Oliner, J.D.; Pietenpol, J.A.; Thiagalingam, S.; Gyuris, J.; Kinzler, K.W.; Vogelstein, B. Oncoprotein MDM2 conceals the activation domain of tumour suppressor p53. *Nature,* **1993**, *362*(6423), 857-860. [http://dx.doi.org/10.1038/362857a0] [PMID: 8479525]

[50] Haupt, Y.; Maya, R.; Kazaz, A.; Oren, M. Mdm2 promotes the rapid degradation of p53. *Nature,* **1997**, *387*(6630), 296-299. [http://dx.doi.org/10.1038/387296a0] [PMID: 9153395]

[51] Shvarts, A.; Bazuine, M.; Dekker, P.; Ramos, Y.F.; Steegenga, W.T.; Merckx, G.; van Ham, R.C.; van der Houven van Oordt, W.; van der Eb, A.J.; Jochemsen, A.G. Isolation and identification of the human homolog of a new p53-binding protein, Mdmx. *Genomics,* **1997**, *43*(1), 34-42. [http://dx.doi.org/10.1006/geno.1997.4775] [PMID: 9226370]

[52] Wade, M.; Li, Y.C.; Wahl, G.M. MDM2, MDMX and p53 in oncogenesis and cancer therapy. *Nat. Rev. Cancer,* **2013**, *13*(2), 83-96. [http://dx.doi.org/10.1038/nrc3430] [PMID: 23303139]

[53] Martins, C.P.; Brown-Swigart, L.; Evan, G.I. Modeling the therapeutic efficacy of p53 restoration in tumors. *Cell,* **2006**, *127*(7), 1323-1334. [http://dx.doi.org/10.1016/j.cell.2006.12.007] [PMID: 17182091]

[54] Ventura, A.; Kirsch, D.G.; McLaughlin, M.E.; Tuveson, D.A.; Grimm, J.; Lintault, L.; Newman, J.; Reczek, E.E.; Weissleder, R.; Jacks, T. Restoration of p53 function leads to tumour regression *in vivo. Nature,* **2007**, *445*(7128), 661-665. [http://dx.doi.org/10.1038/nature05541] [PMID: 17251932]

[55] Xue, W.; Zender, L.; Miething, C.; Dickins, R.A.; Hernando, E.; Krizhanovsky, V.; Cordon-Cardo, C.; Lowe, S.W. Senescence and tumour clearance is triggered by p53 restoration in murine liver carcinomas. *Nature,* **2007**, *445*(7128), 656-660. [http://dx.doi.org/10.1038/nature05529] [PMID: 17251933]

[56] Muller, P.A.J.; Vousden, K.H. Mutant p53 in cancer: new functions and therapeutic opportunities. *Cancer Cell,* **2014**, *25*(3), 304-317. [http://dx.doi.org/10.1016/j.ccr.2014.01.021] [PMID: 24651012]

[57] Maslon, M.M.; Hupp, T.R. Drug discovery and mutant p53. *Trends Cell Biol.,* **2010**, *20*(9), 542-555. [http://dx.doi.org/10.1016/j.tcb.2010.06.005] [PMID: 20656489]

[58] Marine, J.C. MDM2 and MDMX in cancer and development. *Curr. Top. Dev. Biol.,* **2011**, *94*, 45-75. [http://dx.doi.org/10.1016/B978-0-12-380916-2.00003-6] [PMID: 21295684]

[59] Shi, X.; Zhao, Y.; Jiao, Y.; Shi, T.; Yang, X. ROS-dependent mitochondria molecular mechanisms underlying antitumor activity of *Pleurotus abalonus* acidic polysaccharides in human breast cancer MCF-7 cells. *PLoS One,* **2013**, *8*(5)e64266 [http://dx.doi.org/10.1371/journal.pone.0064266] [PMID: 23691187]

[60] Aleem, E. The Mushroom Extract Schizophyllan Reduces Cellular Proliferation and Induces G2/M Arrest in MCF-7 Human Breast Cancer Cells. *Life Sci. J.,* **2011**, *8*(4), 777-784.

[61] Reza, M.A.; Hossain, M.A.; Lee, S.J.; Yohannes, S.B.; Damte, D.; Rhee, M.H.; Jo, W.S.; Suh, J.W.; Park, S.C. Dichlormethane extract of the jelly ear mushroom Auricularia auricula-judae (higher Basidiomycetes) inhibits tumor cell growth in vitro. *Int. J. Med. Mushrooms,* **2014**, *16*(1), 37-47. [http://dx.doi.org/10.1615/IntJMedMushr.v16.i1.40] [PMID: 24940903]

[62] Chang, Y.C.; Hsiao, Y.M.; Wu, M.F.; Ou, C.C.; Lin, Y.W.; Lue, K.H.; Ko, J.L. Interruption of lung cancer cell migration and proliferation by fungal immunomodulatory protein FIP-fve from *Flammulina velutipes. J. Agric. Food Chem.,* **2013**, *61*(49), 12044-12052. [http://dx.doi.org/10.1021/jf4030272] [PMID: 24274472]

[63] Ji, Z.; Tang, Q.; Hao, R.; Zhang, J.; Pan, Y. Induction of apoptosis in the SW620 colon carcinoma cell line by triterpene-enriched extracts from *Ganoderma lucidum* through activation of caspase-3. *Oncol. Lett.,* **2011**, *2*(3), 565-570. [http://dx.doi.org/10.3892/ol.2011.275] [PMID: 22866120]

[64] Zhao, S.; Ye, G.; Fu, G.; Cheng, J.X.; Yang, B.B.; Peng, C. *Ganoderma lucidum* exerts anti-tumor effects on ovarian cancer cells and enhances their sensitivity to cisplatin. *Int. J. Oncol.,* **2011**, *38*(5), 1319-1327. [PMID: 21399867]

[65] Sliva, D. Medicinal mushroom *Phellinus linteus* as an alternative cancer therapy. *Exp. Ther. Med.,* **2010**, *1*(3), 407-411. [http://dx.doi.org/10.3892/etm_00000063] [PMID: 22993555]

[66] Froufe, H.J.; Abreu, R.M.; Ferreira, I.C.F.R. Virtual screening of low molecular weight mushrooms compounds as potential Mdm2 inhibitors. *J. Enzyme Inhib. Med. Chem.,* **2013**, *28*(3), 569-575. [http://dx.doi.org/10.3109/14756366.2012.658787] [PMID: 22380771]

[67] Lee, H.S.; Kim, E.J.; Kim, S.H. Ethanol extract of *Innotus obliquus* (Chaga mushroom) induces G1 cell cycle arrest in HT-29 human colon cancer cells. *Nutr. Res. Pract.,* **2015**, *9*(2), 111-116. [http://dx.doi.org/10.4162/nrp.2015.9.2.111] [PMID: 25861415]

[68] Proestos, C. Superfoods: Recent Data on their Role in the Prevention of Diseases. *Curr. Res. Nutr. Food Sci.,* **2018**, *6*(3) [http://dx.doi.org/10.12944/CRNFSJ.6.3.02]

[69] Valverde, M.E.; Hernández-Pérez, T.; Paredes-López, O. Edible mushrooms: improving human health and promoting quality life. *Int. J. Microbiol.,* **2015**, *2015*376387 [http://dx.doi.org/10.1155/2015/376387] [PMID: 25685150]

[70] Patel, S.; Goyal, A. Recent developments in mushrooms as anti-cancer therapeutics: a review *3 Biotech,* **2012**, *2*(1), 1-15.

[71] Sanders, K.; Moran, Z.; Shi, Z.; Paul, R.; Greenlee, H. Natural products for cancer prevention: clinical update 2016. *Semin. Oncol. Nurs.,* **2016**, *32*(3), 215-240. [http://dx.doi.org/10.1016/j.soncn.2016.06.001] [PMID: 27539278]

[72] Donaldson, M.S. Nutrition and cancer: a review of the evidence for an anti-cancer diet. *Nutr J.,* **2004**, *20;3*, 19. [http://dx.doi.org/10.1186/1475-2891-3-19]

[73] Tao, J.; Li, Y.; Li, S.; Li, H.B. Plant foods for the prevention and management of colon cancer. *J. Funct. Foods,* **2018**, *42*, 95-110. [http://dx.doi.org/10.1016/j.jff.2017.12.064]

[74] Cao, S.; Li, Y.; Meng, X.; Yhao, C.N.; Li, S.; Gan, R.Y.; Li, H.B. Dietary natural products and lung cancer: Effects and mechanisms of action. *J. Funct. Foods,* **2019**, *52*, 316-331. [http://dx.doi.org/10.1016/j.jff.2018.11.004]

[75] Hara, M.; Hanaoka, T.; Kobayashi, M.; Otani, T.; Adachi, H.Y.; Montani, A.; Natsukawa, S.; Shaura, K.; Koizumi, Y.; Kasuga, Y.; Matsuzawa, T.; Ikekawa, T.; Sasaki, S.; Tsugane, S. Cruciferous vegetables, mushrooms, and gastrointestinal cancer risks in a multicenter, hospital-based case-control

study in Japan. *Nutr. Cancer,* **2003**, *46*(2), 138-147. [http://dx.doi.org/10.1207/S15327914NC4602_06] [PMID: 14690789]

[76] Zhang, M.; Huang, J.; Xie, X.; Holman, C.D. Dietary intakes of mushrooms and green tea combine to reduce the risk of breast cancer in Chinese women. *Int J Cancer.,* **2009**, *15;124*(6), 1404-1408. [http://dx.doi.org/10.1002/ijc.24047]

[77] Shin, A.; Kim, J.; Lim, S.Y.; Kim, G.; Sung, M.K.; Lee, E.S.; Ro, J. Dietary mushroom intake and the risk of breast cancer based on hormone receptor status. *Nutr. Cancer,* **2010**, *62*(4), 476-483. [http://dx.doi.org/10.1080/01635580903441212] [PMID: 20432168]

[78] Mohsenzadegan, M.; Seif, F.; Farajollahi, M.M.; Khoshmirsafa, M. Anti-oxidants as chemopreventive agents in prostate cancer: a gap between preclinical and clinical studies. *Recent Patents Anticancer Drug Discov.,* **2018**, *13*(2), 224-239. [http://dx.doi.org/10.2174/1574892813666180213164700] [PMID: 29446748]

[79] Pan, S.Y.; Zhou, J.; Gibbons, L.; Morrison, H.; Wen, S.W. Antioxidants and breast cancer risk- a population-based case-control study in Canada. *BMC Cancer,* **2011**, *11*(11), 372. [http://dx.doi.org/10.1186/1471-2407-11-372] [PMID: 21864361]

[80] Serafini, M.; Bellocco, R.; Wolk, A.; Ekström, A.M. Total antioxidant potential of fruit and vegetables and risk of gastric cancer. *Gastroenterology,* **2002**, *123*(4), 985-991. [http://dx.doi.org/10.1053/gast.2002.35957] [PMID: 12360458]

[81] Ferreira, I.C.; Barros, L.; Abreu, R.M. Antioxidants in wild mushrooms. *Curr. Med. Chem.,* **2009**, *16*(12), 1543-1560. [http://dx.doi.org/10.2174/092986709787909587] [PMID: 19355906]

[82] Feeney, M.J.; Dwyer, J.; Hasler-Lewis, C.M.; Milner, J.A.; Noakes, M.; Rowe, S.; Wach, M.; Beelman, R.B.; Caldwell, J.; Cantorna, M.T.; Castlebury, L.A.; Chang, S.T.; Cheskin, L.J.; Clemens, R.; Drescher, G.; Fulgoni, V.L., III; Haytowitz, D.B.; Hubbard, V.S.; Law, D.; Myrdal Miller, A.; Minor, B.; Percival, S.S.; Riscuta, G.; Schneeman, B.; Thornsbury, S.; Toner, C.D.; Woteki, C.E.; Wu, D. Mushrooms and Health Summit proceedings. *J. Nutr.,* **2014**, *144*(7), 1128S-1136S. [http://dx.doi.org/10.3945/jn.114.190728] [PMID: 24812070]

[83] Wasser, S.P. Current findings, future trends, and unsolved problems in studies of medicinal mushrooms. *Appl. Microbiol. Biotechnol.,* **2011**, *89*(5), 1323-1332. [http://dx.doi.org/10.1007/s00253-010-3067-4] [PMID: 21190105]

[84] Gao, Y.; Zhou, S.; Jiang, W.; Huang, M.; Dai, X. Effects of ganopoly (a *Ganoderma lucidum* polysaccharide extract) on the immune functions in advanced-stage cancer patients. *Immunol. Invest.,* **2003**, *32*(3), 201-215. [http://dx.doi.org/10.1081/IMM-120022979] [PMID: 12916709]

[85] Zhou, X.W.; Su, K.Q.; Zhang, Y.M. Applied modern biotechnology for cultivation of Ganoderma and development of their products. *Appl. Microbiol. Biotechnol.,* **2012**, *93*(3), 941-963. [http://dx.doi.org/10.1007/s00253-011-3780-7] [PMID: 22170106]

[86] Fortes, R.C.; Recôva, V.L.; Melo, A.L.; Novaes, M.R. Effects of dietary supplementation with medicinal fungus in fasting glycemia levels of patients with colorectal cancer: a randomized, double-blind, placebo-controlled clinical study. *Nutr. Hosp.,* **2008**, *23*(6), 591-598. [PMID: 19132268]

[87] Baek, J.; Roh, H.S.; Baek, K.H.; Lee, S.; Lee, S.; Song, S.S.; Kim, K.H. Bioactivity-based analysis and chemical characterization of cytotoxic constituents from Chaga mushroom (*Inonotus obliquus*) that induce apoptosis in human lung adenocarcinoma cells. *J. Ethnopharmacol.,* **2018**, *224*(5), 63-75. [http://dx.doi.org/10.1016/j.jep.2018.05.025] [PMID: 29800742]

[88] Zhong, X.H.; Wang, L.B.; Sun, D.Z. Effects of inotodiol extracts from inonotus obliquus on proliferation cycle and apoptotic gene of human lung adenocarcinoma cell line A549. *Chin. J. Integr. Med.,* **2011**, *17*(3), 218-223. [http://dx.doi.org/10.1007/s11655-011-0670-x] [PMID: 21359924]

[89] Wang, Q.; Mu, H.; Zhang, L.; Dong, D.; Zhang, W.; Duan, J. Characterization of two water-soluble lignin metabolites with antiproliferative activities from *Inonotus obliquus*. *Int. J. Biol. Macromol.*, **2015**, *74*, 507-514.
[http://dx.doi.org/10.1016/j.ijbiomac.2014.12.044] [PMID: 25583019]

[90] Wu, S.H.; Lin, Y.T.; Chern, C.L.; Ke, S.T. *Inonotus taiwanensis* sp. nov. (Basidiomycota) from Taiwan. *Mycoscience,* **2018**.
[http://dx.doi.org/10.1016/j.myc.2017.07.003]

[91] Chao, T.L.; Wang, T.Y.; Lee, C.H.; Yiin, S.J.; Ho, C.T.; Wu, S.H.; You, H.L.; Chern, C.L. Anti-cancerous effect of Inonotus taiwanensis polysaccharide extract on human acute monocytic leukemia cells through ROS-independent intrinsic mitochondrial pathway *Int. J. Mol. Sci.,* **2018**, *29,19*(2), e 393.

[92] Wang, F.F.; Shi, C.; Yang, Y.; Fang, Y.; Sheng, L.; Li, N. Medicinal mushroom *Phellinus igniarius* induced cell apoptosis in gastric cancer SGC-7901 through a mitochondria-dependent pathway. *Biomed. Pharmacother.*, **2018**, *102*, 18-25.
[http://dx.doi.org/10.1016/j.biopha.2018.03.038] [PMID: 29549725]

[93] Chen, X.Q.; Chen, L.X.; Zhao, J.; Tang, Y.P.; Li, S.P. Nortriterpenoids from the Fruiting Bodies of the Mushroom *Ganoderma resinaceum. Molecules,* **2017**, *22*(7)E1073
[http://dx.doi.org/10.3390/molecules22071073] [PMID: 28657576]

[94] Sedky, N.K.; El Gammal, Z.H.; Wahba, A.E.; Mosad, E.; Waly, Z.Y.; El-Fallal, A.A.; Arafa, R.K.; El-Badri, N. The molecular basis of cytotoxicity of α-spinasterol from *Ganoderma resinaceum*: Induction of apoptosis and overexpression of p53 in breast and ovarian cancer cell lines. *J. Cell. Biochem.,* **2018**, *119*(5), 3892-3902.
[http://dx.doi.org/10.1002/jcb.26515] [PMID: 29143969]

[95] Elkhateeb, W.A.; Zaghlol, G.M.; El-Garawani, I.M.; Ahmed, E.F.; Rateb, M.E.; Abdel Moneim, A.E. *Ganoderma applanatum* secondary metabolites induced apoptosis through different pathways: *in vivo* and *in vitro* anticancer studies. *Biomed. Pharmacother.*, **2018**, *101*, 264-277.
[http://dx.doi.org/10.1016/j.biopha.2018.02.058] [PMID: 29494964]

[96] Nowacka-Jechalke, N.; Nowak, R.; Juda, M.; Malm, A.; Lemieszek, M.; Rzeski, W.; Kaczyński, Z. New biological activity of the polysaccharide fraction from *Cantharellus cibarius* and its structural characterization. *Food Chem.,* **2018**, *268*, 355-361.
[http://dx.doi.org/10.1016/j.foodchem.2018.06.106] [PMID: 30064769]

[97] Vasdekis, E.; Karkabounas, A.; Giannakopoulos, I.; Savvas, D.; Lekka, M. Screening of mushrooms bioactivity: piceatannol was identified as a bioactive ingredient in the order Cantharellales. *Eur. Food Res. Technol.,* **2018**, *244*(5), 861-871.
[http://dx.doi.org/10.1007/s00217-017-3007-y]

[98] Finimundy, T.C.; Abreu, R.M.V.; Bonetto, N.; Scariot, F.J.; Dillon, A.J.P.; Echeverrigaray, S.; Barros, L.; Ferreira, I.C.F.R.; Henriques, J.A.P.; Roesch-Ely, M. Apoptosis induction by *Pleurotus sajor-caju* (Fr.) Singer extracts on colorectal cancer cell lines. *Food Chem. Toxicol.,* **2018**, *112*, 383-392.
[http://dx.doi.org/10.1016/j.fct.2018.01.015] [PMID: 29337231]

[99] Yap, H.Y.; Muria-Gonzalez, M.J.; Kong, B.H.; Stubbs, K.A.; Tan, C.S.; Ng, S.T.; Tan, N.H.; Solomon, P.S.; Fung, S.Y.; Chooi, Y.H. Heterologous expression of cytotoxic sesquiterpenoids from the medicinal mushroom *Lignosus rhinocerotis* in yeast. *Microb. Cell Fact.,* **2017**, *16*(1), 103.
[http://dx.doi.org/10.1186/s12934-017-0713-x] [PMID: 28606152]

[100] Yap, H.Y.Y.; Tan, N.H.; Ng, S.T.; Tan, C.S.; Fung, S.Y. Molecular attributes and apoptosis-inducing activities of a putative serine protease isolated from Tiger Milk mushroom *(Lignosus rhinocerus) sclerotium against breast cancer cells in vitro. PeerJ,* **2018**, *5,6*, e4940.

[101] Lee, S.R.; Roh, H-S.; Lee, S.; Park, H.B.; Jang, T.S.; Ko, Y-J.; Baek, K-H.; Kim, K.H. Bioactivity-guided isolation and chemical characterization of antiproliferative constituents from morel mushroom (*Morchella esculent*) in human lung adenocarcinoma cells. *J. Funct. Foods,* **2018**, *40*, 249-260.

[http://dx.doi.org/10.1016/j.jff.2017.11.012]

[102] Lau, B.F.; Abdullah, N. Bioprospecting of *Lentinus squarrosulus* Mont., an underutilized wild edible mushroom, as a potential source of functional ingredients: A review. *Trends Food Sci. Technol.,* **2017**, *61*, 116-131.
[http://dx.doi.org/10.1016/j.tifs.2016.11.017]

[103] Prateep, A.; Sumkhemthong, S.; Suksomtip, M.; Chanvorachote, P.; Chaotham, C. Peptides extracted from edible mushroom: *Lentinus squarrosulus* induces apoptosis in human lung cancer cells. *Pharm. Biol.,* **2017**, *55*(1), 1792-1799.
[http://dx.doi.org/10.1080/13880209.2017.1325913] [PMID: 28532227]

[104] Zhou, R.; Han, Y.J.; Zhang, M.H.; Zhang, K.R.; Ng, T.B.; Liu, F. Purification and characterization of a novel ubiquitin-like antitumour protein with hemagglutinating and deoxyribonuclease activities from the edible mushroom *Ramaria botrytis. AMB Express,* **2017**, *7*(1), 47.
[http://dx.doi.org/10.1186/s13568-017-0346-9] [PMID: 28229436]

[105] Tešanović, K.; Pejin, B.; Šibul, F.; Matavulj, M.; Rašeta, M.; Janjušević, L.; Karaman, M. A comparative overview of antioxidative properties and phenolic profiles of different fungal origins: fruiting bodies and submerged cultures of *Coprinus comatus* and *Coprinellus truncorum. J. Food Sci. Technol.,* **2017**, *54*(2), 430-438.
[http://dx.doi.org/10.1007/s13197-016-2479-2] [PMID: 28242942]

[106] Zhang, P.; Li, K.; Yang, G.; Xia, C.; Polston, J.E.; Li, G. Cytotoxic protein from the mushroom Coprinus comatus possesses a unique mode for glycan binding and specificity *Proc Natl Acad Sci U S A,* **2017**, *22;114*(34), 8980-8985.

[107] Zhang, A.; Deng, J.; Yu, S.; Zhang, F.; Linhardt, R.J.; Sun, P. Purification and structural elucidation of a water-soluble polysaccharide from the fruiting bodies of the *Grifola frondosa. Int. J. Biol. Macromol.,* **2018**, *115*, 221-226.
[http://dx.doi.org/10.1016/j.ijbiomac.2018.04.061] [PMID: 29660454]

[108] Zhao, F.; Wang, Y.F.; Song, L.; Jin, J.X.; Zhang, Y.Q.; Gan, H.Y.; Yang, K.H. Synergistic apoptotic effect of D-fraction from *Grifola frondosa* and vitamin C on hepatocellular carcinoma SMMC-7721 cells. *Integr. Cancer Ther.,* **2017**, *16*(2), 205-214.
[http://dx.doi.org/10.1177/1534735416644674] [PMID: 27151580]

[109] Petrović, J.; Glamočlija, J.; Stojković, D.; Nikolić, M.; Ćirić, A.; Fernandes, A.; Ferreira, I.C.F.R.; Soković, M. Bioactive composition, antimicrobial activities and the influence of *Agrocybe aegerita* (Brig.) Sing on certain quorum-sensing-regulated functions and biofilm formation by *Pseudomonas aeruginosa. Food Funct.,* **2014**, *5*(12), 3296-3303.
[http://dx.doi.org/10.1039/C4FO00819G] [PMID: 25367459]

[110] Landi, N.; Pacifico, S.; Ragucci, S.; Iglesias, R.; Piccolella, S.; Amici, A.; Di Giuseppe, A.M.A.; Di Maro, A. Purification, characterization and cytotoxicity assessment of Ageritin: The first ribotoxin from the basidiomycete mushroom *Agrocybe aegerita. Biochim. Biophys. Acta, Gen. Subj.,* **2017**, *1861* 5 Pt A, 1113-1121.
[http://dx.doi.org/10.1016/j.bbagen.2017.02.023] [PMID: 28232091]

[111] Chang, C.T.; Korivi, M.; Huang, H.C.; Thiyagarajan, V.; Lin, K.Y.; Huang, P.J.; Liu, J.Y.; Hseu, Y.C.; Yang, H.L. Inhibition of ROS production, autophagy or apoptosis signaling reversed the anticancer properties of *Antrodia salmonea* in triple-negative breast cancer (MDA-MB-231) cells. *Food Chem. Toxicol.,* **2017**, *103*, 1-17.
[http://dx.doi.org/10.1016/j.fct.2017.02.019] [PMID: 28219700]

[112] Chang, C.T.; Hseu, Y.C.; Thiyagarajan, V.; Huang, H.C.; Hsu, L.S.; Huang, P.J.; Liu, J.Y.; Liao, J.W.; Yang, H.L. Antrodia salmonea induces G_2 cell-cycle arrest in human triple-negative breast cancer (MDA-MB-231) cells and suppresses tumor growth in athymic nude mice. *J. Ethnopharmacol.,* **2017**, *196*(196), 9-19.
[http://dx.doi.org/10.1016/j.jep.2016.12.018] [PMID: 27986611]

[113] Wu, T.R.; Huang, T.T.; Martel, J.; Liau, J.C.; Chiu, C.Y.; Leu, Y.L.; Jian, W.T.; Chang, I.T.; Lu, C.C.; Ojcius, D.M.; Ko, Y.F.; Lai, H.C.; Young, J.D. Pinicolol B from *Antrodia cinnamomea* induces apoptosis of nasopharyngeal carcinoma cells. *J. Ethnopharmacol.*, **2017**, *201*(201), 117-122. [http://dx.doi.org/10.1016/j.jep.2017.02.008] [PMID: 28167294]

[114] Wang, J.J.; Wu, C.C.; Lee, C.L.; Hsieh, S.L.; Chen, J.B.; Lee, C.I. Antimelanogenic, antioxidant and antiproliferative effects of *Antrodia camphorata* fruiting bodies on B16-F0 melanoma cells. *PLoS One,* **2017**, *12*(1)e0170924 [http://dx.doi.org/10.1371/journal.pone.0170924] [PMID: 28125738]

[115] Kaygusuz, O.; Kaygusuz, M.; Dodurga, Y.; Seçme, M.; Herken, E.N.; Gezer, K. Assessment of the antimicrobial, antioxidant and cytotoxic activities of the wild edible mushroom *Agaricus lanipes* (F.H. Møller & Jul. Schäff.) Hlaváček. *Cytotechnology,* **2017**, *69*(1), 135-144. [http://dx.doi.org/10.1007/s10616-016-0045-4] [PMID: 28058568]

[116] Mocan, A.; Fernandes, Â.; Barros, L.; Crişan, G.; Smiljković, M.; Soković, M.; Ferreira, I.C.F.R. Chemical composition and bioactive properties of the wild mushroom Polyporus squamosus (Huds.) Fr: a study with samples from Romania. *Food Funct.*, **2018**, *9*(1), 160-170. [http://dx.doi.org/10.1039/C7FO01514C] [PMID: 29168866]

[117] Manna, D.; Pust, S.; Torgersen, M.L.; Cordara, G.; Künzler, M.; Krengel, U.; Sandvig, K. *Polyporus squamosus* Lectin 1a (PSL1a) Exhibits Cytotoxicity in Mammalian Cells by Disruption of Focal Adhesions, Inhibition of Protein Synthesis and Induction of Apoptosis. *PLoS One,* **2017**, *12*(1)e0170716 [http://dx.doi.org/10.1371/journal.pone.0170716] [PMID: 28114329]

[118] Kim, S.; Min, S.O.H.; Roh, H.S.; Kim, J.; Sik, Yu. J.; Lee, S. Vulpinic acid contributes to the cytotoxicity of *Pulveroboletus ravenelii* to human cancer cells by inducing apoptosis. *RSC Advances,* **2017**, *7*, 35297. [http://dx.doi.org/10.1039/C7RA05059C]

[119] Teng, J-F.; Lee, C-H.; Hsu, T-H.; Lo, H-C. Potential activities and mechanisms of extracellular polysaccharopeptides from fermented *Trametes versicolor* on regulating glucose homeostasis in insulin-resistant HepG2 cells. *PLoS One,* **2018**, *13*(7)e0201131 [http://dx.doi.org/10.1371/journal.pone.0201131] [PMID: 30024975]

[120] Ricciardi, M.R.; Licchetta, R.; Mirabilii, S.; Scarpari, M.; Parroni, A.; Fabbri, A.A.; Cescutti, P.; Reverberi, M.; Fanelli, C.; Tafuri, A. Preclinical antileukemia activity of tramesan: a newly identified bioactive fungal metabolite. *Oxid. Med. Cell. Longev.*, **2017**, *2017*5061639 [http://dx.doi.org/10.1155/2017/5061639] [PMID: 29270245]

[121] Stojković, D.S.; Barros, L.; Calhelha, R.C.; Glamočlija, J.; Ćirić, A.; van Griensven, L.J.; Soković, M.; Ferreira, I.C.F.R. A detailed comparative study between chemical and bioactive properties of *Ganoderma lucidum* from different origins. *Int. J. Food Sci. Nutr.*, **2014**, *65*(1), 42-47. [http://dx.doi.org/10.3109/09637486.2013.832173] [PMID: 24020451]

[122] Dai, J.; Miller, M.A.; Everetts, N.J.; Wang, X.; Li, P.; Li, Y.; Xu, J.H.; Yao, G. Elimination of quiescent slow-cycling cells via reducing quiescence depth by natural compounds purified from *Ganoderma lucidum. Oncotarget,* **2017**, *8*(8), 13770-13781. [http://dx.doi.org/10.18632/oncotarget.14634] [PMID: 28099150]

[123] Dan, X.; Liu, W.; Wong, J.H.; Ng, T.B. A ribonuclease isolated from wild *Ganoderma lucidum* suppressed autophagy and triggered apoptosis in colorectal cancer cells. *Front. Pharmacol.*, **2016**, *7*, 217. [http://dx.doi.org/10.3389/fphar.2016.00217] [PMID: 27504094]

[124] Wan-Mohtar, W.A.; Young, L.; Abbott, G.M.; Clements, C.; Harvey, L.M.; McNeil, B. Antimicrobial properties and cytotoxicity of sulfated (1,3)-β-D-Glucan from the mycelium of the mushroom *Ganoderma lucidum. J. Microbiol. Biotechnol.*, **2016**, *26*(6), 999-1010. [http://dx.doi.org/10.4014/jmb.1510.10018] [PMID: 26907757]

[125] Ruan, W.; Wei, Y.; Popovich, D.G. Distinct responses of cytotoxic *Ganoderma lucidum* triterpenoids in human carcinoma cells. *Phytother. Res.,* **2015**, *29*(11), 1744-1752. [http://dx.doi.org/10.1002/ptr.5426] [PMID: 26292672]

[126] Soković, M.; Ćirić, A.; Glamočlija, J.; Nikolić, M.; van Griensven, L.J. *Agaricus blazei* hot water extract shows anti quorum sensing activity in the nosocomial human pathogen *Pseudomonas aeruginosa. Molecules,* **2014**, *19*(4), 4189-4199. [http://dx.doi.org/10.3390/molecules19044189] [PMID: 24705563]

[127] Hetland, G.; Eide, D.M.; Tangen, J.M.; Haugen, M.H.; Mirlashari, M.R.; Paulsen, J.E. The *Agaricus blazei*-based mushroom extract, Andosan™, protects against intestinal tumorigenesis in the A/J Min/+ Mouse. *PLoS One,* **2016**, *11*(12)e0167754 [http://dx.doi.org/10.1371/journal.pone.0167754] [PMID: 28002446]

[128] Shimizu, T.; Kawai, J.; Ouchi, K.; Kikuchi, H.; Osima, Y.; Hidemi, R. Agarol, an ergosterol derivative from *Agaricus blazei*, induces caspase-independent apoptosis in human cancer cells. *Int. J. Oncol.,* **2016**, *48*(4), 1670-1678. [http://dx.doi.org/10.3892/ijo.2016.3391] [PMID: 26893131]

[129] Fernando, D.; Adhikari, A.; Nanayakkara, C.; de Silva, E.D.; Wijesundera, R.; Soysa, P. Cytotoxic effects of ergone, a compound isolated from *Fulviformes fastuosus. BMC Complement. Altern. Med.,* **2016**, *16*(1), 484. [http://dx.doi.org/10.1186/s12906-016-1471-8] [PMID: 27887609]

[130] Chen, S.Y.; Chang, C.L.; Chen, T.H.; Chang, Y.W.; Lin, S.B. Colossolactone H, a new Ganoderma triterpenoid exhibits cytotoxicity and potentiates drug efficacy of gefitinib in lung cancer. *Fitoterapia,* **2016**, *114*, 81-91. [http://dx.doi.org/10.1016/j.fitote.2016.08.015] [PMID: 27575325]

[131] Eroğlu, C.; Seçme, M.; Atmaca, P.; Kaygusuz, O.; Gezer, K.; Bağcı, G.; Dodurga, Y. Extract of *Calvatia gigantea* inhibits proliferation of A549 human lung cancer cells. *Cytotechnology,* **2016**, *68*(5), 2075-2081. [http://dx.doi.org/10.1007/s10616-016-9947-4] [PMID: 26820971]

[132] Majumder, R.; Banik, S.P.; Khowala, S. AkP from mushroom *Termitomyces clypeatus* is a proteoglycan specific protease with apoptotic effect on HepG2. *Int. J. Biol. Macromol.,* **2016**, *91*, 198-207. [http://dx.doi.org/10.1016/j.ijbiomac.2016.05.034] [PMID: 27180294]

[133] Kostić, M.; Smiljković, M.; Petrović, J.; Glamočlija, J.; Barros, L.; Ferreira, I.C.F.R.; Ćirić, A.; Soković, M. Chemical, nutritive composition and a wide range of bioactive properties of honey mushroom *Armillaria mellea* (Vahl: Fr.) Kummer. *Food Funct.,* **2017**, *8*(9), 3239-3249. [http://dx.doi.org/10.1039/C7FO00887B] [PMID: 28812768]

[134] Chen, Y.J.; Chen, C.C.; Huang, H.L. Induction of apoptosis by *Armillaria mellea* constituent armillarikin in human hepatocellular carcinoma. *OncoTargets Ther.,* **2016**, *9*, 4773-4783. [http://dx.doi.org/10.2147/OTT.S103940] [PMID: 27536140]

[135] Zhang, Y.; Wang, P.; Xiao, Y.; Wang, X.; Yang, S.; Liu, Q. Chemical compositions and antiproliferation activities of the chloroform fraction from *Pyropolyporus fomentarius* in K562 cells. *Hum. Exp. Toxicol.,* **2015**, *34*(7), 732-743. [http://dx.doi.org/10.1177/0960327114558888] [PMID: 25403175]

[136] Li, Y.; Zhou, Y.; Wang, X.; Wang, P.; Xiao, Y.; Cheng, X.; Zhang, Y.; Liu, Y.; Liu, Q. Fruit extract from *Pyropolyporus fomentarius* (L. ex Fr.) Teng induces mitochondria-dependent apoptosis in leukemia cells but enhances immunomodulatory activities of splenic lymphocytes. *Nutr. Cancer,* **2016**, *68*(4), 708-717. [http://dx.doi.org/10.1080/01635581.2016.1158290] [PMID: 27115601]

[137] Zhang, Y.; Xiao, Y.; Wang, P.; Liu, Q. Compositions and anti-tumor activity of *Pyropolyporus fomentarius* petroleum ether fraction *in vitro* and *in vivo. PLoS One,* **2014**, *9*(10)e109599

[http://dx.doi.org/10.1371/journal.pone.0109599] [PMID: 25302783]

[138] Reis, F.S.; Barros, L.; Martins, A.; Vasconcelos, M.H.; Morales, P.; Ferreira, I.C.F.R. *Leccinum molle* (Bon) Bon and *Leccinum vulpinum* Watling: The First Study of Their Nutritional and Antioxidant Potential. *Molecules,* **2016**, *21*(2), 246. [http://dx.doi.org/10.3390/molecules21020246] [PMID: 26907239]

[139] Reis, F.S.; Sousa, D.; Barros, L.; Martins, A.; Morales, P.; Ferreira, I.C.F.R.; Vasconcelos, M.H. *Leccinum vulpinum* Watling induces DNA damage, decreases cell proliferation and induces apoptosis on the human MCF-7 breast cancer cell line. *Food Chem. Toxicol.,* **2016**, *90*, 45-54. [http://dx.doi.org/10.1016/j.fct.2016.02.005] [PMID: 26854920]

[140] Wang, Y.; Chen, Y.; Zhang, X.; Cai, G.; An, S.; Wang, X.; Teng, L.; Wang, D. *Tricholoma matsutake* Aqueous Extract Induces Hepatocellular Carcinoma Cell Apoptosis via Caspase-Dependent Mitochondrial Pathway. *BioMed Res. Int.,* **2016**, *2016*9014364 [http://dx.doi.org/10.1155/2016/9014364] [PMID: 28018916]

[141] Li, W.; Zhou, W.; Kim, E.J.; Shim, S.H.; Kang, H.K.; Kim, Y.H. Isolation and identification of aromatic compounds in Lion's Mane Mushroom and their anticancer activities. *Food Chem.,* **2015**, *170*, 336-342. [http://dx.doi.org/10.1016/j.foodchem.2014.08.078] [PMID: 25306354]

[142] Jiao, C.; Xie, Y-Z.; Yang, X.; Li, H.; Li, X-M.; Pan, H-H.; Cai, M.H.; Zhong, H.M.; Yang, B.B. Anticancer activity of *Amauroderma rude. PLoS One,* **2013**, *8*(6)e66504 [http://dx.doi.org/10.1371/journal.pone.0066504] [PMID: 23840494]

[143] Li, X.; Wu, Q.; Xie, Y.; Ding, Y.; Du, W.W.; Sdiri, M.; Yang, B.B. Ergosterol purified from medicinal mushroom *Amauroderma rude* inhibits cancer growth *in vitro* and *in vivo* by up-regulating multiple tumor suppressors. *Oncotarget,* **2015**, *6*(19), 17832-17846. [http://dx.doi.org/10.18632/oncotarget.4026] [PMID: 26098777]

[144] Chou, S.M.; Lai, W.J.; Hong, T.W.; Lai, J.Y.; Tsai, S.H.; Chen, Y.H.; Yu, S.H.; Kao, C.H.; Chu, R.; Ding, S.T.; Li, T.K.; Shen, T.L. Synergistic property of cordycepin in cultivated *Cordyceps militaris*-mediated apoptosis in human leukemia cells. *Phytomedicine,* **2014**, *21*(12), 1516-1524. [http://dx.doi.org/10.1016/j.phymed.2014.07.014] [PMID: 25442260]

[145] Liao, Y.; Ling, J.; Zhang, G.; Liu, F.; Tao, S.; Han, Z.; Chen, S.; Chen, Z.; Le, H. Cordycepin induces cell cycle arrest and apoptosis by inducing DNA damage and up-regulation of p53 in Leukemia cells. *Cell Cycle,* **2015**, *14*(5), 761-771. [http://dx.doi.org/10.1080/15384101.2014.1000097] [PMID: 25590866]

[146] Suh, W.; Nam, G.; Yang, W.S.; Sung, G.H.; Shim, S.H.; Cho, J.Y. Chemical Constituents Identified from Fruit Body of *Cordyceps bassiana* and Their Anti-Inflammatory Activity. *Biomol. Ther. (Seoul),* **2017**, *25*(2), 165-170. [http://dx.doi.org/10.4062/biomolther.2016.063] [PMID: 27530115]

[147] Kim, J.H.; Lee, Y.; Sung, G.H.; Kim, H.G.; Jeong, D.; Park, J.G. Antiproliferative and apoptosis-inducing activities of 4-isopropyl-2,6-bis(1-phenylethyl)phenol isolated from butanol fraction of *Cordyceps bassiana. e CAM,* **2015**, 739874.

[148] Wang, W.; Chen, K.; Liu, Q.; Johnston, N.; Ma, Z.; Zhang, F.; Zheng, X. Suppression of tumor growth by *Pleurotus ferulae* ethanol extract through induction of cell apoptosis, and inhibition of cell proliferation and migration. *PLoS One,* **2014**, *9*(7)e102673 [http://dx.doi.org/10.1371/journal.pone.0102673] [PMID: 25029345]

[149] Arora, R.; Yates, C.; Gary, B.D.; McClellan, S.; Tan, M.; Xi, Y.; Reed, E.; Piazza, G.A.; Owen, L.B.; Dean-Colomb, W. Panepoxydone targets NF-kB and FOXM1 to inhibit proliferation, induce apoptosis and reverse epithelial to mesenchymal transition in breast cancer. *PLoS One,* **2014**, *9*(6)e98370 [http://dx.doi.org/10.1371/journal.pone.0098370] [PMID: 24896091]

[150] Chen, Y.; Hu, M.; Wang, C.; Yang, Y.; Chen, J.; Ding, J.; Guo, W. Characterization and *in vitro* antitumor activity of polysaccharides from the mycelium of *Sarcodon aspratus. Int. J. Biol.*

Macromol., **2013**, *52*, 52-58.
[http://dx.doi.org/10.1016/j.ijbiomac.2012.09.005] [PMID: 22982812]

[151] Han, J.; Sohn, E.J.; Kim, B.; Kim, S.; Won, G.; Yoon, S.; Lee, J.; Kim, M.J.; Lee, H.; Chung, K.; Kim, S.H. Upregulation of death receptor 5 and activation of caspase 8/3 play a critical role in ergosterol peroxide induced apoptosis in DU 145 prostate cancer cells. *Cancer Cell Int.,* **2014**, *14*(1), 117.
[http://dx.doi.org/10.1186/s12935-014-0117-5] [PMID: 25506265]

[152] Stojković, D.; Kovačević-Grujičić, N.; Reis, F.; Davidović, S.; Barros, L.; Popović, J.; Petrović, I.; Pavić, A.; Glamočlija, J.; Ćirić, A.; Stevanović, M.; Ferreira, I.C.F.R.; Soković, M. Chemical composition of the mushroom *Meripilus giganteus* Karst. and bioactive properties of its methanolic extract. *LWT - Food. Sci. Tech. (Paris),* **2017**, *79*, 454-462.

[153] Petrovic, I.P.; Kovacevic-Grujicic, N.R.; Stojkovic, D.S.; Davidovic, S.B.; Glamoclija, J.M.; Ciric, A.D.; Sokovic, M.D.; Stevanovic, M.J. *Meripilus giganteus* in prevention of cancer: Phenolic profile, biological potential and antitumor effect via upregulation of p53 and SOX1 expression in HeLa cells (Meeting Abstract). *Eur. J. Cancer,* **2014**, *50* Suppl. 5, S194.
[http://dx.doi.org/10.1016/S0959-8049(14)50709-5]

[154] Smiljkovic, M.; Stanisavljevic, D.; Stojkovic, D.; Petrovic, I.; Marjanovic Vicentic, J.; Popovic, J.; Golic Grdadolnik, S.; Markovic, D.; Sankovic-Babice, S.; Glamoclija, J.; Stevanovic, M.; Soković, M. Apigenin-7-O-glucoside versus apigenin: Insight into the modes of anticandidal and cytotoxic actions. *EXCLI J.,* **2017**, *16*, 795-807.
[PMID: 28827996]

[155] Reis, F.S.; Barreira, J.C.M.; Calhelha, R.C.; van Griensven, L.J.L.D.; Ćirić, A.; Glamočlija, J.; Soković, M.; Ferreira, I.C.F.R. Chemical characterization of the medicinal mushroom *Phellinus linteus* (Berkeley & Curtis) Teng and contribution of different fractions to its bioactivity. *Lebensm. Wiss. Technol.,* **2014**, *58*(2), 478-485.
[http://dx.doi.org/10.1016/j.lwt.2014.04.013]

[156] Stojković, D.; Reis, F.S.; Barros, L.; Glamočlija, J.; Ćirić, A.; van Griensven, L.J.; Soković, M.; Ferreira, I.C.F.R. Nutrients and non-nutrients composition and bioactivity of wild and cultivated *Coprinus comatus* (O.F.Müll.) Pers. *Food Chem. Toxicol.,* **2013**, *59*, 289-296.
[http://dx.doi.org/10.1016/j.fct.2013.06.017] [PMID: 23793036]

[157] Petrović, J.; Stojković, D.; Reis, F.S.; Barros, L.; Glamočlija, J.; Ćirić, A.; Ferreira, I.C.F.R.; Soković, M. Study on chemical, bioactive and food preserving properties of *Laetiporus sulphureus* (Bull.: Fr.) Murr. *Food Funct.,* **2014**, *5*(7), 1441-1451.
[http://dx.doi.org/10.1039/C4FO00113C] [PMID: 24810655]

[158] Stojković, D.; Reis, F.S.; Glamočlija, J.; Ćirić, A.; Barros, L.; Van Griensven, L.J.L.D.; Ferreira, I.C.F.R.; Soković, M. Cultivated strains of Agaricus bisporus and A. brasiliensis: chemical characterization and evaluation of antioxidant and antimicrobial properties for the final healthy product--natural preservatives in yoghurt. *Food Funct.,* **2014**, *5*(7), 1602-1612.
[http://dx.doi.org/10.1039/c4fo00054d] [PMID: 24881564]

[159] Vieira, V.; Fernandes, Â.; Barros, L.; Glamočlija, J.; Ćirić, A.; Stojković, D.; Martins, A.; Soković, M.; Ferreira, I.C.F.R. Wild *Morchella conica* Pers. from different origins: a comparative study of nutritional and bioactive properties. *J. Sci. Food Agric.,* **2016**, *96*(1), 90-98.
[http://dx.doi.org/10.1002/jsfa.7063] [PMID: 25546397]

[160] Glamočlija, J.; Ćirić, A.; Nikolić, M.; Fernandes, Â.; Barros, L.; Calhelha, R.C.; Ferreira, I.C.F.R.; Soković, M.; van Griensven, L.J.L.D. Chemical characterization and biological activity of Chaga (*Inonotus obliquus*), a medicinal "mushroom". *J. Ethnopharmacol.,* **2015**, *162*, 323-332.
[http://dx.doi.org/10.1016/j.jep.2014.12.069] [PMID: 25576897]

[161] Stanisavljevic, D.; Petrovic, I.; Vukovic, V.; Schwirtlich, M.; Gredic, M.; Stevanovic, M.; Popovic, J. SOX14 activates the p53 signaling pathway and induces apoptosis in a cervical carcinoma cell line. *PLoS One,* **2017**, *12*(9)e0184686
[http://dx.doi.org/10.1371/journal.pone.0184686] [PMID: 28926586]

CHAPTER 6

Health Related Enzyme Inhibiting Natural Products from Medicinal Plants

Athar Ata[1], **Samina Naz**[1], **Kenneth Friesen**[1] and **Bilge Sener**[2,*]

[1] *Department of Chemistry, Richardson College for the Environmental and Science Complex, The University of Winnipeg, 599 Portage Avenue, Winnipeg, Manitoba R3B 2G3, Canada*

[2] *Department of Pharmacognosy, Faculty of Pharmacy, Gazi University, Ankara, Turkey*

Abstract: Natural product chemistry is an important class of organic chemistry that contributes novel organic compounds to the chemical literature and is considered as one of the successful sources of supplying lead bioactive compounds to the drug discovery. One of the aspects of drug discovery is the identification of small molecules with enzyme inhibiting activities. Enzymes play an important role in all aspects of health in life and their overexpression and hyperactivation is involved in the pathogenesis of various diseases. For instance, anti-acetylcholinesterase (AChE) compounds are potential candidates for curing Alzheimer's Disease (AD). During the past years, we are involved in discovering new enzyme inhibiting natural products from medicinally important plants. This chapter describes the identification of new anti-α-glucosidase, anti-renin, anti-glutathione transferase (GST) and anti-AChE compounds from medicinally important plants. Additionally, structure-activity relationships (SAR) and determination of active pharmacophores of newly discovered bioactive natural products exhibiting aforementioned bioactivities are also discussed.

Key words: Alzheimer's Disease, α-glucosidase, Glutathione Transferase (GST), Acetylcholinesterase, Natural Products, Diabetes, Hypertension, Chemo-enzymatic Synthesis.

INTRODUCTION

Natural products are organic compounds that provide lead compounds to the drug discovery program with novel carbon skeletons. This is due to the enormous structural diversity of natural products that is difficult to achieve through traditional chemical synthesis and other genomic approaches. The huge structural diversity of natural products might be attributed to the harsh environmental conditions that these living organisms resist to survive [1]. Recent studies suggest that over 50% of prescribed pharmaceuticals are of natural product origin

* **Corresponding author Bilge Sener:** Department of Pharmacognosy, Faculty of Pharmacy, Gazi University, Ankara, Turkey; Tel/Fax: +90-3122133921; E-mail: bilgesen@gazi.edu.tr

and nearly half of them are of plant natural products [1 - 4].

Unexplored sources of drug repository in medicinal plants have marvelous therapeutic potential and are helpful in achieving new challenges of novel drug lead targets for the treatment of cancer, diabetes, neurological disorders and autoimmune diseases. Advancement in research increased the knowledge of humanbeings in the field of plants having medicinal value. It is observed that even the great interest in molecular modelling, combinatorial chemistry and advanced techniques for synthetic chemistry; the natural products are a significant source for discovering of novel therapeutically active compounds [5]. However, among the estimated 250,000-400,000 plant species, only 6% of them have been studied for biological activity and about 15% of them have been investigated phytochemically [6, 7]. This shows a need for activity guided phytopharmacological evaluation of herbal drugs.

A lot of effort and investments have been made to investigate pharmacological potential of the medicinal plants.One aspect of the drug discovery process is the identification of small molecules with enzyme-inhibiting activities. Malfunctioning of enzymes often leads to diseases that can be caused either by their dysfunction, overexpression, or hyper-activation. Certain enzymes known as purified human enzymes are necessary as molecular targets for drug discovery. In this procedure, measurement of product formation is realized by spectroscopic methods and the results are compared by using standard clinically used inhibitors [8, 9]. Many therapeutic strategies are developed for the major health problems and the key enzyme inhibitory theory is one of the most applied approaches. A wide variety of therapeutics used against a number of diseases are inhibitiors of clinically relevant enzymes. Most of the inhibitors interact with particular enzymes by blocking their activity towards their corresponding physiological natural substances without disturbing other enzymes. For instance, some secondary metabolites exhibit interesting anti-acetylcholinesterase (anti-AChE) activity, an enzyme involved in the pathogenesis of Alzheimer's Disease (AD) [10, 11]. Tyrosinase is also a multifunctional enzyme catalyzing the hydroxylation of L-tyrosine to 3,4-dihydroxyphenylalanine and by the oxidation of L-DOPA to dopaquinone to give rise to melatonin. α-Tyrosinase is another key enzyme in melatonin biosynthesis by preventing of skin disorders as well as Parkinson's Disease. Neurodegenerative diseases involve the cholinergic, dopaminergic neuronal loss in the brain and the aggregation of β-amyloid peptides which results in the creation of neurotoxic forms of β-amyloid peptides generated by γ-secretase mediated sequential cleavages of amyloid precursor protein and β-secretase (BACE1). In addition, the inhibitors of tau-induced neurotoxicity (glycogen synthase kinase-3-enzyme inhibitors) are also important focuses for drug design.

Phosphodiesterase inhibitors are known for their pharmacological properties including vasodilator, antidepressant, smooth muscle relaxant, anti-inflammatory and enhancer of cognitive functions.

α-Glucosidase and α-amylase are also key enzymes for the catabolism of carbohydrates by decreasing blood glucose levels. *Helicobacter pylori* infection and ulcer is caused by increased concentration of Urease enzymes. Ureases have great acerbity influence concerned in the focalization of urinary stones, hepatic coma and other infections. Urea is hydrolyzed by urease enzyme to carbon dioxide and ammonia.

Besides, serine proteases are among the most targeted enzymes for the development of therapeutics against diseases such as thrombosis, angina, hepatitis C-virus infection, inflammation, pancreatitis, cancer, gastrointestinal disorders and diabetes etc. Serine proteases such as chymotrypsin and trypsin are responsible for digestion of certain fibrous proteins. These enzymes are thought to be essential for viral replication and has been identified as a target for the development of anti-HCV drugs.

During the last few years, we have identified natural products from medicinally important plants exhibiting anti-enzymatic activity having applications in curing diabetes, AD, hypertension and over coming the drug resistance problems in cancer chemotherapy. In this chapter, structures of novel health related enzyme inhibitors and their structure-activity relationships (SAR) will be discussed.

Naturally Occurring α-Glucosidase Inhibitors

α-Glucosidase, a membrane bound intestinal enzyme, digests carbohydrates by cleaving glycosidic bonds to liberate free glucose. The resulting glucose is a source of an exaggerated rise in blood sugar causing postprandial hyperglycemia. This causes type 2 diabetes mellitus that affects nearly 21 billion people worldwide [12, 13]. Potent α-glucosidase inhibitors prevent the breakdown of carbohydrates in small intestine and prolong the absorption of glucose or carbohydrates in blood. These compounds may be used as chemotherapeutic agents in clinics for the treatment of diabetes. Due to the catalytic role of α-glucosidase in carbohydrate digestion, these inhibitors may also be used as therapeutic target for other carbohydrate mediated diseases including viral infections, cancer, HIV, obesity and hepatitis [14 - 16].

Our chemical investigation of the methanolic extract of *Drypetes gossweileri*, of South African origin resulted in the identification of *N*-β-D-glucopyranosyl-*p*-hydroxyphenylacetamide (**1**), *p*-hydroxyphenylacetic acid (**2**), *p*-hydroxyphenyl-acetonitrile (**3**), *p*-hydroxyacetophenone (**4**), 3,4,5-trimethoxyphenol (**5**), dolichandroside A (**6**), and *β*-amyrone (**7**) given in Figs. (**1** and **2**). Compounds **1-7** were active in *α*-glucosidase inhibition assay with IC_{50} values of 12, 50, 48, 50, 56, 20 and 25 µM, respectively [17]. Compound **1**, a first example of the plant natural product containing *N*-glucose moiety incorporated in its structure, was significantly more active than the rest of the isolates. We decided to carry out the acidic hydrolysis of this compound that yielded compounds **2** and **8**. The latter was also weakly active in our *α*-glucosidase inhibition assay (IC_{50} = 60.0 µM). This bioactivity data suggested that the higher potency of compound **1**,compared to the rest of the isolates, was due to the presence of the *N*-glucose moiety.

Compounds **1** and **7** were also active in anti-fungal assay against *Candida albicans* with minimum inhibitory concentrations (MIC) of 8.0 and 16 µg/ml, respectively. Compound **2** was weakly active in this bioassay with MIC value of 32 µg/ml, again suggesting that the *N*-glucose moiety was responsible for the higher potency of compound **1**. In order to study the structure-activity relationships of compound **7** for anti-fungal activity, it was reacted with *m*-chloroperbenzoic acid to afford 12,13-epoxy analogues of compound **7** (**9** and **10**). Both of these compounds were further reacted with 20% ammonium hydroxide solution to give compound **11** and **12** [18]. Compounds **9-12** were evaluated for their potential to inhibit the growth of *C. albicans* and were found to be active with MIC values of 4.0, 8.0, 8.0 and ≤2.0 µg/ml. Compounds **9-12** were also active in *α*-glucosidase inhibition assay with IC_{50} values of 4.0, 10.0, 1.0 and 10.0 µM, respectively. The bioactivity data of compounds **9-12** suggested that the presence of *β*-oriented C-12/C-13 epoxy functionality and an amino group at C-12 in these compounds are responsible for their enhanced anti-fungal and anti-*α*-glucosidase activities. It was also discovered that C-12/*α*-amino C-13/*β*-OH groups play a significant role in these aforemen- tioned bioactivities.

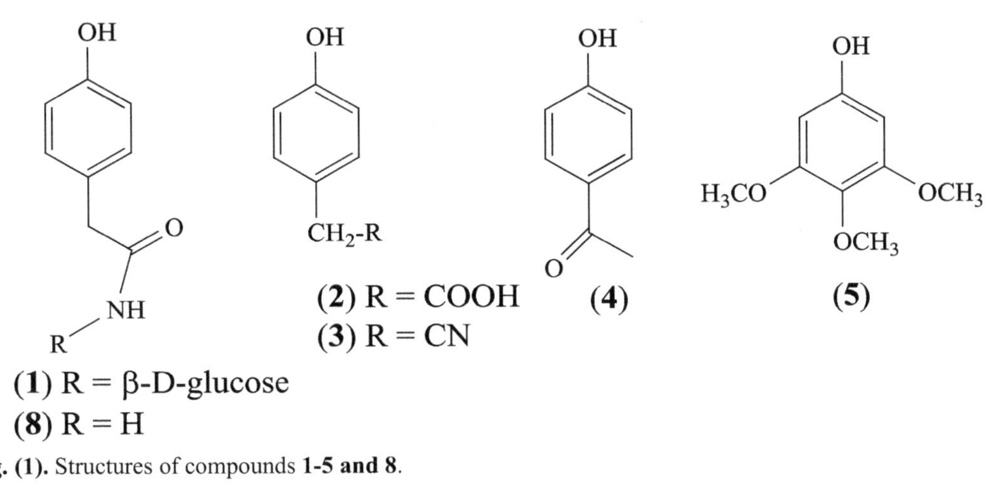

Fig. (1). Structures of compounds **1-5 and 8**.

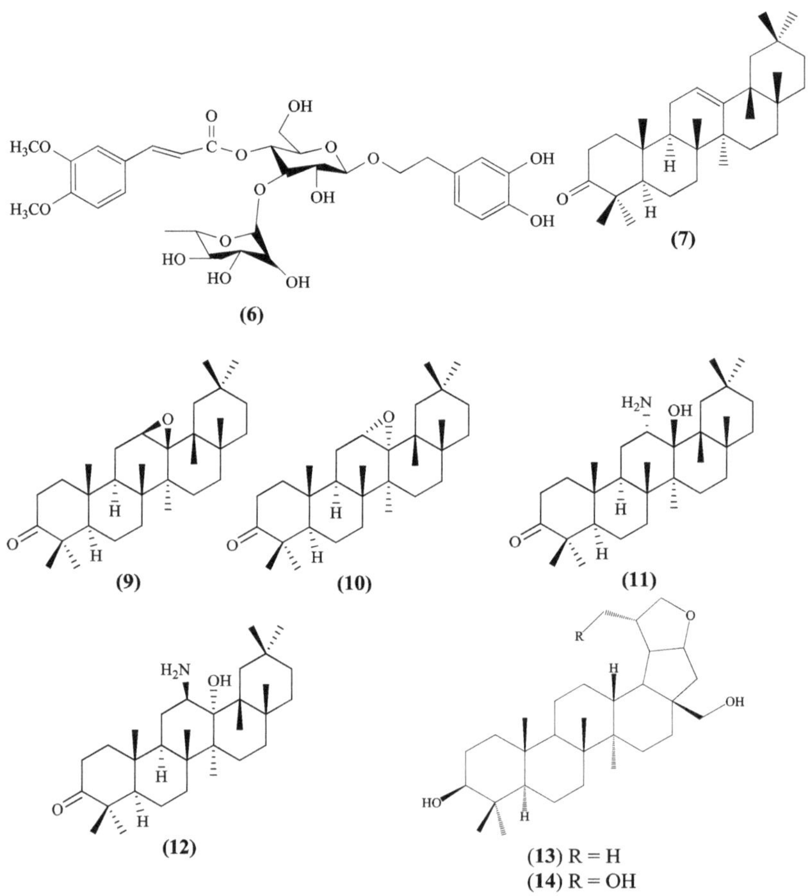

Fig. (2). Structures of compounds **6-14**.

Our α-glucosidase directed phytochemical studies on *Epilobium angustifolium,* collected from Manitoba, afforded two novel compounds **13** and **14** exhibiting potent anti-α-glucosidase (yeast) activity with IC_{50} values of 120 and 122 nM, respectively. Both of these compounds were a minor secondary metabolites of *E. angustifolium.* In order to study the *in-vivo* bioactivity, we have developed chemo-enzymatic approach to scale up compound **13** using a commercially available betulin (**15**). To achieve this goal, we reacted compound **15** with tri-methylsilyl chloride (TMSCl) in the presence of 4-dimethylaminopyridine (DMAP) to yield compound **16**, the C-3 and C-28 silyl ether analogues of compound **15**. Incubation of compound **16** in liquid whole cell culture of *Cunninghamella blakesleeana* afforded 21-hydroxybetulin (**17**). The latter on reaction with $Hg(CF_3COO)_2$ and $NaBH_4$ followed by treatment with HF provided compound **13** [19]. The chemo-enzymatic synthesis of **13** is outlined in Scheme (**1**).

Our chemical invesitgation of the chloroform fraction of *Swertia corymbosa* of Indian origin, resulted in the isolation of five bioactive xanthones, namely, 3-allyl-2,8-dihydroxy-1,6-dimethoxy xanthen-9-one (**18**), gentiacaulein (**19**), norswertianin (**20**), 1,3,6,8-tetrahydroxyxanthone (**21**), and 1,3-dihydroxy-xanthone (**22**). Structures of these compounds are shown in Fig. (**3**). All of the isolates (**18-22**) exhibited anti-α-glucosidase activities with IC_{50} values of 26.3, 44.5, 23.2, 39.0 and 35.2 μM, respectively [15].

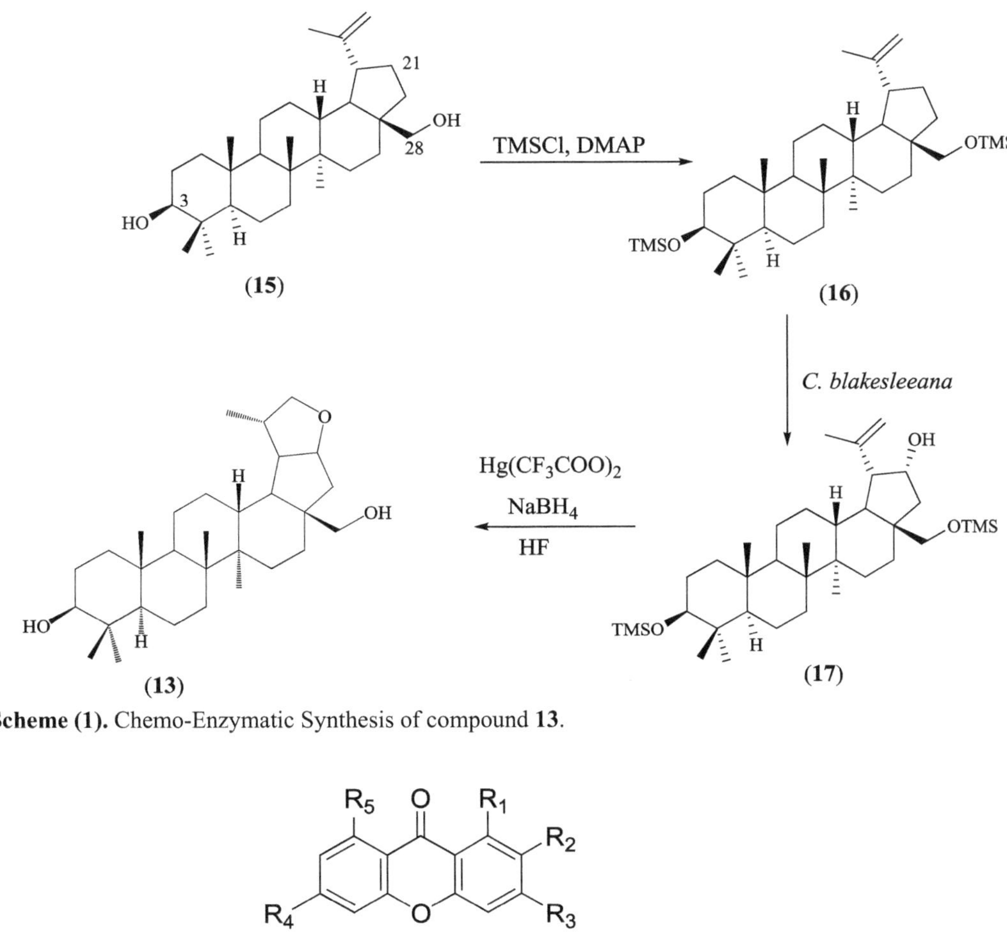

Scheme (1). Chemo-Enzymatic Synthesis of compound **13**.

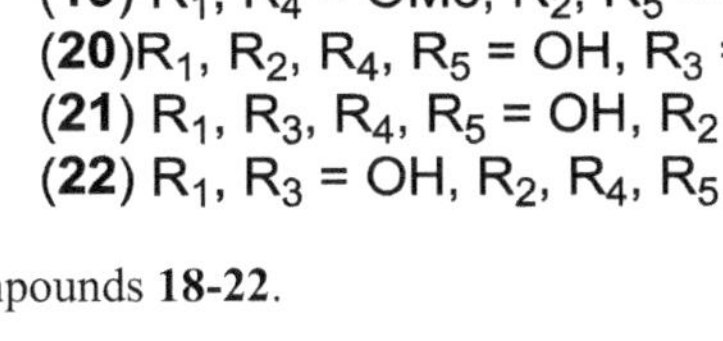

(**18**) R_1, R_4 = OMe, R_2, R_5 = OH, R_3 = Allyl,
(**19**) R_1, R_4 = OMe, R_2, R_5 = OH, R_3 = H,
(**20**)R_1, R_2, R_4, R_5 = OH, R_3 = H
(**21**) R_1, R_3, R_4, R_5 = OH, R_2 = H
(**22**) R_1, R_3 = OH, R_2, R_4, R_5 = H

Fig. (3). Structures of compounds **18-22**.

Phytochemical studies on *Muraya koenigii* afforded five novel carbazole alkaloids, namely bisgerayafolines A-D (**23-26**) and bismahanimbinol (**27**) along with four known alkaloids, bispyrayafoline (**28**), *O*-methylmahanine (**29**), *O*-methylmukonal (**30**) and mahanine (**31**). Compounds **23-28** are members of dimeric class of carbazole alkaloids while compounds **29-31** belong to monomeric class carbazole alkaloids. The configuration of biphenyl groups in compounds **23**, **24** and **26** was *aR* while compounds **25** and **27** had *aS* configuration which was determined with the aid of ECD spectroscopic studies. Biphenyl groups with *aR* configuration exhibit negative Cotton effect at 235 nm and positive Cotton effect at 218 nm in ECD spectra while the biphenyl groups with *aS* configuration show mirror image couplet compared to *aR* biphenyl groups. Compounds **23-31** exhibited α-glucosidase inhibitory activity with IC_{50} values of 45.4, 41.2, 69.0, 38.7, 51.3, 29.1, 46.1, 77.5 and 21.4 μM, respectively [16, 20]. The bioactivity of compounds **23**, **24** and **26** was higher than compounds **25** and **27** indicating that biphenyls having *aR* configuration were more active than the biphenyls of *aS* configuration. Furthermore, compounds **28** and **31** were significantly active with IC_{50} values of 29.1 and 21.4 μM compared to the rest of the isolates. A structural comparison of **28** and **31** revealed that the higher potency of **31** might be due to presence of C-9/OH which might be interacting with α-glucosidase through hydrogen bonding [20]. From this bioactivity data, it was also observed that dimeric carbazole alkaloids were less bioactive than their monomer analogues, possibly due to the poor fit of dimeric carbazole alkaloids in the binding site of the enzyme.

All of these isolates were also evaluated for anti-cancer properties using DNA binding assay. DNA is a remarkable bioreceptor for a large number of small molecules and it is a major biological target for designing and discovering new anti-cancer leads. A number of DNA-intercalating agents including ellipticine, rebeccamycin and anthracyclines etc. are in clinics for the treatment of cancer. Ellipticine and rebeccamycin are naturally occurring class of carbazole alkaloids and we decided to evaluate all of these isolates for DNA binding activity. All of these compounds exhibited different level of bioactivity in this bioassay and compounds **1** and **31** were found to be significantly active compared to the rest of the isolates. This higher affinity might be due to the presence of C-9"/OH and C-8"/ OH in compounds **1** and **31**, respectively. These OH groups might be involved in the hydrogen bonding with the base pairs of DNA. These intercalators represent an important class of antitumoral DNA binders and are characterized by the insertion of planar aromatic or heteroaromatic rings in between DNA base pairs. Structures of compounds (**23-31**) are shown in Fig. (**4**).

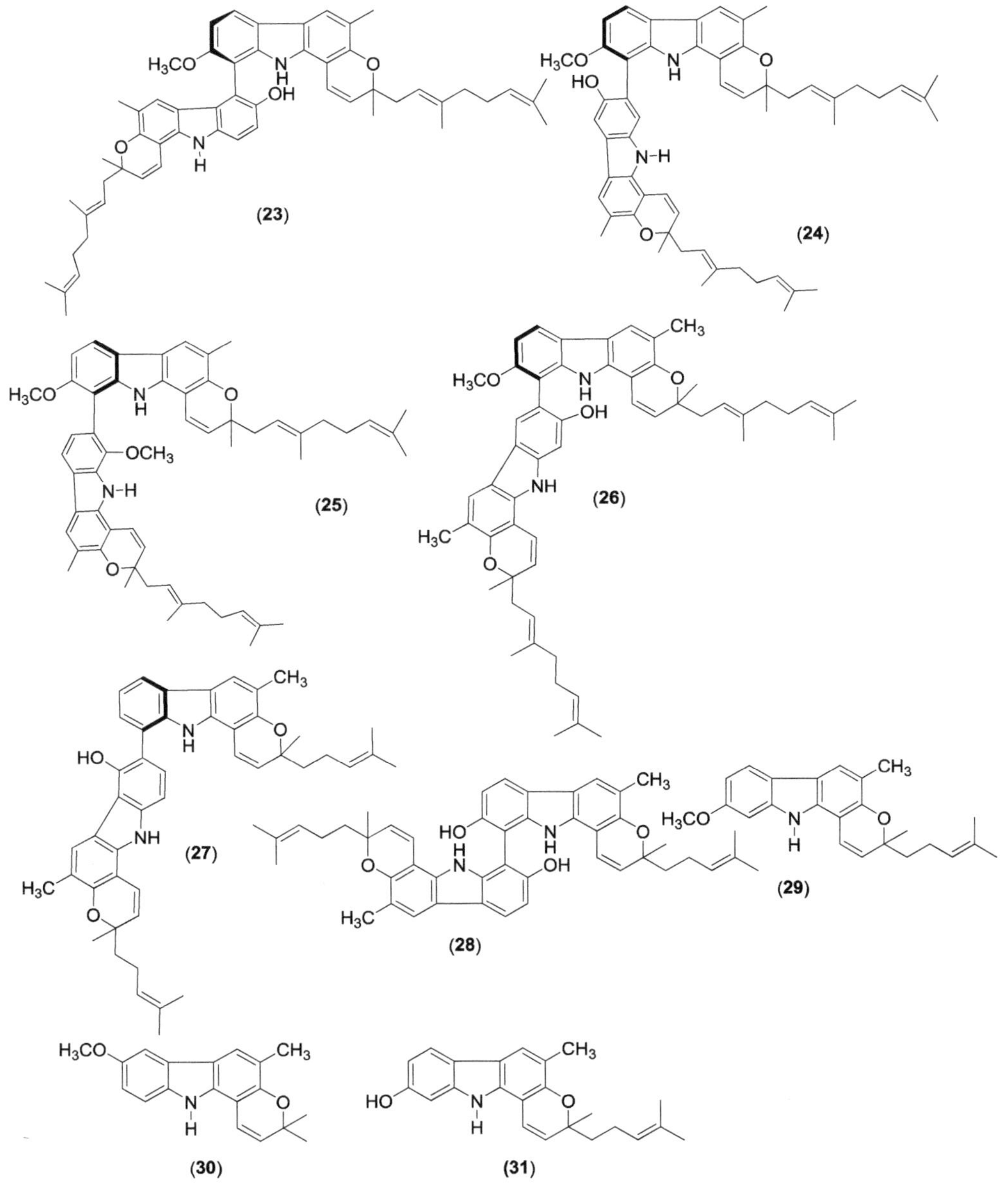

Fig. (4). Structures of compounds **23-31**.

Naturally Occurring Acetylcholinesterase Inhibitors

Alzheimer's disease (AD) is a neurodegenerative disorder that causes severe health problems including memory loss in elderly people [21]. One of the major causes of AD is the deficiency of acetylcholine in the brain [22]. Accordingly, enhancement of acetylcholine levels in the brain is currently used to treat AD [23,

24]. This task can be accomplished by using potent AChE inhibitors. AChE inhibitors also play a role in preventing pro-aggregating activity of AChE leading to the deposition of β-amyloid, another cause of AD [24]. AChE inhibitors also have applications in treating senile dementia, ataxia, myasthenia gravis and Parkinson's disease [4, 25]. Two types of AChE inhibition assays (microplate reader and TLC based assays) are used to screen plant extracts and pure natural products [8]. Microplate reader bioassays are more accurate and reliable in order to determine the accurate potency of pure natural products while TLC based bioassays can be used to guide the bioactivity and to determine chromatographic properties of bioactive fractions.Four AChE inhibitors, tacrine (**32**), donepezil (**33**), galanthamine (**34**) and rivastigmine (**35**) are approved by FDA, USA to be used in clinics [4,26]. These compounds have limited effectiveness and a number of side effects. For instance, tacrine shows hepatotoxic lability and rivastigmine has a short half-life.

In this area, a few natural products exhibiting potent AChE inhibitory activity are reported in the literature. Hopeahainol (**36**), isolated from *Hopea hainanensis*, has been reported as a potent AChE inhibitor (IC_{50} value of 4.33 μM) and its potency is almost the same as that of huperzine A (**37**) (IC_{50} value of 1.6 μM), a prescribed drug used to treat AD [27]. Similarly, other natural products including *N*-allylnorgalanthamine (**38**), and *N*(14-methylallyl)norgalanthamine (**39**) have shown anti-AChE activity with IC_{50} values of 0.18 and 0.17 μM, respectively [28]. Compounds **38** and **39** are found to be more potent than galanthamine (**34**) (IC_{50} = 1.82 μM) shown in Fig. (**5**).

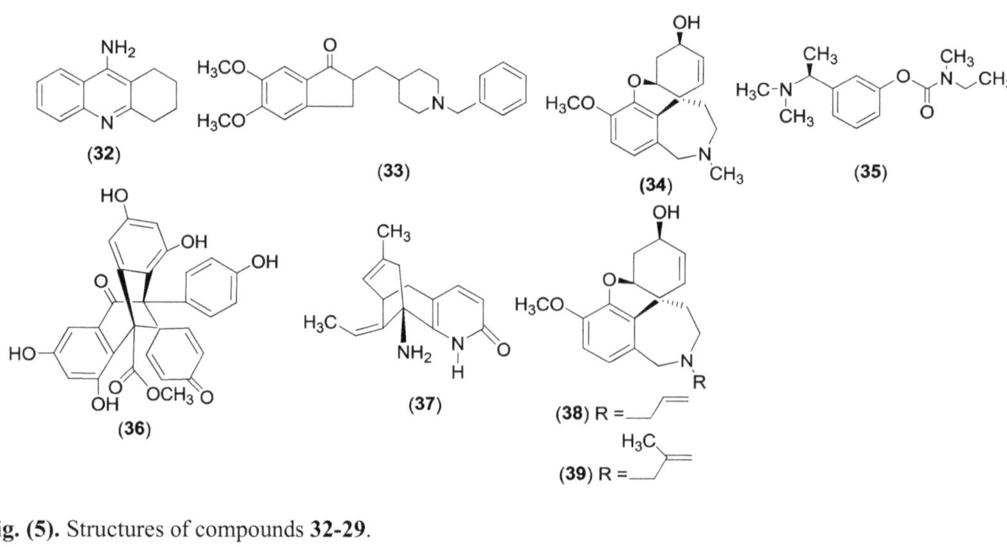

Fig. (5). Structures of compounds **32-29**.

The aglycone of helicid (**40**) was isolated from from *Helicia nilagirica* and showed potent GABA transaminase activity with an IC_{50} value of 4.1 μg/ml. Its structure-activity relationships revealed that the aldehyde group on the benzene ring is responsible for the aforementioned bioactivity [29]. Song's group reported a weak AChE inhibitory activity with an IC_{50} value of 37.8 mM of this aglycone. These authors prepared three derivatives (**41-43**) of compound **40**. These derivatives exhibit potent anti-AChE activity with IC_{50} values of 0.45, 0.49 and 0.20 μM, respectively. Similarly, compound **45**, a synthetic analog of berberine (**44**) is a potent AChE inhibitor (IC_{50} value of 0.097 μM). Its potency is better than galanthamine (**34**) [30]. In this compound, berberine (**44**) is linked with phenol by 4-carbon spacers. The SAR studies suggest that higher potency of **45** is due to the functional group present at the end of the chain and the length of the connecting tether. Structures of compounds **40-45** are shown in Fig. (**6**).

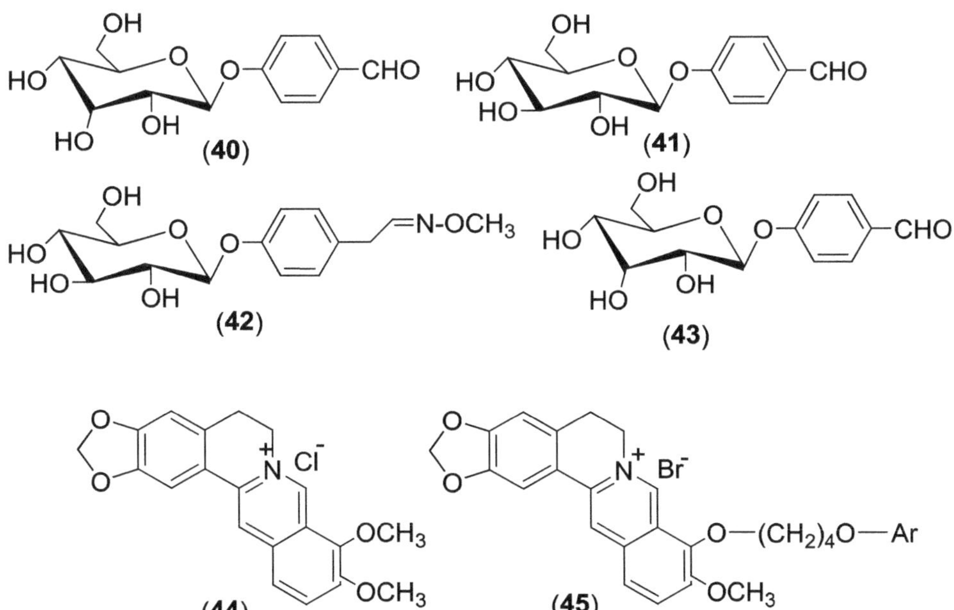

Fig. (6). Structures of compounds **40-45**.

In this area, we have investigated genus *Buxus* for the identification of steroidal alkaloids exhibiting anti-AChE activity [31 - 39]. *O*^{6}-Buxafurandiene (**46**) and 7-deoxy-*O*^{6}-buxafurandiene (**47**), steroidal alkaloids purified from *Buxus hyrcana*, exhibited this bioactivity with IC_{50} values 17.0 and 13.0 μM, respectively [39].

These results prompted us to collect *Buxus natalesis* and *B. macowanii* from South Africa based on their ethnomedicinal use to enhance memory in elderly people by local traditional healers [40, 41]. The crude methanolic extract of *B. natalensis* and *B. macowanii* were active in AChE inhibition assay with IC_{50} values of 28 and 30 μg/ml, respectively. Our AChE-inhibition guided phytochemical investigation of *B. natalensis* resulted in the isolation of two new bioactive natural products, O^2-natafuranamine (**48**), and O^{10}-natafuranamine (**49**) along with two known steroidal bases buxafuranamide (**50**) and buxalongifolamidine (**51**). All of these compounds exhibited anti-AChE activity with IC_{50} values of 3.0, 8.5, 14 and 30.2 μμ, respectively [40]. Phytochemical studies on *B. macowanii* resulted in the isolation of five novel bioactive alkaloids, 31-hydroxybuxatrienone (**52**), macowanioxazine (**53**), 16α-hydroxymacowanitriene (**54**), macowanitriene (**55**), and macowamine (**56**) along with two know steroidal bases, N_b-demethylpapillotrienine (**57**), and moenjodaramine (**58**). Compounds **52-58** exhibited anti-AChE activity with IC_{50} values of 17, 32.5, 11.4, 10.8, 45, 19 and 27 μM, respectively. Compounds **52** and **58** were also moderately active in BACE1 inhibitory assay [41]. Structures of all of the compounds (**46-58**) are shown in Fig. (**7**).

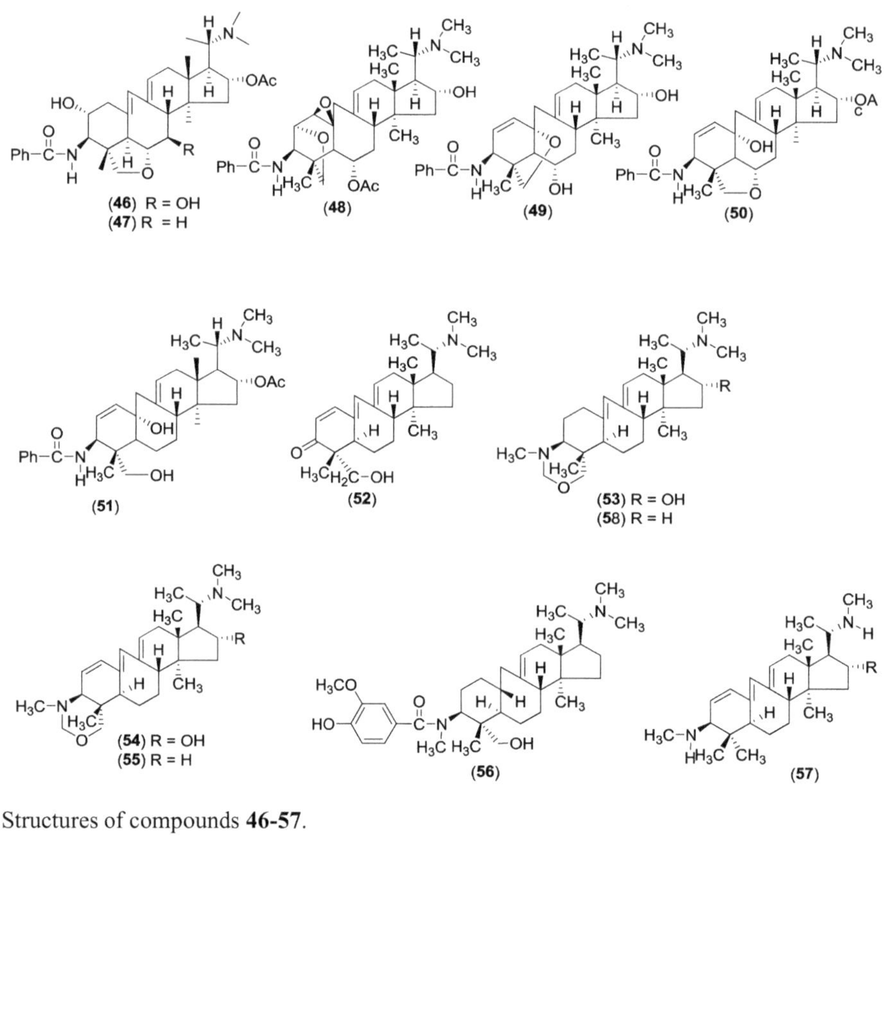

Fig. (7). Structures of compounds **46-57**.

The anti-AChE potency of compound **48** was almost identical to huperzine A. Compounds **49**, **50**, **53** and **58** were equally potent in AChE inhibition assays, suggesting the bioactivity of these compounds might be due to the presence of tetrahydrofuran or tetrahydrooxazine rings incorporated in their structures. A very careful structural analysis of these compounds also revealed that the location of an ether linkage in these compounds does not play any role in enzyme inhibition assays, as **49** contains an ether linkage between C-31 and C-10, and **50** has an ether linkage between C-31 and C-6. Compounds **53** and **58** have a tetrahydrooxazine ring. Compound **48** has an ether linkage between C-31 and C-2 and an epoxy functionality at C-1/C-10. The higher potency of this compound was assumed to be due to the presence of these two functionalities.

Buxus alkaloids are assumed to be derived in nature from cycloartenol type triterpenoids and to the best of our knowledge no experimental report on the biosynthesis of these alkaloids is reported. Our phytochemical studies on *Artocarpus* species have resulted in the isolation of 4,4,14-trimethyl-9*β*,19-cyclopregnane-3,20-dione (**59**) as a new natural product which is hypothesized to be a putative intermediate involved in the biosynthesis of *Buxus* alkaloids [42]. In order to confirm this hypothesis, we incorporated tritium at the C-21 methyl group by using a chemo-enzymatic approach. For this task, compound **59** was incubated with the liquid culture of *Cunninghamella echinulata* to produce the C-21/OH analogue of **59** (**60**). Intermediate **60** upon reaction with trimethylsilyl iodide (TMSI) using a mixture of methanol and tritiated water (^3H_2O) afforded compound **61** [43]. Chemo-enzymatic synthesis of **61** is shown in Scheme (**2**).

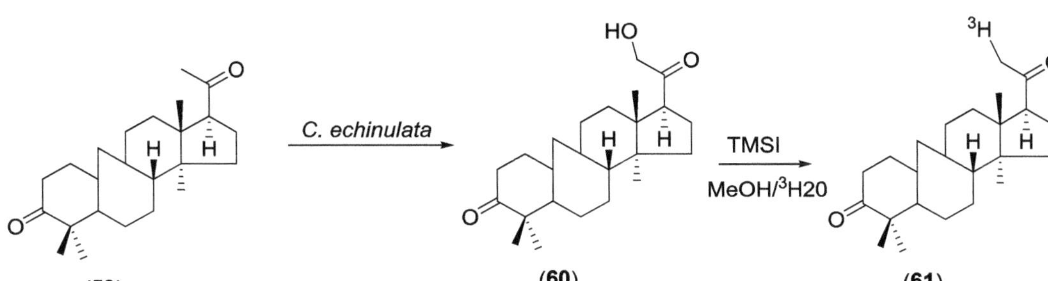

Scheme (2). Chemo-Enzymatic Synthesis of compound **61**.

Our synthesized compound **61** was fed to the fresh leaves of *B*uxus *natalaensis* and investigation of these leaves, after two weeks, afforded C-21 tritium labeled compounds **48**-**51**. During these studies, we have also identified compound **(51)** as a putative intermediate involved in the biosynthesis of compound **48** (Scheme **3**). We are working on the biosynthesis of these compounds to elucidate the mechanism for the incorporation of amino group at C-3 and C-20, opening of

9*β*,10*β* cyclopropane ring to afford 9(10→19) *abeo* diene system, and substitution of other functional groups. These biosynthetic studies will help us to gain knowledge about the key enzymes involved in the biosynthesis of *Buxus* alkaloids. This information will be used to purify key enzymes and clone them into a suitable vector, *E. coli*, for designing a biotechnological method to scale up these minor plant metabolites for carrying out in-vivo AChE inhibition assays.

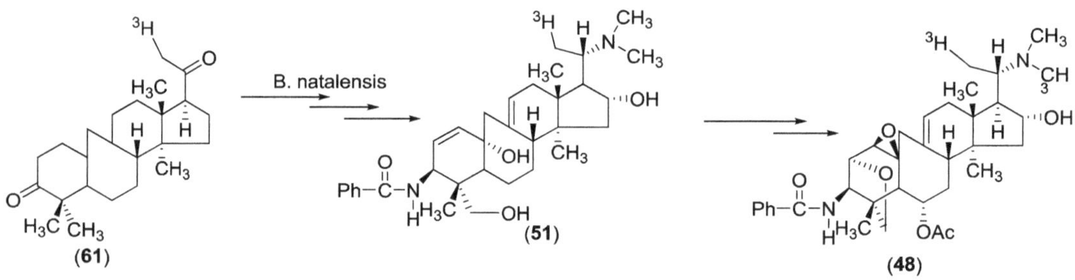

Scheme (3). Biosynthesis of compound **48 and 51**.

Naturally Occurring Glutathione S-Transferase (GST) Inhibitors

Glutathione *S*-transferase (EC 2.3.1.18), a multifunctional enzyme, helps to prevent cells from cytotoxic and genotoxic stresses. This enzyme is involved in catalysing a reaction between cytotoxic agents containing electrophilic centers and glutathione to afford a chemically inert water soluable adduct that can be excreted from the body. Based on these facts, this enzyme is also refered as phase II detoxification system. Due to the catalysis of a xenobiotic and glutathione reaction to make a removable adduct by GST, this enzyme is assumed to be involved in the acquired drug resistance for curing cancer and parasitic diseases. Anti-cancer and anti-parasitic therapeutic agents contain electrophilic centers incorporated in their structures and considered as xenobiotics by the human body. GST plays a catalytic role in producing their water soluble adducts with glutathione to remove them from the body. This would decrease the concentrations of these therapeutical agents in the body and results in lowering the efficiency of anti-cancer and anti-parasitic chemotherapeutic agents [44, 45]. GSTs are over expressed in various human cancer cells compared to normal tissues [46, 47]. A 2-fold increase in GST activity has been observed in lymphocytes isolated from chronic lymphocytic leukemia (CLL) patients that were resistant to chlorambucil when compared with untreated CLL patients [48, 49]. These studies suggest that the use of GST inhibitors as adjuvants during cancer and parasitic chemotherapy can help to overcome the acquired drug resistance problems.

The field of natural products for discovering new GST inhibitors is underpopulated and it would be worthwhile to discover new naturally occurring GST inhibitors as currently used GST inhibitors are synthetic compounds that exhibit either severe *in-vivo* toxicity or are inactive *in-vivo*. In this area, we have screened several medicinally important plants, collected from various parts of the world, for their potential to inhibit GST activity. These efforts led us to discover a few medicinal plants including *Caesalpinia bonduc*, *Artocarpus nobilis, Nauclea latifolia* and *Barleria prionitis*. Their crude extracts exhibited anti-GST activity with IC_{50} values of 83.0, 125, 10.5 and 160 μg/ml, respectively. GST Inhibition-directed phytochemical studies on these medicinally important plants were performed in order to isolate GST inhibitors present in them. These studies are summarized as follows.

Our chemical studies on the bioactive fractions of *Caesalpinia bonduc* resulted in identification of 17-hydroxycompesta-4,6-dien-3-one (**62**), 13,14-*seco*-stigmasta-5,14-dien-3*α*-ol (**63**), 13,14-*seco*-9(11),14-dien-3a-ol (**64**), caesaldekarin J (**65**), neocaesalpin P (**66**), neocaesalpin H (**67**), cordylane A (**68**), caesalpinin B (**69**), caesalpinianone (**70**), 6-*O*-methylcaesalpinianone (**71**), and hematoxylol (**72**) [50 - 52]. Structures of these compounds are shown in Fig. (**8**). Compounds **62-72** were active in GST inhibition assays with IC_{50} values of 380, 230, 248, 259, 200, 218, 250, 350, 16.5, 17.1 and 23.6 μM, respectively. The bioactivity data of all of these compounds indicated that compounds **70**, **71** and **72** were significantly active compared to the rest of the isolated phytochemicals. We used ethacrynic acid, a standard GST inhibitor, as a positive control in these studies and it was active with an IC_{50} value of 16 μM. A comparison of bioactivity data of compounds **70** and **71** with our positive control suggested that homoisoflavanoids have more or less the same potency of inhibiting GST activity as that of ethacrynic acid.

Our bioassay-directed phytochemical studies on the ethanolic extract of *Artocarpus nobilis* of Sri Lankan origin resulted in the identification of four known triterpenoids, cyclolaudenyl acetate (**72**), lupeol acetate (**73**), *β*-amyrine acetate (**74**), and zizphursolic acid (**75**) along with five known flavonoids, artonins E (**76**), artobiloxanthone (**77**) artoindonesianin U (**78**), cyclocommunol (**79**) and multiflorins A (**80**). Structures of compounds **72-80** are shown in Fig. (**9**). The anti-GST activity of compounds **72-80** was found to be in a wide range from weak to strong with IC_{50} values of 195.1, 146.1, 251.0, 68.5, 2.0, 1.0, 6.0, 3.0 and 14.0 μM, respectively. Again, flavonoids (**76-80**) were significantly more active than the rest of the isolates, especially **76-79** were more possibly due to the presence of the prenyl group in these compounds [53].

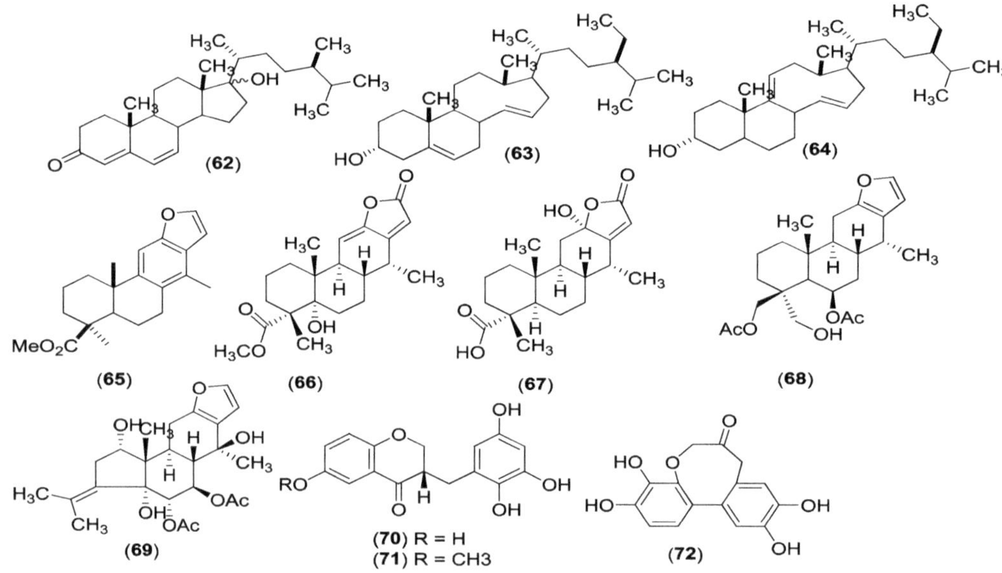

Fig. (8). Structures of compounds **62-72**.

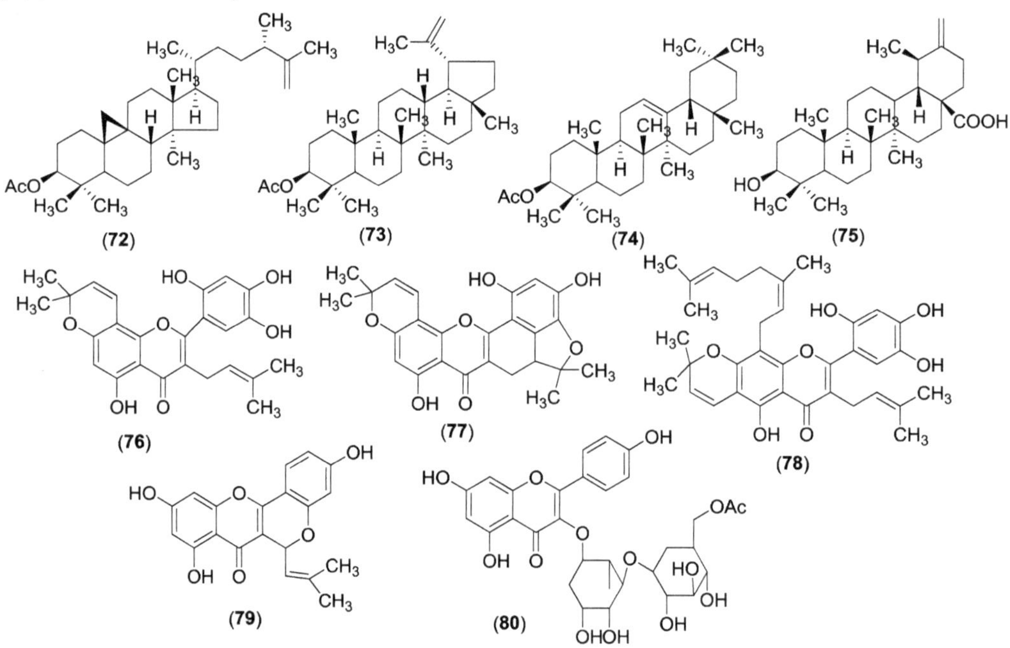

Fig. (9). Structures of compounds **72-80**.

Nauclea latifolia exhibits various biological activities including GST inhibitory, anti-malarial and anti-hypertensive activities. In order to identify natural products responsible for these individual bioactivities, it is important to carry out bioassay-directed phytochemical studies on this plant. This plant was active in our GST inhibition screening assays and we carried out GST-inhibition directed phytochemical studies that resulted in the isolation of five known compounds, strictosamide (**81**), naucleamides A (**82**), naucleamide F (**83**), quinovic acid-3-*O*-β-rhamnosylpyranoside (**84**), and quinovic acid 3-*O*-*β*-fucosylpyranoside (**85**) (Fig. **10**) [54]. All of these isolates (**81-85**) exhibited GST inhibitory activity with IC_{50} values of 20.3, 27.2, 23.6, 143.8, and 53.5 μM, respectively. Compound **81** was significantly active in our anti-GST assay and was isolated in a large quantity. We carried out SAR studies by synthesizing its different analogues by using a microbial reaction approach. For this goal, we screened five different fungi, namely *Mucor plumbeus* (ATCC 4740), *Cunninghamella blakesleeana* (ATCC 9245), *C. echinulata* (ATCC 9244), *Curvularia lunata* (ATCC 12017), *Rhizopus circinans* (ATCC 1225) and *Aspergillus niger* (ATCC 1004), for their capability to metabolize compound **81**. During these biotransformation experiments, we discovered that *R. circinans* metabolized compound **81** into 10-hydroxy-strictosamide (**86**), 10-*β*-glucosyloxyvincoside lactam (**87**) and 16,17-dihydro-10-*β*-glucosyloxyvincoside lactam (**88**). These metabolites appeared to follow the sequence for the formation of compounds **86** to **88**. A time-dependent biotransformation experiment was performed in order to confirm the order of formation of these metabolites. This experiment was carried out by incubating compound **81** in the liquid culture of *Rhizopus circinans*; this afforded compounds **86** and **87**. Incubation of compound **87** with liquid culture of this fungus afforded compound **88**. These results indicated that *R. circinans* initially performed microbial hydroxylation at C-10 of compound **81** to yield compound **86**. This metabolite further underwent glycosylation, followed by reduction of the $\Delta^{16\text{-}17}$ double bond to give compounds **87** and **88**, respectively [54]. Compounds **86-88** also exhibited anti-GST activity with IC_{50} values of 18.6, 12.3 and 16.6 μM, respectively.

Our chemical investigation of *Barleria prionitis,* collected from Sri Lanka, afforded seven natural products, barlerinoside (**89**), shanzhiside methyl ester (**90**), 6-*O*-*trans*-*p*-coumaroyl-8-*O*-acetylshanzhiside methyl ester (**91**), barlerin (**92**), acetylbarlerin (**93**), 7-methoxydiderroside (**94**), and lupulinoside (**95**). Compound **89** belongs to the class of phenylethanoids while compounds **90-95** are members of the iridioid class of natural products. Structures of these compounds are shown in Fig. (**11**). All of these phytochemicals **89-95** exhibited anti-GST activity with IC_{50} values of 12.4, 49.2, 22.9, 38.9, 40.6, 122.0 and 134.0 μM, respectively [55]. These studies suggested that phenylethanoids have potential to inhibit the activity of GST.

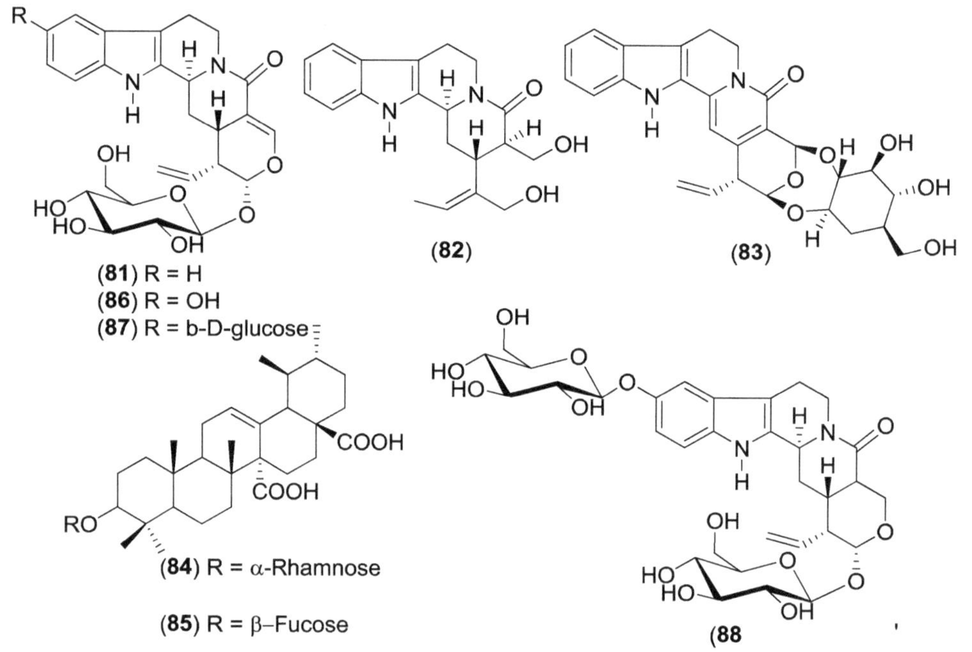

Fig. (10). Structures of compounds **81-87**.

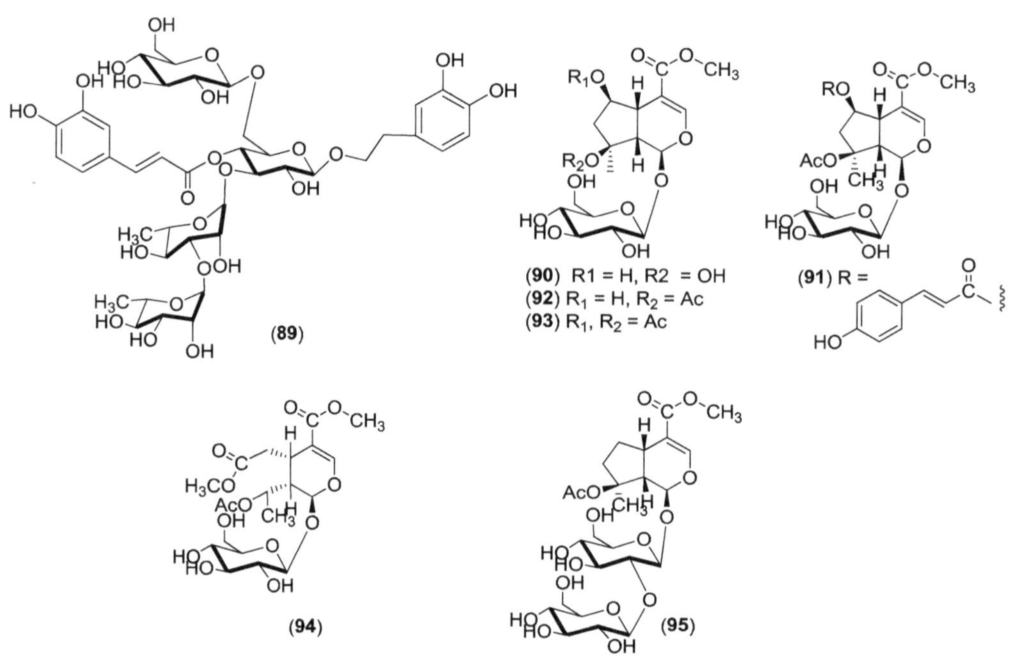

Fig. (11). Structures of compounds **89-95**.

A very careful examination of the structures of all GST inhibiting natural products (**62-95**) revealed that all of these compounds contain a common functional group *i.e.* α, β–unsaturated carbonyl group which is assumed to be a required pharmacophore for the expression of this bioactivity. The α, β-unsaturated carbonyl group may form a glutathione adduct of these compounds through Michael addition to inhibit the activity of GST.

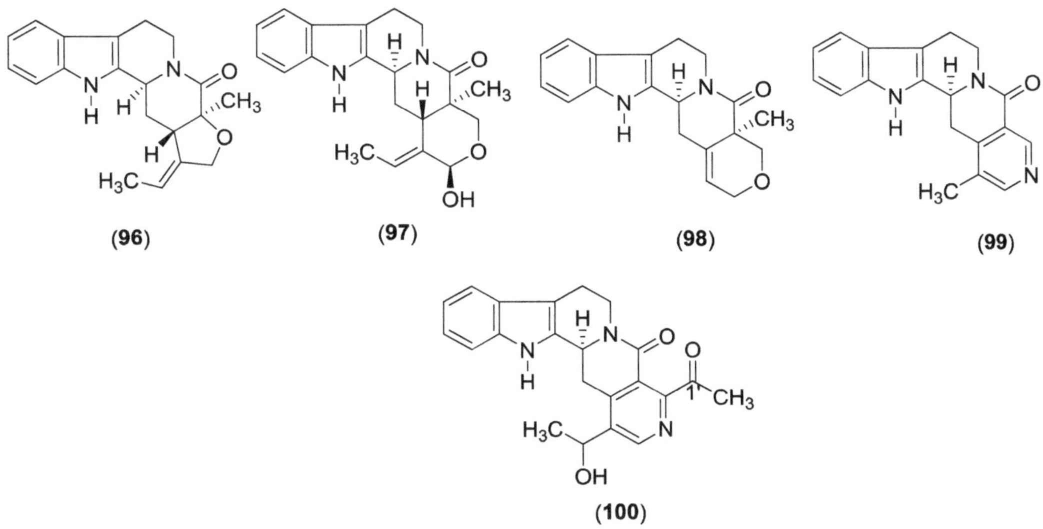

Fig. (12). Structures of compounds **96-100**.

Naturally Occurring Renin Inhibitors

The main cause of hypertension is abnormal blood pressure of the body. The renin-angiotensin system (RAS) helps in controlling and maintaining blood pressure in animals [56]. Renin (EC 3.4.23.15), an enzyme, is produced by the epithelial cells of the kidney and released into the circulation system by various stimuli. This enzyme generates the *deca*-peptide angiotensin I (AI), an inactive peptide, by cleaving the *N*-terminus of angiotensinogen. It is a rate-limiting step in RAS. AI is converted to angiotensin II (AII) by the angiotensin converting enzyme (ACE). AII lies on the arterial smooth muscle cells to maintain blood pressure and stimulates the synthesis and release of aldosterone from the adrenal cortex. Its overexpression leads to the abnormalities of blood pressure causing hypertension. RAS inhibition activity is an ideal target to discover new drugs against hypertension. *Nauclea latifolia* is reported to exhibit anti-hypertensive activity [57] and our anti-renin directed phytochemical studies on methanolic extract of this plant resulted in the identification of five bioactive indole alkaloids, latifoliamide A-E (**96-100**). Fig. (**12**) lists the structures of compounds **96-100**. These phytochemicals (**96-100**) showed anti-renin activity with IC_{50} values of

32.6, 11.3, 95.0, 94.5, and 16.3 μM, respectively [58]. This anti-renin activity was very weak compared to the currently used anti-hypertensive drug, alkisiren (IC_{50} = 0.6 nM) which works by inhibiting the RAS activity [59]. Alkisiren has several side effects and it is worthwhile to explore natural products for discovering novel anti-renin lead compounds. Our phytochemical results suggest that natural products have potential for discovering lead anti-renin compounds with fewer side effects.

CONCLUDING REMARKS

A wide variety of therapeutics used against a number of diseases are inhibitors of clinically relevant enzymes. Most of the inhibitors interact with particular enzymes by blocking their activity towards their corresponding physiological natural substances without disturbing other enzymes. At present, AChE inhibitors are the first group of drugs such as galanthamine approved by FDA to treat mild to moderate AD. Application of antioxidants is also significant in the prevention of some health problems along with enzyme inhibitors.

Our phytochemical studies have resulted in the discovery of new bioactive natural products that might have potential in developing new biomedical agents. For instance, compounds **1**, **13**, **14**, **20** have shown significant *in-vitro* anti-*α*-glucosidase activity. *Buxus* alkaloids, especially compound **48**, have shown potent anti-AChE activity as its potency is nearly the same as that of currently used pharmaceuticals (huperzine and galantamine) in clinics to cure AD. The phenylethanoids and flavonoids have shown potent *in-vitro* anti-GST activity and these compounds have potential to overcome drug resistance problem during cancer chemotherapy. Also, we have discovered that the *α,β*-unsaturated carbonyl group is required to be present in lead compounds as an active pharmacophore against GST. This information is very helpful in designing new biomedical agents against GST. We have found that natural products have potential for "discovering" new anti-renine lead compounds. These compounds need to be screened for *in-vivo* anti-enzymatic assays to develop them as pharmaceuticals. If these compounds are weakly active or inactive in *in-vivo* bioassays then SAR studies can help to improve their bioactivities. Our chemo-enzymatic approach for the synthesis of minor bioactive natural products from commercially available natural products is helpful to scaleup the minor bioactive natural products for *in-vivo* studies. We have also confirmed the hypothesis that cycloartenol type terpenoids are the biosynthetic precursors of *Buxus* alkaloids. Further biosynthetic studies on these compounds can help to design and develop new biotechnological methods for the production of bioactive *Buxus* alkaloids.

CONSENT FOR PUBLICATION

Not applicable.

CONFLICT OF INTEREST

The authors confirm that this chapter contents have no conflict of interest.

ACKNOLWDGEMENTS

We would like to thank all of our undergraduate and graduate students as well as our collaborators who were involved in discovering new anti-enzymatic compounds and their names are cited in the references. Funding provided by the University of Winnipeg and Natural Sciences and Engineering Research Council of Canada is gratefully acknowledged.

REFERENCES

[1] Annang, F.; Genilloud, O.; Vicente, F. Contribution of natural products to drug discovery in tropical diseases. *Drug Discovery in Infectious Diseases,* **2016**, *7*, 75-104. [http://dx.doi.org/10.1002/9783527694082.ch3]

[2] Cheuka, P. M.; Mayoka, G.; Mutai, P.; Chibale, K. The role of natural products in drug discovery and development against neglected tropical diseases. *Molecules,* **2017**, *22*(1), 58/1-58/41.

[3] Hong, J. Natural product synthesis at the interface of chemistry and biology. *Chemistry,* **2014**, *20*(33), 10204-10212. [http://dx.doi.org/10.1002/chem.201402804] [PMID: 25043880]

[4] Ata, A. Novel plant –derived biomedical agents and their biosynthetic origin. In: *Studies in Natural Products Chemistry*; Elsevier Science Publishers: New York, **2012**; 38, . 225

[5] Newman, D.J.; Cragg, G.M. Natural Products as Sources of New Drugs from 1981 to 2014. *J. Nat. Prod.,* **2016**, *79*(3), 629-661. [http://dx.doi.org/10.1021/acs.jnatprod.5b01055] [PMID: 26852623]

[6] Simmonds, M.S.J. Opportunities and challenges for ethnobotany at the start of twenty-first century.*Plant-Derived Natural Products: Synthesis, Function and Applications*; Osbourn, A.E.; Lanzolti, V., Eds.; Springer Dordrecht Heidelberg: London, **2009**, pp. 97-125. [http://dx.doi.org/10.1007/978-0-387-85498-4_5]

[7] Yun, U.W.; Yan, Z.; Amir, R.; Hong, S.; Jin, Y.W.; Lee, E.K.; Loake, G.J. Plant natural products: history, limitations and the potential of cambial meristematic cells. *Biotechnol. Genet. Eng. Rev.,* **2012**, *28*, 47-59. [http://dx.doi.org/10.5661/bger-28-47] [PMID: 22616481]

[8] Ata, A.; Van Den Bosch, S.A.; Harwanik, D.J.; Pidwinski, G.E. Glutathione S-transferase and acetylcholinesterase inhibiting natural products from medicinally important plants. *Pure Appl. Chem.,* **2007**, *79*(12), 2269-2276. [http://dx.doi.org/10.1351/pac200779122269]

[9] Yap, A.K.L.; Luscombe, D.K. Rapid and inexpensive enzyme inhibition assay of methotrexate. *J. Pharmacol. Methods,* **1986**, *16*(2), 139-150. [http://dx.doi.org/10.1016/0160-5402(86)90019-7] [PMID: 3528670]

[10] Goschorska, M.; Baranowska-Bosiacka, I.; Gutowska, I.; Tarnowski, M.; Piotrowska, K.; Metryka, E.; Safranow, K.; Chlubek, D. Effect of acetylcholinesterase inhibitors donepezil and rivastigmine on the

activity and expression of cyclooxygenases in a model of the inflammatory action of fluoride on macrophages obtained from THP-1 monocytes. *Toxicology,* **2018**, *406-407*, 9-20. [http://dx.doi.org/10.1016/j.tox.2018.05.007] [PMID: 29777723]

[11] Eleti, S. Drugs in Alzheimer's disease Dementia: An overview of current pharmacological management and future directions. *Psychiatr. Danub.,* **2016**, *28* Suppl. 1, 136-140. [PMID: 27663824]

[12] Atta-ur-Rahman, ; Zareen, S.; Choudhary, M.I.; Akhtar, M.N.; Khan, S.N. α-Glucosidase inhibitory activity of triterpenoids from Cichorium intybus. *J. Nat. Prod.,* **2008**, *71*(5), 910-913. [http://dx.doi.org/10.1021/np800001v] [PMID: 18341288]

[13] Ata, A. Novel bioactive compounds from endophytic fungi of aboriginal medicinal plants. *Planta Med.,* **2015**, *81*(11), 875. [http://dx.doi.org/10.1055/s-0035-1556183]

[14] Ata, A.; Alhazmi, H. Bioactive natural products and their structure-activity relationships studies.*Asymmetric Synthesis of Drugs and Natural Products*; Nag, A., Ed.; CRC Press: Boca Raton, FL, **2018**, pp. 189-201.

[15] Uvarani, C.; Arumugasamy, K.; Chandraprakash, K.; Sankaran, M.; Ata, A.; Mohan, P.S. A new DNA-intercalative cytotoxic allylic xanthone from *Swertia corymbosa. Chem. Biodivers.,* **2015**, *12*(3), 358-370. [http://dx.doi.org/10.1002/cbdv.201400055] [PMID: 25766909]

[16] Uvarani, C.; Sankaran, M.; Jaivel, N.; Chandraprakash, K.; Ata, A.; Mohan, P.S. Bioactive dimeric carbazole alkaloids from *Murraya koenigii. J. Nat. Prod.,* **2013**, *76*(6), 993-1000. [http://dx.doi.org/10.1021/np300464t] [PMID: 23691929]

[17] Ata, A.; Tan, D.S.; Matochko, W.L.; Adesanwo, J.K. Chemical constituents of *Drypetes gossweileri* and their enzyme inhibitory and anti-fungal activities. *Phytochem. Lett.,* **2011**, *4*(1), 34-37. [http://dx.doi.org/10.1016/j.phytol.2010.10.007]

[18] Ata, A.; Naz, S.; Elias, E.M. Naturally Occurring enzyme inhibitors and their pharmaceutical applications. *Pure Appl. Chem.,* **2011**, *83*(9), 1741-1749. [http://dx.doi.org/10.1351/PAC-CON-10-11-16]

[19] Khan, M.S. Novel α-Glucosidase Inhibiting Triterpenoids from *Epilobium angustifolium* and their Chemo-Enzymatic Synthesis. *.Sc. Thesis, University of Manitoba: Winnipeg, July,* **2015**.

[20] Uvarani, C.; Jaivel, N.; Sankaran, M.; Chandraprakash, K.; Ata, A.; Mohan, P.S. Axially chiral biscarbazoles and biological evaluation of the constituents from *Murraya koenigii. Fitoterapia,* **2014**, *94*, 10-20. [http://dx.doi.org/10.1016/j.fitote.2014.01.004] [PMID: 24444889]

[21] Ata, A.; Conci, L.J.; Orhan, I. Mucoralactone A: an unusual steroid from the liquid culture of *Mucor plumbeus. Heterocycles,* **2006**, *68*, 2097-2106. [http://dx.doi.org/10.3987/COM-06-10829]

[22] Rosenberry, T.L. Acetylcholinesterase. *Adv. Enzymol. Relat. Areas Mol. Biol.,* **1975**, *43*, 103-218. [PMID: 891]

[23] Enz, A.; Amstutz, R.; Boddeke, H.; Gmelin, G.; Malanowski, J. Brain selective inhibition of acetylcholinesterase: a novel approach to therapy for Alzheimer's disease. *Prog. Brain Res.,* **1993**, *98*, 431-438. [http://dx.doi.org/10.1016/S0079-6123(08)62429-2] [PMID: 8248533]

[24] Fang, L.; Chen, Y.; Zhang, Y. Advances in the researches on cholinesterase inhibitors for the treatment of Alzheimer's disease. *Yaoxue Jinzhan,* **2009**, *33*, 289-296.

[25] Tumiatti, V.; Minarini, A.; Bolognesi, M.L.; Milelli, A.; Rosini, M.; Melchiorre, C. Tacrine derivatives and Alzheimer's disease. *Curr. Med. Chem.,* **2010**, *17*(17), 1825-1838. [http://dx.doi.org/10.2174/092986710791111206] [PMID: 20345341]

[26] Ribeiz, S.R.I.; Bassitt, D.P.; Arrais, J.A.; Avila, R.; Steffens, D.C.; Bottino, C.M.C. Cholinesterase inhibitors as adjunctive therapy in patients with schizophrenia and schizoaffective disorder: a review and meta-analysis of the literature. *CNS Drugs,* **2010**, *24*(4), 303-317.
[http://dx.doi.org/10.2165/11530260-000000000-00000] [PMID: 20297855]

[27] Ge, H.M.; Zhu, C.H.; Shi, H.; Zhang, L.D.; Xie, D.Q.; Yang, J.; Ng, S.W.; Tan, R.X.; Hopeahainol, A. Hopeahainol A: an acetylcholinesterase inhibitor from Hopea hainanensis. *Chemistry,* **2008**, *14*(1), 376-381.
[http://dx.doi.org/10.1002/chem.200700960] [PMID: 17943703]

[28] Berkov, S.; Codina, C.; Viladomat, F.; Bastida, J. N-Alkylated galanthamine derivatives: Potent acetylcholinesterase inhibitors from *Leucojum aestivum. Bioorg. Med. Chem. Lett.,* **2008**, *18*(7), 2263-2266.
[http://dx.doi.org/10.1016/j.bmcl.2008.03.008] [PMID: 18356045]

[29] Wen, H.; Lin, C.; Que, L.; Ge, H.; Ma, L.; Cao, R.; Wan, Y.; Peng, W.; Wang, Z.; Song, H. Synthesis and biological evaluation of helicid analogues as novel acetylcholinesterase inhibitors. *Eur. J. Med. Chem.,* **2008**, *43*(1), 166-173.
[http://dx.doi.org/10.1016/j.ejmech.2007.03.018] [PMID: 17574306]

[30] Huang, L.; Luo, Z.; He, F.; Lu, J.; Li, X. Synthesis and biological evaluation of a new series of berberine derivatives as dual inhibitors of acetylcholinesterase and butyrylcholinesterase. *Bioorg. Med. Chem.,* **2010**, *18*(12), 4475-4484.
[http://dx.doi.org/10.1016/j.bmc.2010.04.063] [PMID: 20471843]

[31] Naz, S.; Noor-e-Ain, F.; Ali, R. A.; Choudhary, M. Sener, B.; Turkoz, S. Alkaloids from *Buxus* Species. *Phytochemistry,* **1992**, *31*(8), 2933-2935.

[32] Asif, E.; Ali, S.S.; Nasir, H.; Jamal, A.; Ata, A.; Choudhary M.I.; Sener, B., Turkoz, S. New steroidal alkaloids from the roots of *Buxus papillosa. J. Nat. Prod.,* **1992**, *55*(8), 1063-1066.

[33] Choudhary, M. I; Naz, S.; Ata, A.; Sener, B; Turkoz, S. New Steroidal alkaloids from the roots of *Buxus sempervirens. J. Nat. Prod.,* **1997**, *60*(8), 770-774.
[http://dx.doi.org/10.1021/np970028x]

[34] Ata, A.; Naz, S.; Choudhary, M. I.; Sener, B.; Turkoz, S. New novel triterpenoidal alkaloids from the roots of *Buxus sempervirens. Nat. Prod. Lett.,* **1998**, *12*(4), 299-306.
[http://dx.doi.org/10.1080/10575639808048306]

[36] Atta-ur-Rahman, Au.; Ata, A.; Naz, S.; Choudhary, M.I.; Sener, B.; Turkoz, S. New steroidal alkaloids from the roots of buxus sempervirens. *J. Nat. Prod.,* **1999**, *62*(5), 665-669.
[http://dx.doi.org/10.1021/np980285h] [PMID: 10346940]

[37] Ata, A.; Naz, S.; Choudhary, M.I.; Atta-ur-Rahman, ; Sener, B.; Turkoz, S. New triterpenoidal alkaloids from Buxus sempervirens. *Z. Natforsch. C J. Biosci.,* **2002**, *57*(1-2), 21-28.
[http://dx.doi.org/10.1515/znc-2002-1-204] [PMID: 11926538]

[38] Ata, A.; Iverson, C.D.; Kalhari, K.S.; Akhter, S.; Betteridge, J.; Meshkatalsadat, M.H.; Orhan, I.; Sener, B. Triterpenoidal alkaloids from *Buxus hyrcana* and their enzyme inhibitory, anti-fungal and anti-leishmanial activities. *Phytochemistry,* **2010**, *71*(14-15), 1780-1786.
[http://dx.doi.org/10.1016/j.phytochem.2010.06.017] [PMID: 20655557]

[39] Babar, Z.U.; Ata, A.; Meshkatalsadat, M.H. New bioactive steroidal alkaloids from *Buxus hyrcana. Steroids,* **2006**, *71*(13-14), 1045-1051.
[http://dx.doi.org/10.1016/j.steroids.2006.09.002] [PMID: 17049575]

[40] Matochko, W.L.; James, A.; Lam, C.W.; Kozera, D.J.; Ata, A.; Gengan, R.M. Triterpenoidal alkaloids from Buxus natalensis and their acetylcholinesterase inhibitory activity. *J. Nat. Prod.,* **2010**, *73*(11), 1858-1862.
[http://dx.doi.org/10.1021/np100494u] [PMID: 20954721]

[41] Lam, C.W.; Wakeman, A.; James, A.; Ata, A.; Gengan, R.M.; Ross, S.A. Bioactive steroidal alkaloids

from *Buxus macowanii* Oliv. *Steroids,* **2015**, *95*, 73-79. [http://dx.doi.org/10.1016/j.steroids.2014.12.002] [PMID: 25528196]

[42] Zahid, S.; Ata, A.; Samarasekera, R. New cycloartane-type triterpenoids from *Artocarpus nobilis. Z. Naturforsch. C,* **2007**, *62*(2), 280-284. [http://dx.doi.org/10.1515/znb-2007-0222]

[43] Lam, C.W. Phytochemical Studies on *Buxus macowanii* and Microbial Transformation of Glycyrrhetinic Acid. *M.Sc. Thesis, University of Manitoba: Winnipeg, June,* **2014**.

[44] Ata, A.; Udenigwe, C.C. The discovery and application of inhibitors of glutathione *S*-transferase as therapeutic agents -a review. *Curr. Bioact. Compd.,* **2008**, *4*, 41-50. [http://dx.doi.org/10.2174/157340708784533384]

[45] Ata, A.; Diduck, C.; Udenigwe, C.C.; Zahid, S.; Decken, A. New chemical constituents of *Ambrosia psilostachya. ARKIVOC,* **2007**, *13*, 195-203.

[46] Douglas, K.T. Mechanism of action of glutathione-dependent enzymes. *Adv. Enzymol. Relat. Areas Mol. Biol.,* **1987**, *59*, 103-167. [PMID: 2880477]

[47] Adang, A.E.; Brussee, J.; van der Gen, A.; Mulder, G.J. The glutathione-binding site in glutathione S-transferases. Investigation of the cysteinyl, glycyl and gamma-glutamyl domains. *Biochem. J.,* **1990**, *269*(1), 47-54. [http://dx.doi.org/10.1042/bj2690047] [PMID: 2375757]

[48] Abramovitz, M.; Homma, H.; Ishigaki, S.; Tansey, F.; Cammer, W.; Listowsky, I. Characterization and localization of glutathione-*S*-transferases in rat brain and binding of hormones, neurotransmitters, and drugs. *J. Neurochem.,* **1988**, *50*(1), 50-57. [http://dx.doi.org/10.1111/j.1471-4159.1988.tb13228.x] [PMID: 2891788]

[49] Schisselbauer, J.C.; Silber, R.; Papadopoulos, E.; Abrams, K.; LaCreta, F.P.; Tew, K.D. Characterization of glutathione S-transferase expression in lymphocytes from chronic lymphocytic leukemia patients. *Cancer Res.,* **1990**, *50*(12), 3562-3568. [PMID: 2340505]

[50] Udenigwe, C.C.; Ata, A.; Samarasekera, R. Glutathione S-transferase inhibiting chemical constituents of Caesalpinia bonduc. *Chem. Pharm. Bull. (Tokyo),* **2007**, *55*(3), 442-445. [http://dx.doi.org/10.1248/cpb.55.442] [PMID: 17329887]

[51] Ata, A.; Gale, E.M.; Samarasekera, R. Bioactive chemical constituents of *Caesalpinia bonduc* (Fabaceae). *Phytochem. Lett.,* **2009**, *2*(3), 106-109. [http://dx.doi.org/10.1016/j.phytol.2009.02.002]

[52] Ata, A.; Udenigwe, C.C.; Gale, E.M.; Samarasekera, R. Minor chemical constituents of *Caesalpinia bonduc. Nat. Prod. Commun.,* **2009**, *4*(3), 311-314. [http://dx.doi.org/10.1177/1934578X0900400302] [PMID: 19413105]

[53] Iverson, C.D.; Zahid, S. Li, Y.; Shoqafi, A. H., Ata, A.; Samarasekera, R. Glutathione S-transferase inhibitory, free radical scavenging and anti-leishmanial activities of chemical constituents of *Artocarpus nobilis* and *Matricaria chamomilla. Phytochem. Lett.,* **2010**, *3*(4), 207-211. [http://dx.doi.org/10.1016/j.phytol.2010.07.008]

[54] Ata, A.; Udenigwe, C.C.; Matochko, W.; Holloway, P.; Eze, M.O.; Uzoegwu, P.N. Chemical constituents of *Nauclea latifolia* and their anti-GST and anti-fungal activities. *Nat. Prod. Commun.,* **2009**, *4*(9), 1185-1188. [http://dx.doi.org/10.1177/1934578X0900400905] [PMID: 19831025]

[55] Ata, A.; Kalhari, K.S.; Samarasekeram, R. Chemical constituents of *Barleria prionitis* and their enzyme inhibitory activity and free radical scavenging activities. *Phytochem. Lett.,* **2009**, *2*(1), 37-40. [http://dx.doi.org/10.1016/j.phytol.2008.11.005]

[56] Rusai, K.; Jianxing, C.; Schneider, R.; Struijker-Boudier, H.; Lutz, J.; Heemann, U.; Baumann, M.

Renin inhibition mitigates anti-angiogenesis in spontaneously hypertensive rats. *J. Hypertens.,* **2011**, *29*(2), 266-272.
[http://dx.doi.org/10.1097/HJH.0b013e328340aa72] [PMID: 21045736]

[57] Karou, S.D.; Tchacondo, T.; Ilboudo, D.P.; Simpore, J. Sub-Saharan Rubiaceae: a review of their traditional uses, phytochemistry and biological activities. *Pak. J. Biol. Sci.,* **2011**, *14*(3), 149-169.
[http://dx.doi.org/10.3923/pjbs.2011.149.169] [PMID: 21870639]

[58] Agomuoh, A.A.; Ata, A.; Udenigwe, C.C.; Aluko, R.E.; Irenus, I. Novel indole alkaloids from *Nauclea latifolia* and their renin-inhibitory activities. *Chem. Biodivers.,* **2013**, *10*(3), 401-410.
[http://dx.doi.org/10.1002/cbdv.201200023] [PMID: 23495157]

[59] Kistner, I.; Zeymer, U.; Dechend, R.; Hagedorn, I.; Riemer, T.; Bramlage, P.; Pittrow, D.; Senges, J.; Schmieder, R.E. Benefits and risks of aliskiren treatment in patient with type 2 diabetes: analysis of the 3A registry. *J. Clin. Hypertens. (Greenwich),* **2016**, *18*(10), 1045-1053.
[http://dx.doi.org/10.1111/jch.12828] [PMID: 27094460]

SUBJECT INDEX

A

Atta-ur-Rahman (Ed.)

B

C

D

E

F

G

J

K

L

M

N

O

P

R

S

U

V

W

X

Y

CPSIA information can be obtained
at www.ICGtesting.com
Printed in the USA
BVHW010754030423
661652BV00002B/16

* 9 7 8 9 8 1 1 4 2 3 7 6 5 *